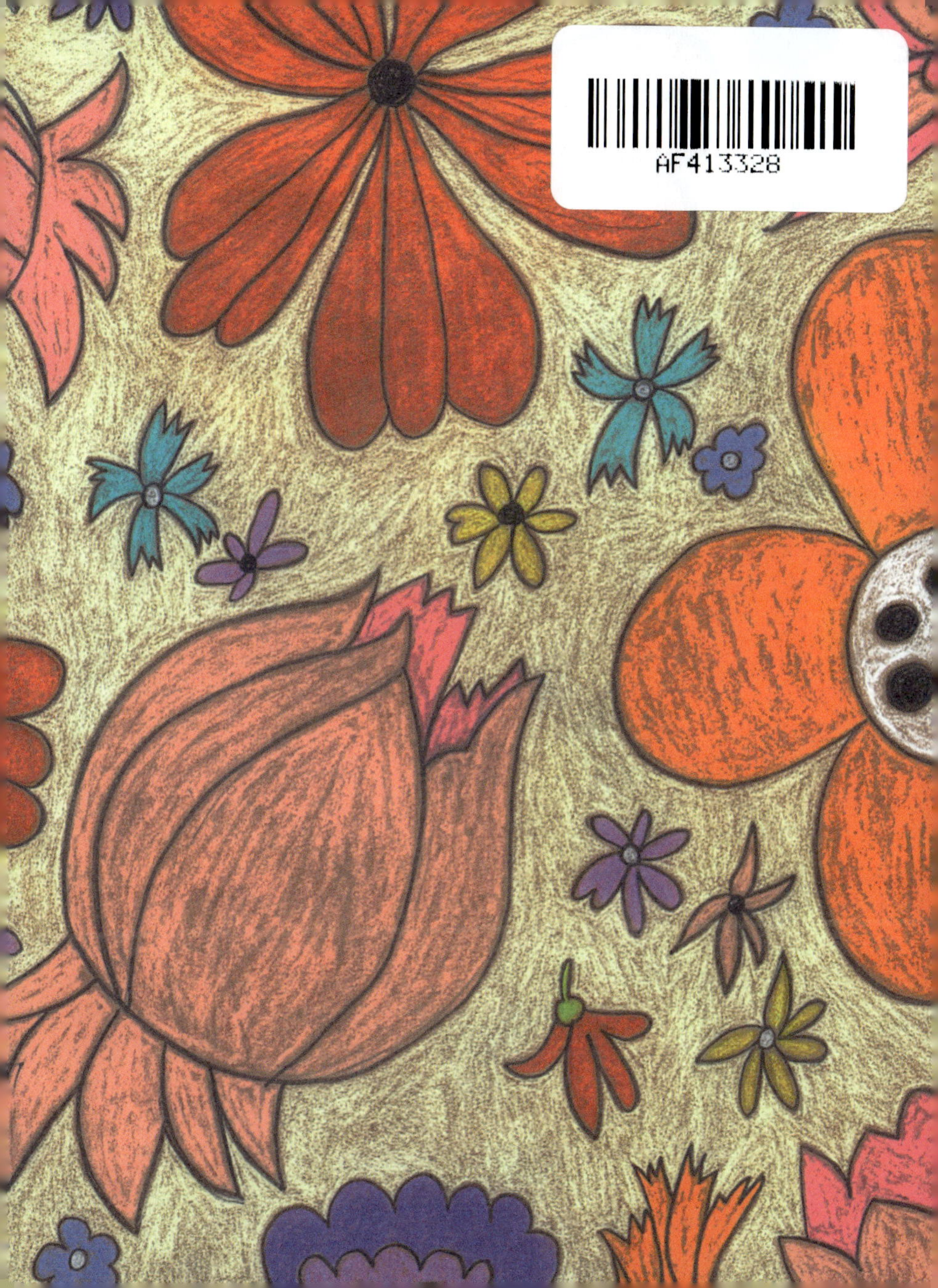
AF413328

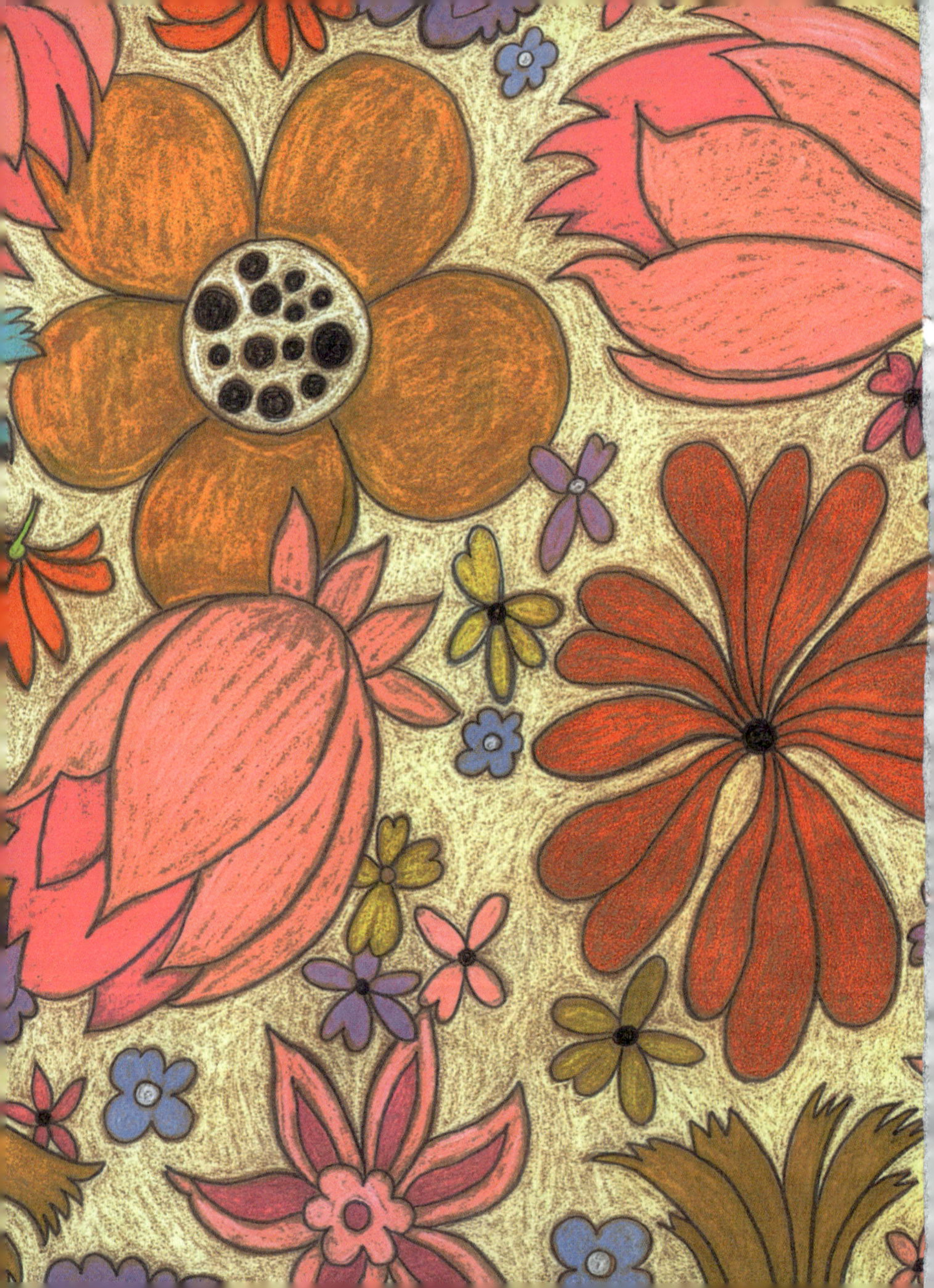

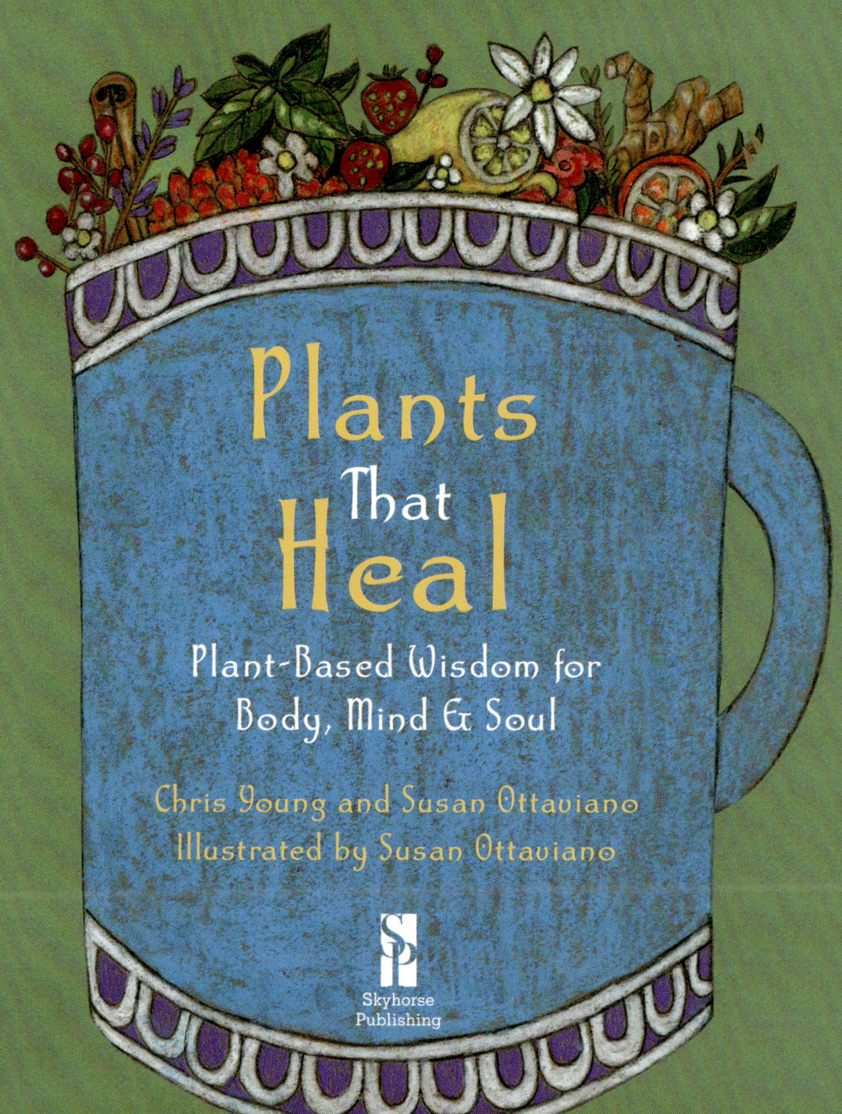

Plants
That
Heal
Plant-Based Wisdom for
Body, Mind & Soul
Chris Young and Susan Ottaviano
Illustrated by Susan Ottaviano
Skyhorse
Publishing

Medical Disclaimer

The information, recipes, and practices in this book are intended for inspirational and general wellness purposes only. They are not a substitute for professional medical advice or treatment.

Always seek the guidance of your physician, pharmacist, or other qualified healthcare provider with any questions you may have regarding a medical condition before making any changes to your health regimen using herbs or plant-based supplements.

All recipes and rituals included herein—such as teas, tonics, baths, scrubs, and other preparations—are plant-based, non-pharmaceutical creations meant to create a deeper connection to nature, and to support mindfulness and relaxation. Individual sensitivities, allergies, and reactions vary; please perform a patch test before applying any topical blend to the skin, and consult your healthcare provider if you are pregnant, nursing, taking medication, or have a chronic condition.

The authors and publishers make no claims to cure, prevent, or treat any disease and assume no responsibility for any adverse reactions resulting from the use or misuse of the information provided.

For Jon Kinnally, Elliott, and Howard.
—Chris

In memory of my dad, who taught me to eat all my vegetables.
—Susan

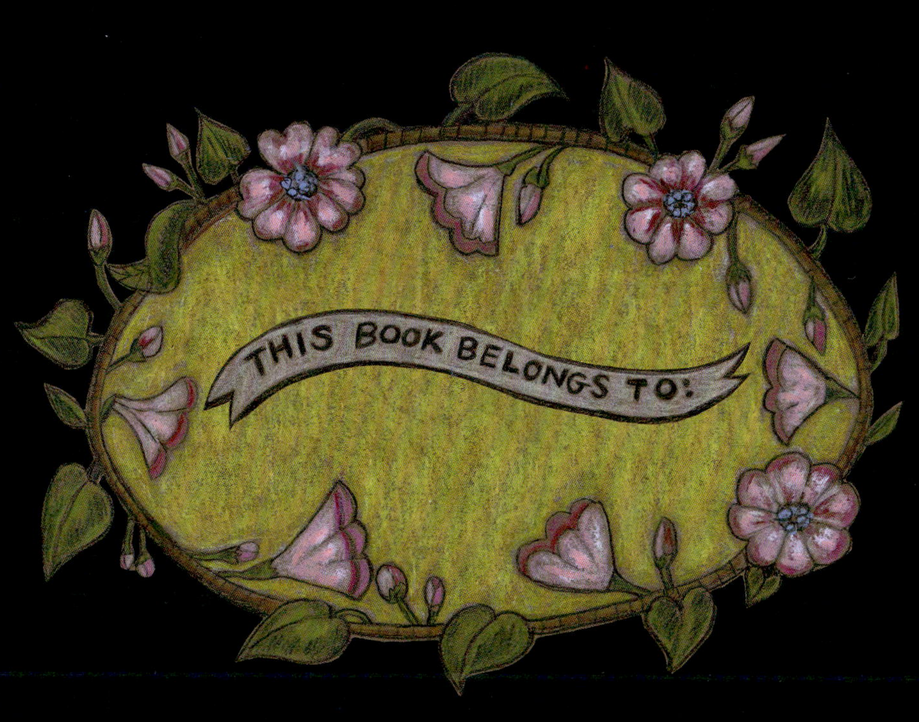

THIS BOOK BELONGS TO:

TABLE OF CONTENTMENTS

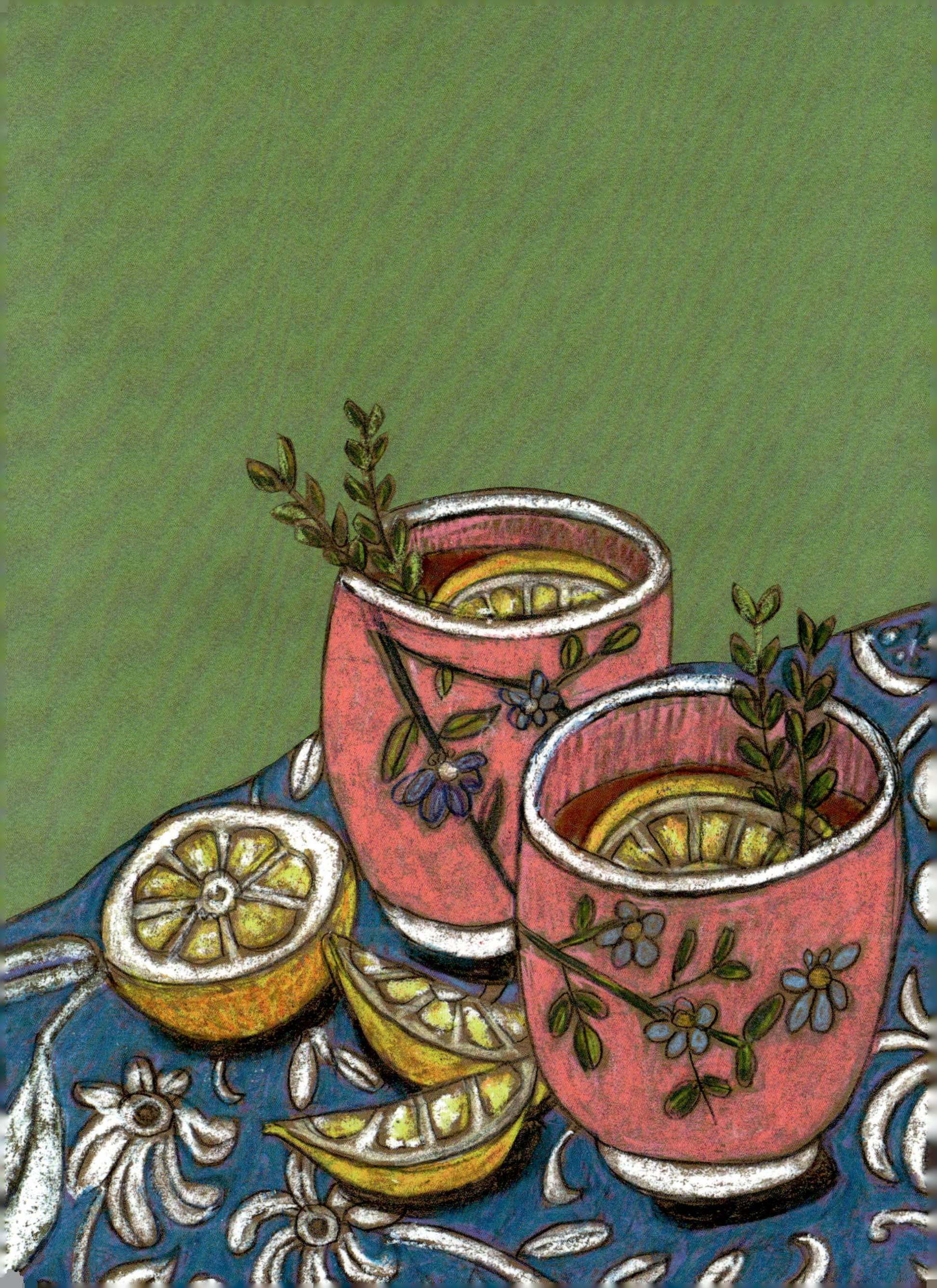

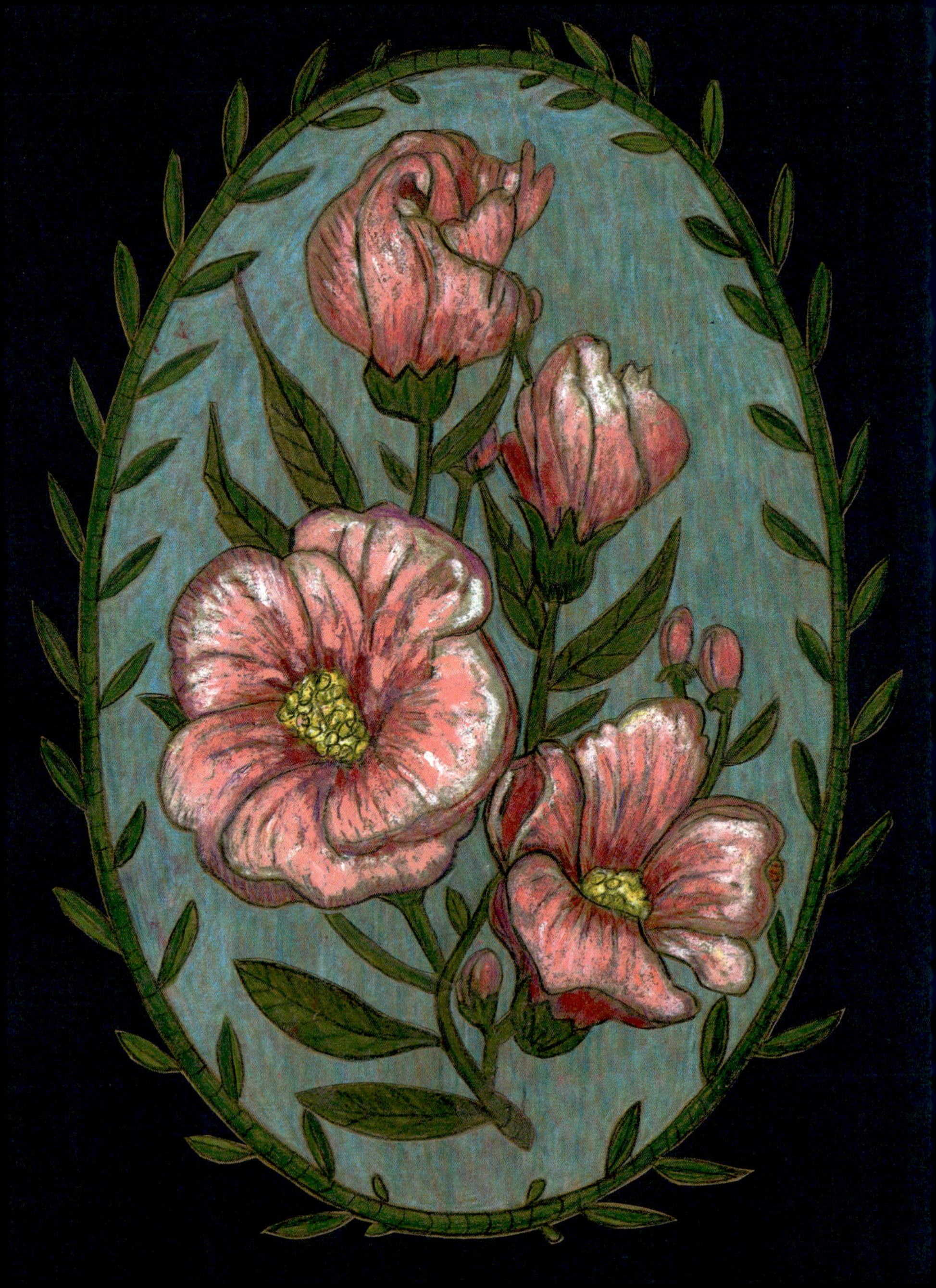

INTRODUCTION

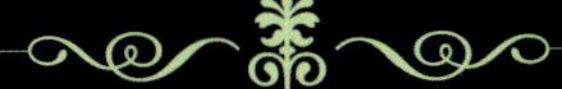

This book is deeply rooted in ancient traditions from cultures around the world. Throughout history, herbs and plants have offered natural healing. Long before modern medicine, people relied on herbal remedies to soothe ailments and support overall well-being. Healers, witches, shamans, and herbalists would gather plants, prepare teas, and make dishes, balms, and blends designed to bring health and comfort to daily life.

Susan and I view mindfulness as an integral part of this book. Mindfulness encourages us to slow down, breathe deeply, and fully experience the present moment. When applied to recipes, mindfulness transforms the simple act of preparing tea or a remedy into an opportunity for grounding and self-care.

We believe that making teas, tinctures, and other plant-based creations is one of the most rewarding, nourishing, and grounding of experiences. These small rituals release stress and provide a space to reset ourselves, despite the hectic pace of the world around us. Always remember: **Intuition is everything!** We encourage you to experiment with different herbs, combinations, and methods to discover what feels best for you.

It is essential to thoughtfully assess the ingredients you use. Whenever possible, choose organic, chemical-free plants so they are safe for consumption. By working with care and intention, you'll create blends that not only taste delicious but also support your health and well-being in the most natural ways. Our wish is that you have fun creating and using the recipes in this book. We certainly had fun creating them for you!

—Chris

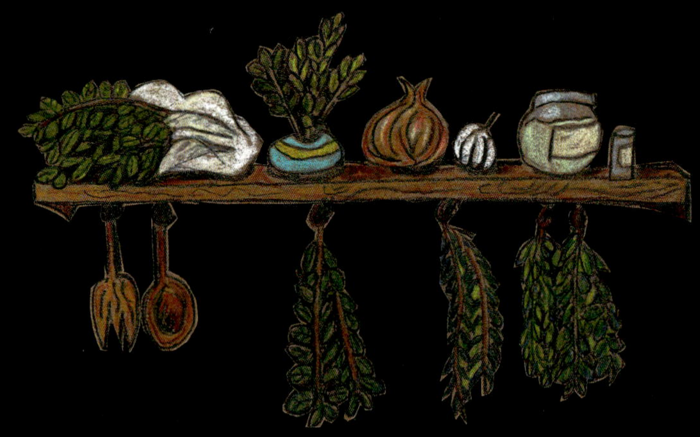

PROCURING AND DRYING YOUR OWN HERBS

Growing and drying your own herbs is one of the most rewarding ways to connect with nature while ensuring that the plants you use for teas, remedies, or cooking are fresh. The most important rule is to always work with herbs that are organic, with no pesticides, herbicides, or synthetic fertilizers, ever! You always want to use the best, most natural ingredients for the health of yourself and your loved ones.

Procuring Herbs

The ideal way to begin is by planting the herbs and plants yourself, whether in a garden bed, patio containers, or even small windowsill boxes or pots. Try to choose organic seeds or starter plants from trusted sources and provide them with sunlight, water, and natural soil. If you cannot grow your own, consider getting your herbs from reputable organic farms, farmers markets, or stores specializing in organic food, such as co-ops. When you pick or purchase herbs, pause a moment to take in their scent and appreciate their texture and beauty.

Harvesting and Drying

Harvest herbs on a dry morning after all the dew has evaporated, but before the sun is too hot, in order to get the best of the plant's essential oils. Always use clean, sharp scissors to clip leaves or sprigs, and collect them in a basket. Tie small bundles of the herbs with twine and hang them upside down in a warm, dark, dry, and well-ventilated space like a pantry.

Drying usually takes one to two weeks. The herbs will be ready when the leaves crumble between your fingers. The next step is to store them in airtight glass jars (we like to recycle old peanut butter or jelly jars), away from heat and light. Always remember to label your jars with the names of the herbs and the date harvested, so you can use them while they're at their very freshest.

As the herbs dry, check on them regularly. When doing so, take a moment for yourself to rub a leaf gently between your fingers and take in its scent.

Using Dried Herbs

Once dried and stored, your herbs are ready for use. Hooray!

Whenever you prepare tea or a recipe with your dried herbs, set an intention for well-being. Give gratitude for the ways these wonderful plants will improve your life. Because they really will.

PLANTS THAT HEAL ESSENTIALS

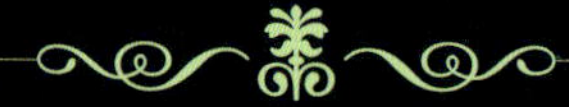

Prep Tools

Mixing bowls in several sizes

Liquid and dry measuring cups

Measuring spoons

Whisk

Stainless steel tongs

Knives—chef's, serrated, and paring

Kitchen scissors for snipping herbs

Zester or rasp-style grater

Box grater

Citrus juicer

Vegetable peeler

Fine mesh sieve strainers—small, medium, and large

Colander

Mortar and pestle for grinding spices and herbs

Appliances

Food processor

Electric hand mixer or stand mixer

Immersion blender

Spice grinder for grinding spices (optional)

Cookware

Small and medium saucepans with lids

Large skillet

Stockpot or Dutch oven

Double boiler (optional; you can use a medium saucepan with a bowl fitted inside)

Pie pan

Loaf pan

Rimmed baking sheet

Parchment paper for lining pans

Serving and Display

Spoons in various shapes and sizes, including wooden and stainless steel

Decorative plates, platters, and bowls for serving

Small wooden or ceramic bowls for spices and herbs

A whimsical pitcher for cool drinks

Decorative cake stand

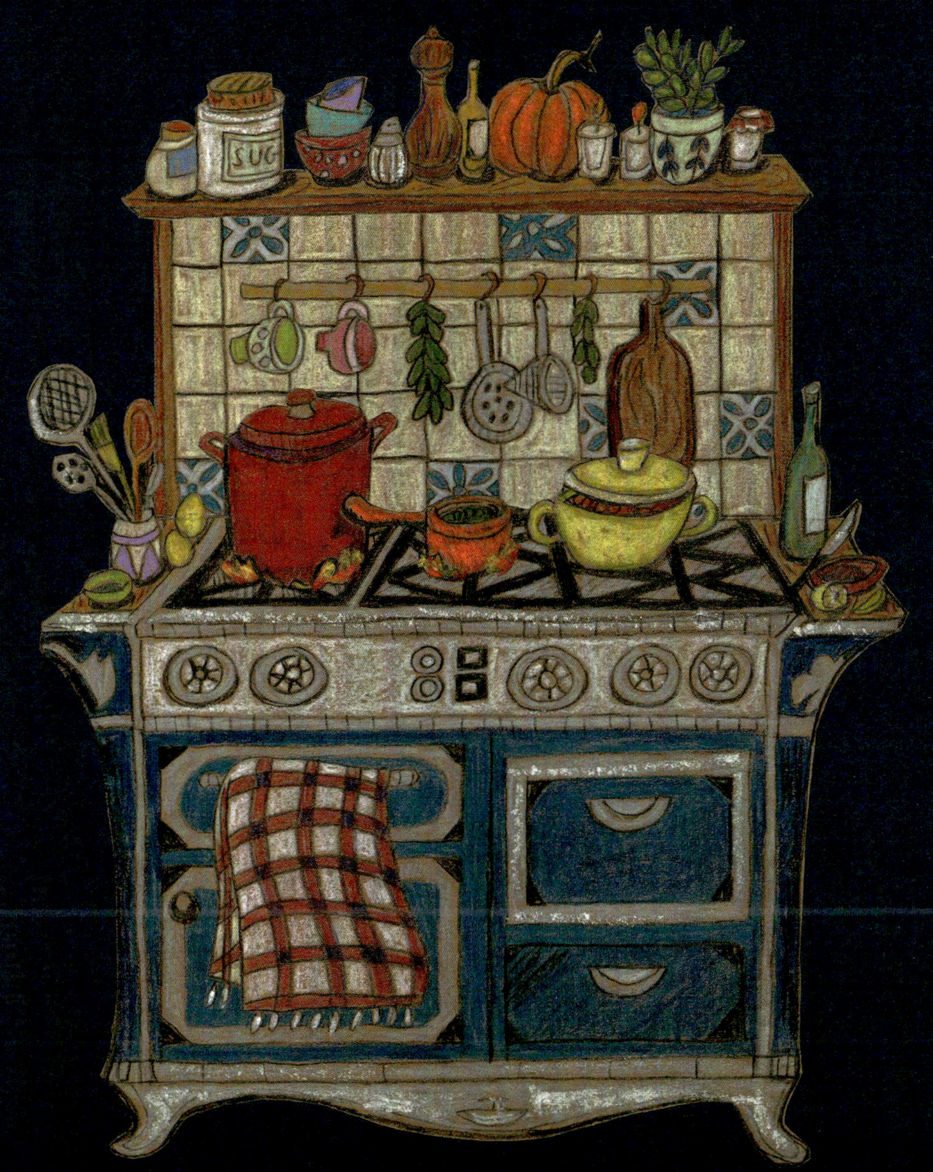

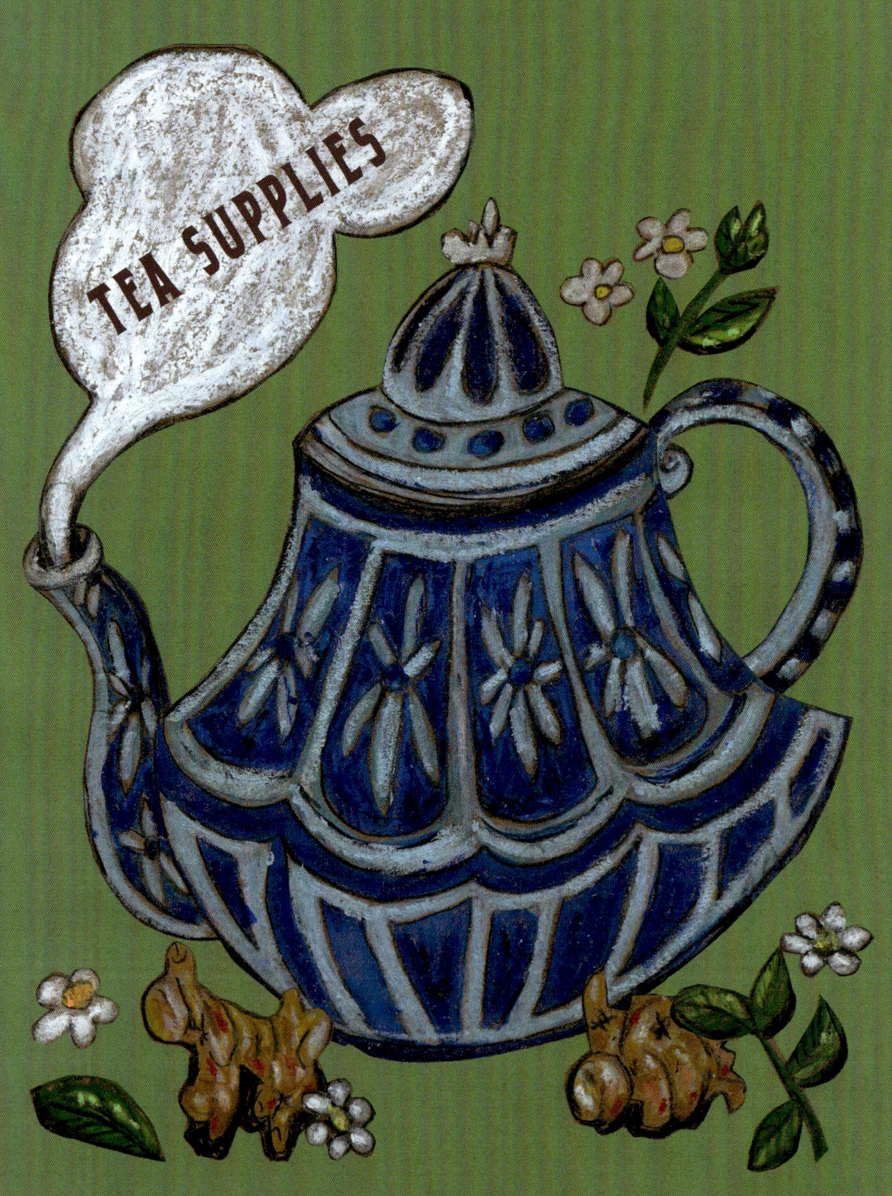
TEA SUPPLIES

Tea Supplies

Tea kettle for heating water

Tea infuser for loose teas

Fine mesh tea or cocktail strainer to strain herbs
   from liquids

Teapots and teacups

Get creative and collect various styles of pots,
cups, saucers, and other teatime accoutrements.
There are many beautiful vintage, modern, and
handmade options to choose from!

More Essentials

Sachet and fabric bags

Cheesecloth

Wood skewers

Cotton kitchen twine

Kitchen matches

Glass jars with tight-fitting lids in various sizes

Glass bottles with screw tops or corks

Spray bottles

Small tins for lip gloss

Decorative jars and bottles for oils and bath salts

Labels for storage containers

Ribbon for decorating your creations

Tissue paper for gift wrapping

Silicone soap molds

Blank journal for your recipes, notes, and journaling

Sourcing Ingredients

For supplies, we like to explore independent businesses in our area, such as kitchen supply places, craft shops, and plant stores, which often carry a variety of essential products. Of course, the internet is also a good source if these types of businesses are unavailable to you. And as usual, always feel free to use recycled items.

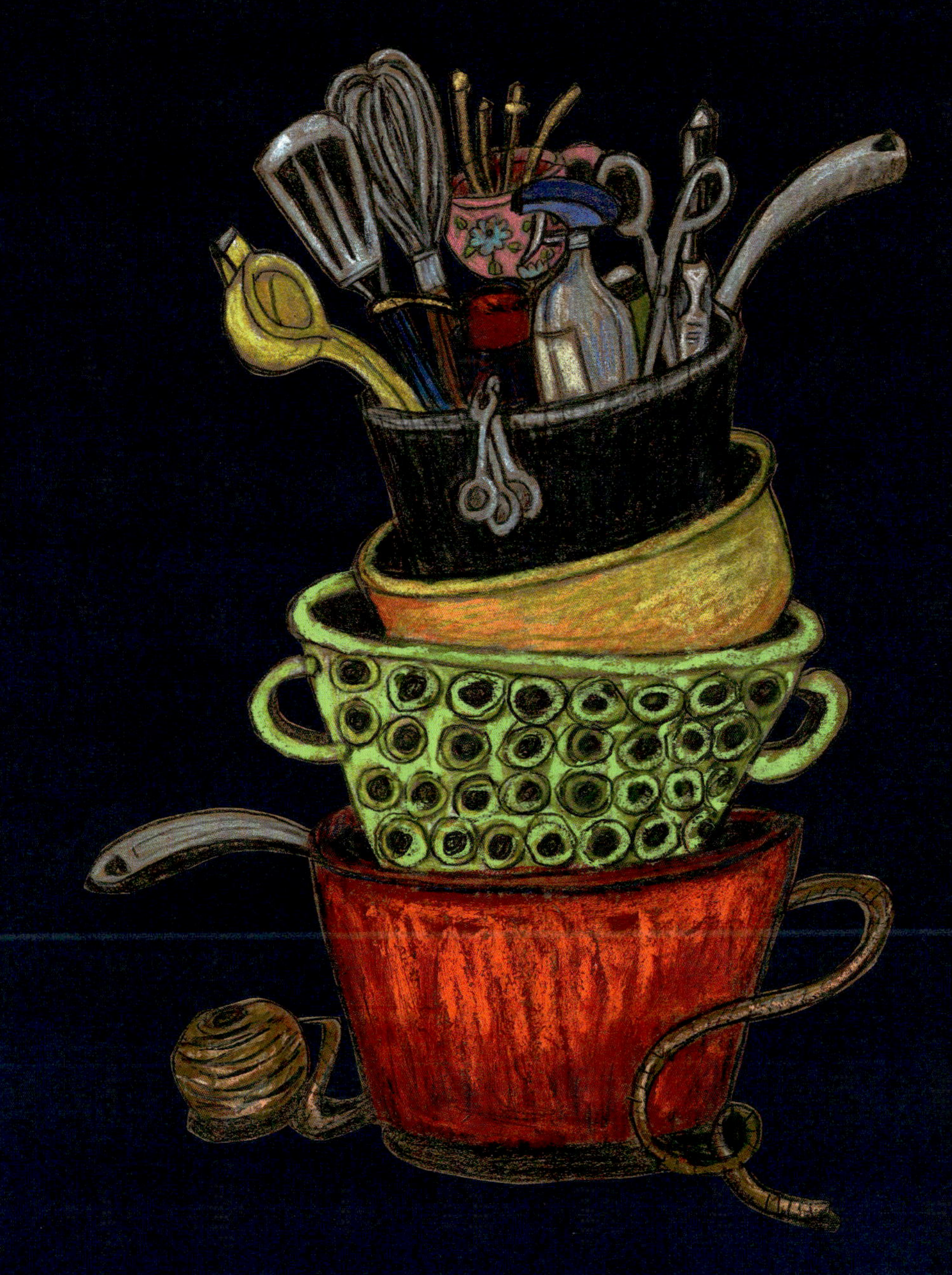

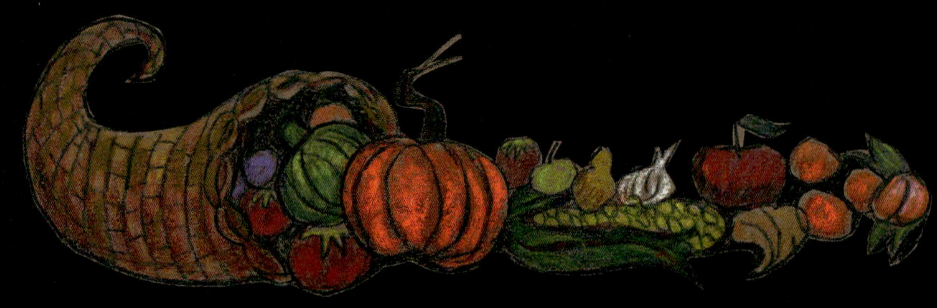

FOOD, LOVE, AND OTHER THINGS PERFECTLY IMPERFECT

Cooking has been my love language for more than thirty years, and it's a deeply fulfilling way for me to express my care for those I cherish. Preparing meals for the people I love feels like giving them a big, warm hug—a way to show just how much they mean to me. The aromas that fill the kitchen and the flavors I create are more than just nourishment; they carry my heart and intention.

Please use our collection of recipes as a guide, but feel free to add your own personal touches. Substitute basil for rosemary if that's what you have in your garden. Try our spinach salad recipe with walnuts and figs in chapter 2, then try it again with a different kind of nut or fruit. Use your imagination to create your own masterpieces. Don't be afraid to find joy in the process of experimentation! You never know what you'll teach yourself.

Just like my experience of creating art, cooking relaxes me and puts me into a wonderful flow state. Cooking with intention means being present; it involves choosing fresh, wholesome ingredients, understanding their flavors and characteristics, and thoughtfully exploring how they can work together to create something extraordinary.

—Susan

We Love to Color Outside the Lines!

All the illustrations in this book are created by hand with colored pencils and Sennelier oil pastels. Then the paintings are cut by hand and attached to the background papers to complete the final art. My work is proudly low-tech!

At a time when so many book illustrations are digital, I love when I can see the artist's hand at work. I appreciate the texture, lines, layers, and evidence of mark-making in art made the old-school way. I love to imagine the person behind the work. Perfection doesn't excite me. Originality does!

We hope our ideas and recipes will inspire you to take time out of your day to care for yourself, and perhaps to share these experiences with someone special.

—Susan

Because this book honors the healing nature of plants, we feel it is important that all our recipes are cruelty-free. For us, this reflects our deep respect for all living beings and the Earth herself. We believe that healing should never come at the expense or harm of another living soul. By carefully keeping each recipe plant-based, organic, and free from animal testing, we know that the recipes we share are infused with compassion, sustainability, and a holistic vision of wellness.

We hope this book becomes a resource you refer to again and again!

—Chris

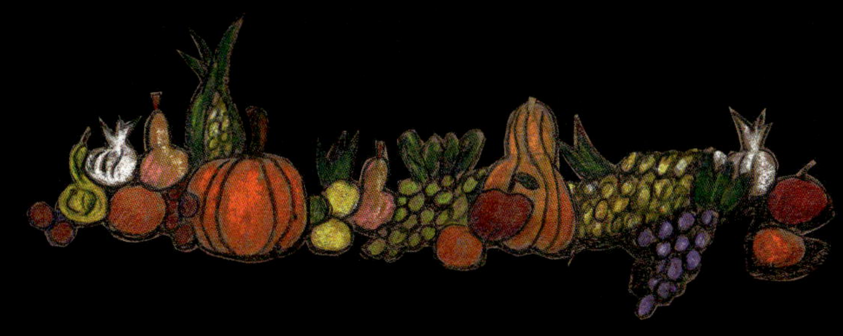

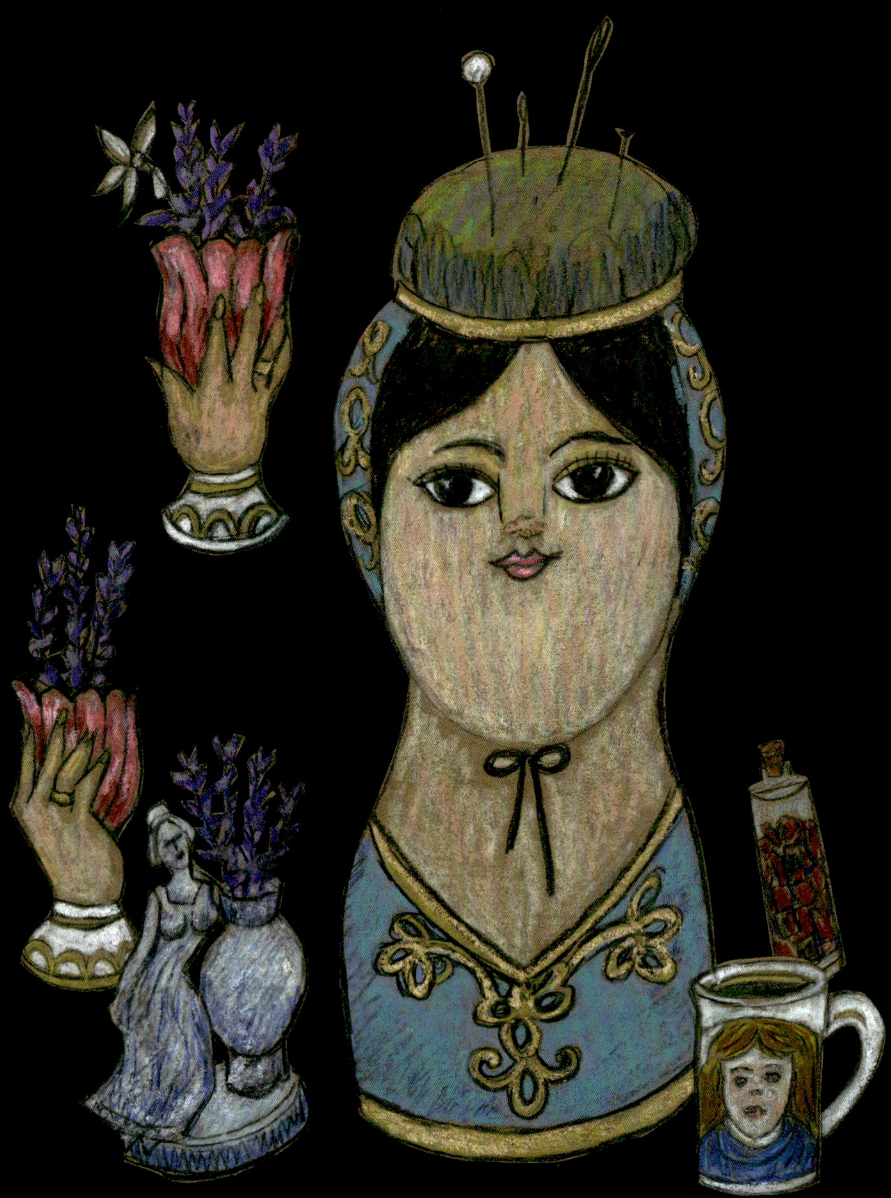

CHAPTER 1

HEAL YOUR BODY

Plants have always been our beloved companions, offering their roots, flowers, and leaves as they guide us toward balance and renewal.

When we brew a cup of tea or stir a soup, we are doing more than cooking. We are performing a simple and essential ritual of healing.

Throughout history, plants have been honored as healers. In the pages ahead, you'll find teas, tonics, soups, soaps, and salves crafted to restore the body and lift the spirit. These are not just remedies; they are also opportunities to practice mindfulness. Wellness is not a destination, but a practice. It's a way of moving through life with self-care and gratitude.

Let this first chapter be your invitation to make healing an integral part of your everyday life.

We'll start with one of our favorite herbs, yarrow. It is so powerful that in ancient times it was said to heal the wounds of warriors. Now it's ready to ease our own headaches with our *Achilles's Yarrow Headache Tea*.

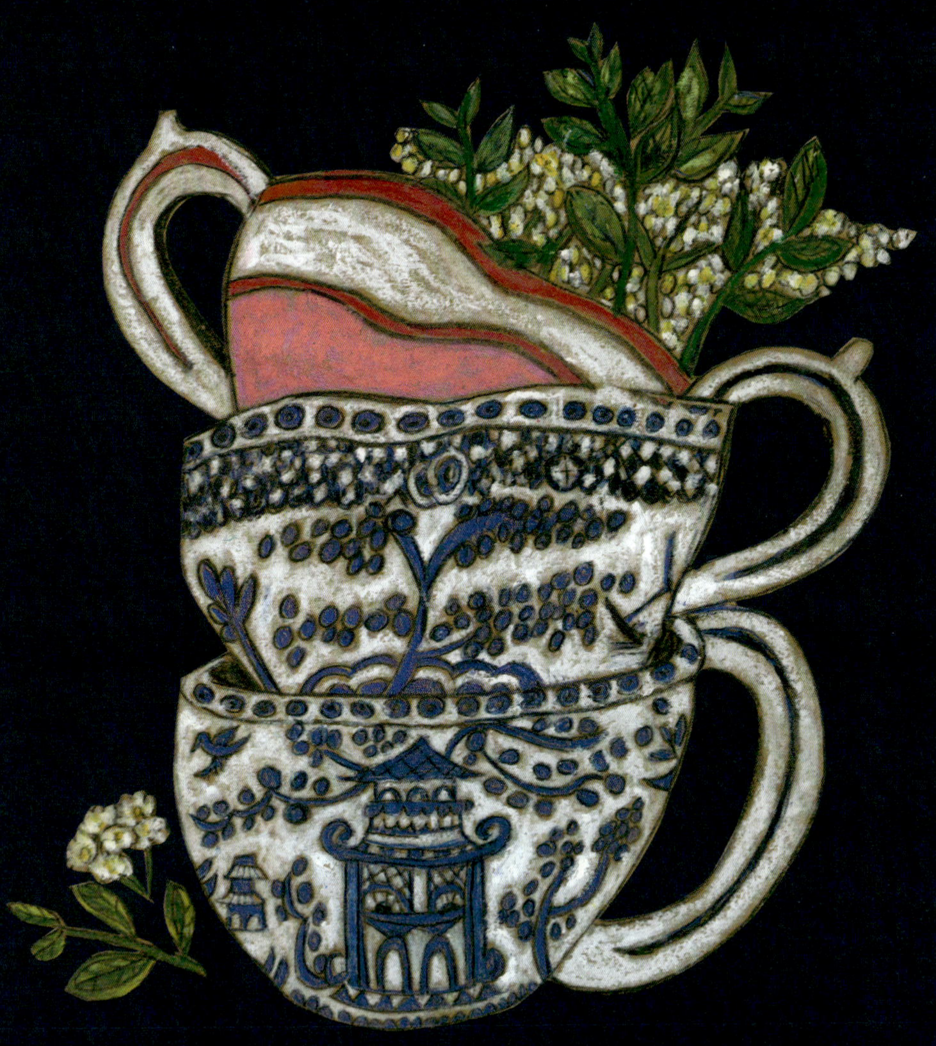

Achilles's Yarrow Headache Tea

(Serves 2)

This soothing herbal tea eases tension, supports digestion, reduces inflammation, and restores calm to the mind.

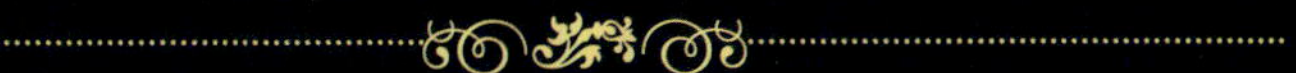

2 cups water
1 tablespoon dried yarrow flowers
1 teaspoon dried peppermint leaves
1 teaspoon dried chamomile flowers
1 teaspoon dried lavender flowers

Bring water to a gentle boil. While waiting, focus on your breath, inhaling deeply and exhaling slowly, cultivating a sense of calm and intention.

Once the water is boiling, reduce the heat to a simmer. Add the dried yarrow, peppermint, chamomile, and lavender to the water. Stir gently and breathe in the aromas as the herbs infuse the water. Let the herbs simmer for 5 to 10 minutes.

Remove the pot from heat and strain the tea through a fine mesh sieve directly into your favorite mugs or teacups. Discard the herbs into your compost bin. Stir your tea slowly, taking note of its transformation. Sip with gratitude.

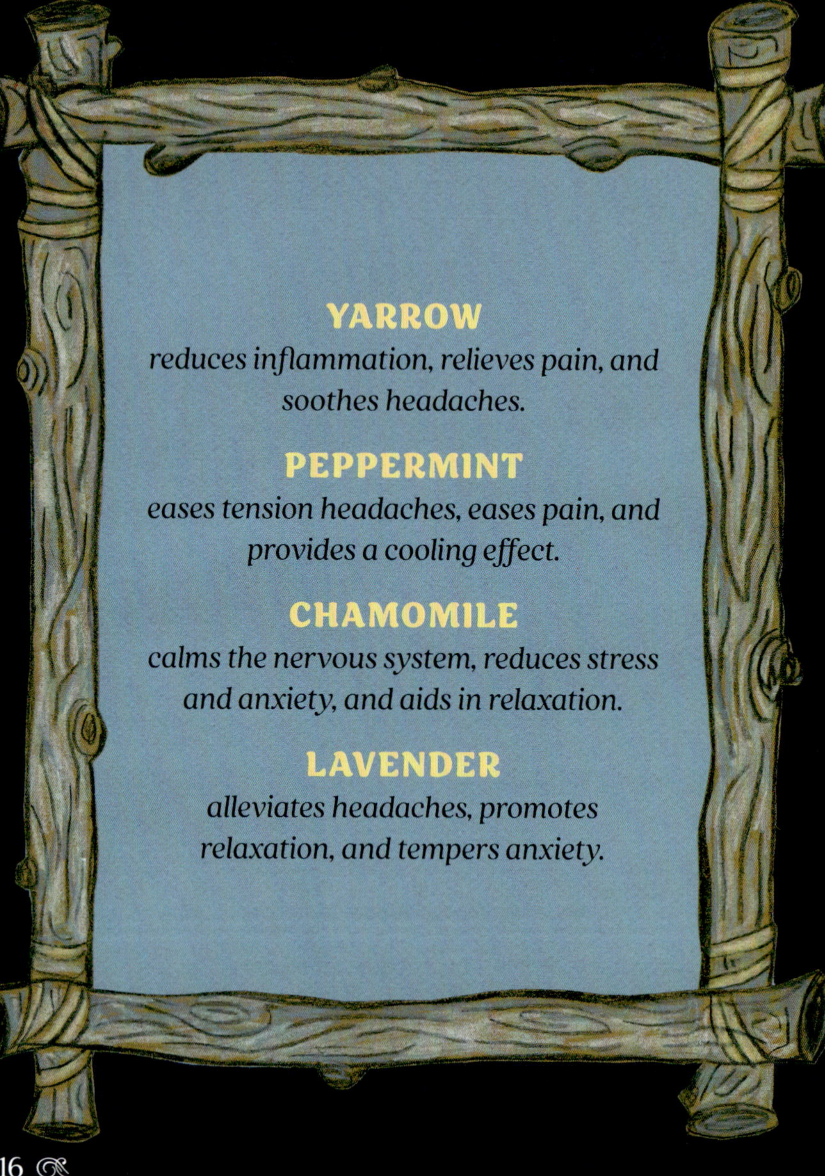

YARROW

reduces inflammation, relieves pain, and soothes headaches.

PEPPERMINT

eases tension headaches, eases pain, and provides a cooling effect.

CHAMOMILE

calms the nervous system, reduces stress and anxiety, and aids in relaxation.

LAVENDER

alleviates headaches, promotes relaxation, and tempers anxiety.

Did You Know?

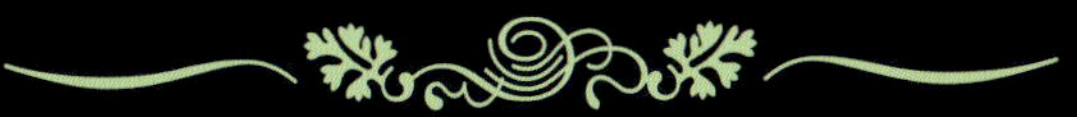

Yarrow (*Achillea millefolium*) is named after the Greek hero Achilles, who used the plant to treat wounds on the battlefield. The legend says that he used yarrow to stop bleeding and aid in healing.

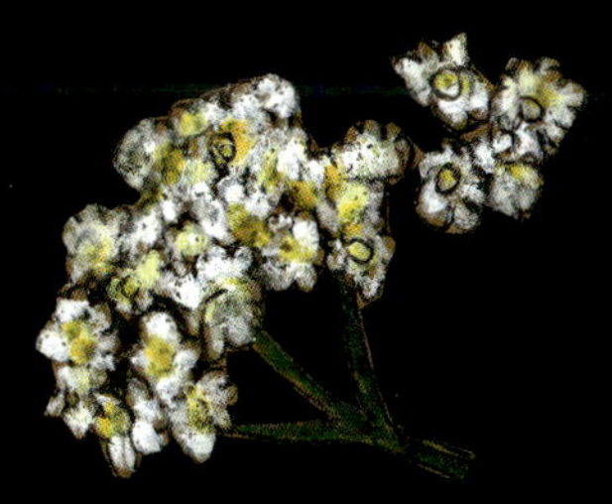

Morgana's Garlic, Lemon, and Ginger Healing Tea

(Serves 2)

**This tea boosts immunity, eases inflammation, and provides
a sense of physical and spiritual balance.**

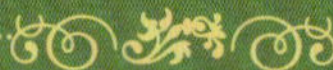

2 cloves fresh garlic
2 cups water
1 piece fresh ginger, about 1 inch, peeled and sliced thinly
Juice from 1 fresh lemon (about 3 tablespoons)

Peel the garlic and crush it gently with the intention of awakening its healing oils.

Bring the water to a boil, taking a moment just to be still. Reduce heat to a gentle simmer. Add crushed garlic and sliced ginger to the pot. Simmer for 10 to 15 minutes to allow the brew to become potent and powerful.

Use this moment to breathe deeply, setting an intention for healing and peace.

Strain the tea through a fine mesh sieve into your favorite mugs. Discard the solids into your compost bin. Stir half the freshly squeezed lemon juice into each mug. Let its brightness awaken the brew.

If you like, float a thin slice of lemon on top.

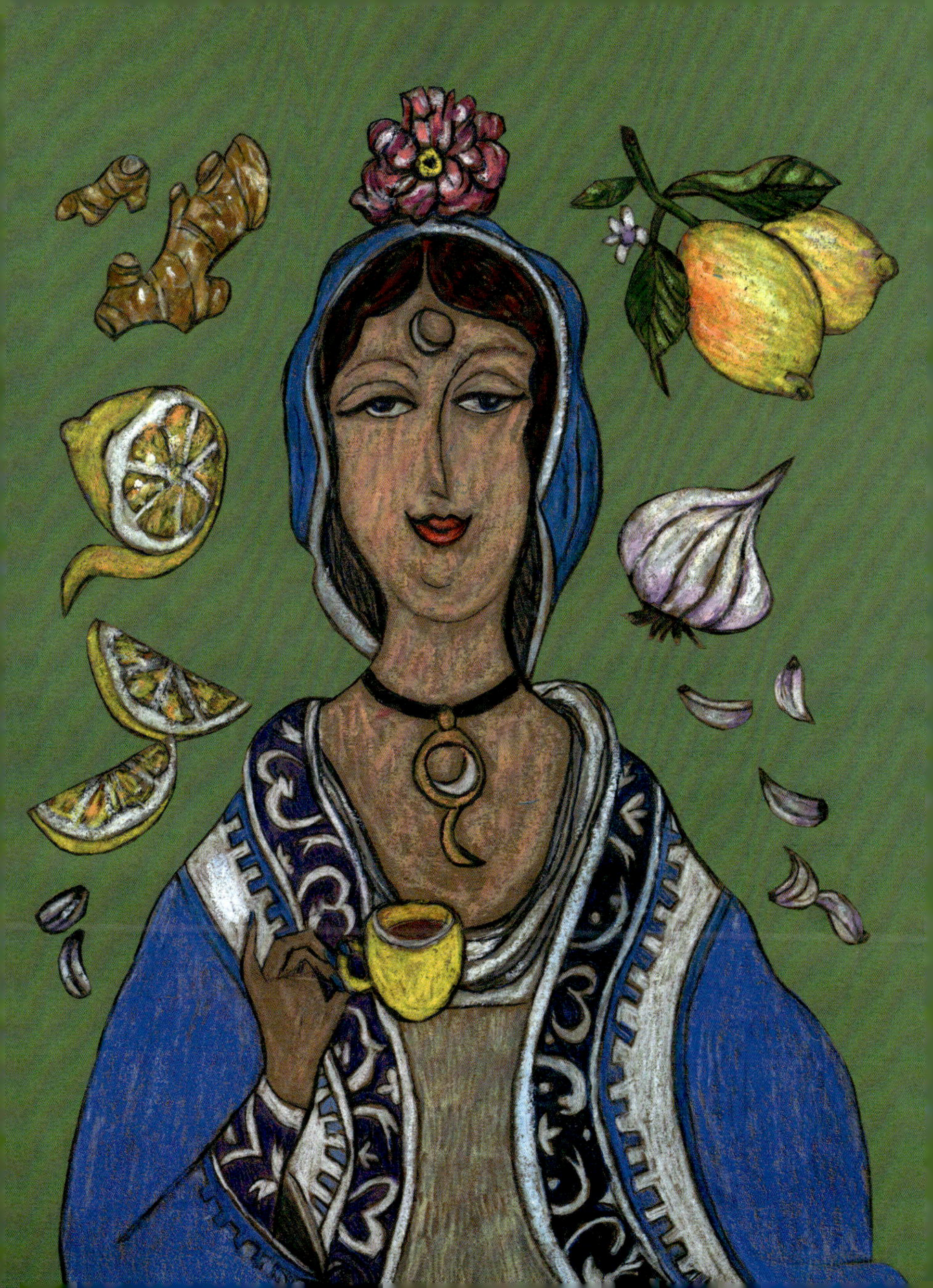

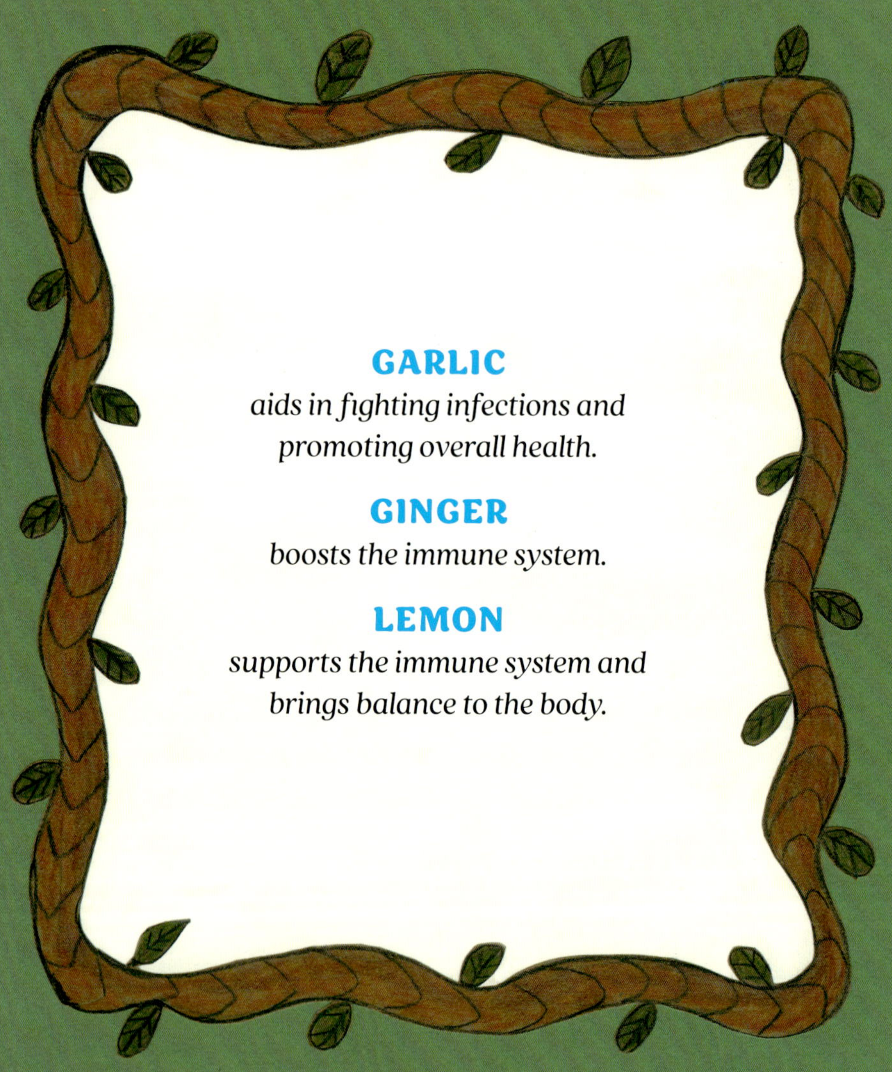

GARLIC

aids in fighting infections and promoting overall health.

GINGER

boosts the immune system.

LEMON

supports the immune system and brings balance to the body.

Did You Know?

Morgana, also known as Morgan le Fay, was King Arthur's half-sister. She was renowned for her extraordinary healing abilities, which were deeply rooted in her extensive knowledge of herbalism.

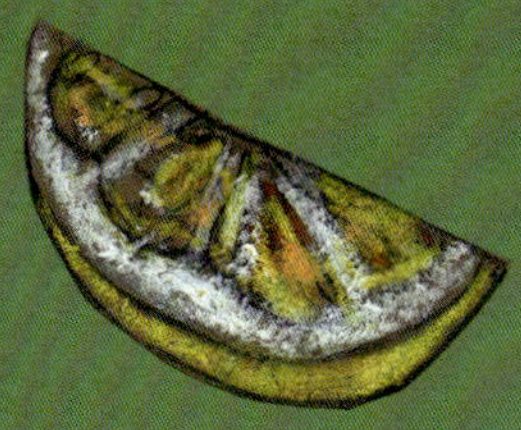

Calendula and Bergamot Anti-Inflammatory Bath Soap

(Makes 6 soap bars)

Calendula is rich in naturally occurring compounds called flavonoids. In this recipe, it's paired with bergamot's calming aroma to create a soap that is a healing ritual for body and spirit.

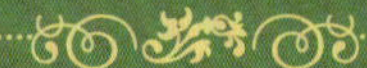

1 pound glycerin melt-and-pour soap base
1 teaspoon calendula essential oil
1 teaspoon bergamot essential oil
2 tablespoons dried calendula petals
Rectangular silicone soap molds

Cut the soap base into small chunks, noticing the texture and clarity of the glycerin as you work. Place the chunks in a microwave-safe container and heat on medium-low in 30-second intervals, stirring at each interval, until fully melted.

Add the calendula and bergamot essential oils, then gently stir in the calendula petals. Carefully pour the mixture into your soap molds, one by one.

Allow the soaps to set for 1 hour. This is a perfect time to sip tea, journal, or simply relax.

Once the soap is completely cool, gently remove the bars from the molds. Congratulations, you've made something healing with your hands and your heart!

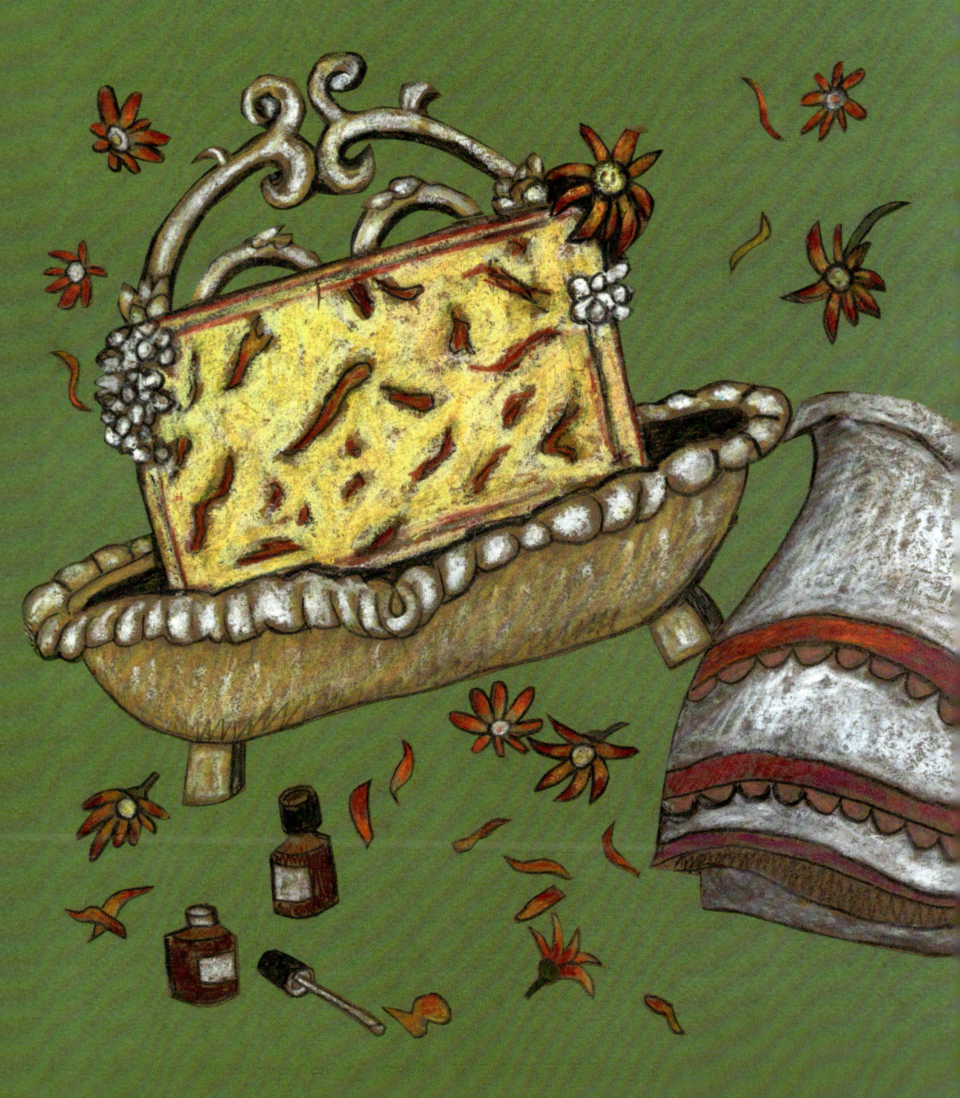

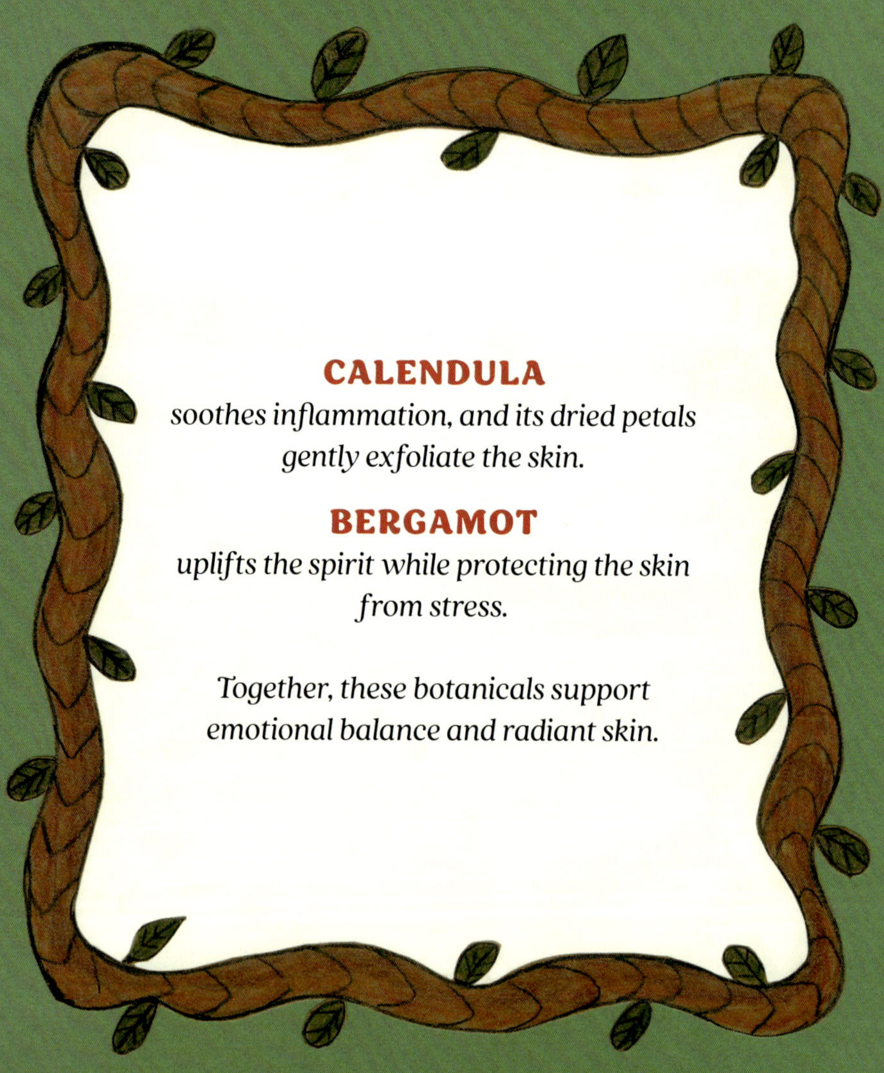

CALENDULA

soothes inflammation, and its dried petals gently exfoliate the skin.

BERGAMOT

uplifts the spirit while protecting the skin from stress.

Together, these botanicals support emotional balance and radiant skin.

Did You Know?

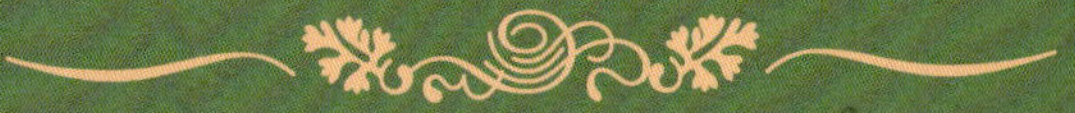

In medieval Europe, calendula was known as the "herb of the sun," believed to draw out sickness, especially fevers and skin infections.

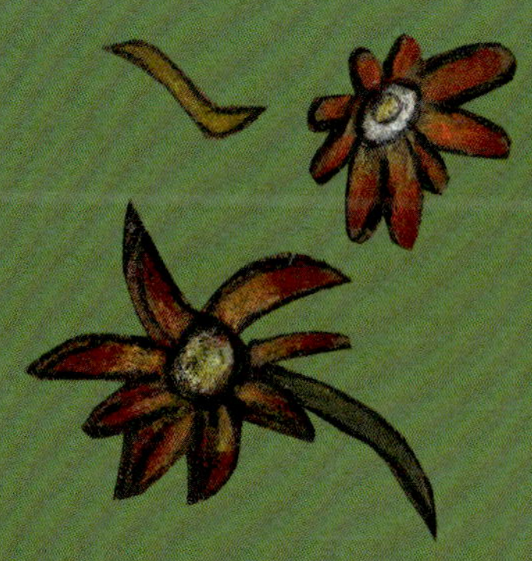

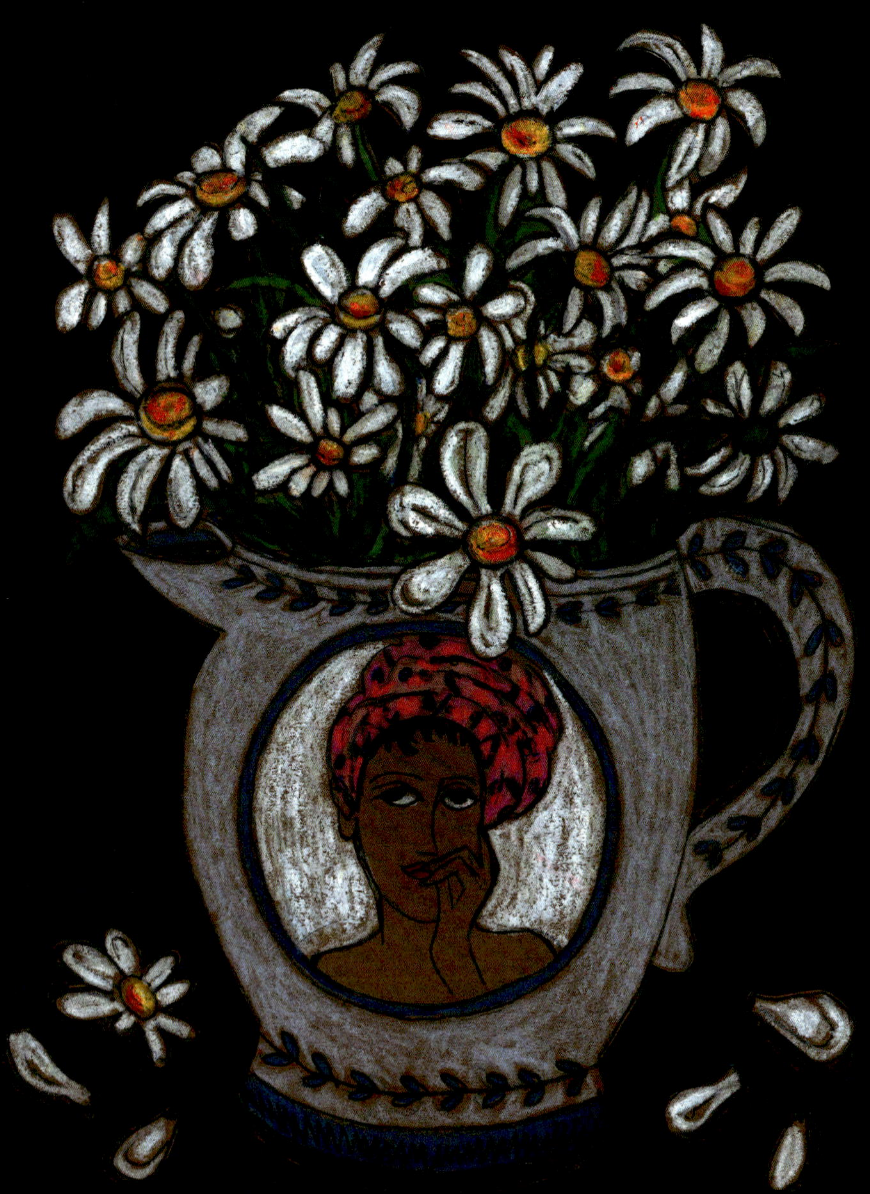

Daisy Salve

(Makes about 4 ounces)

**Daisies are ancient allies in healing. Their essence carries
energies of love, protection, and joy.**

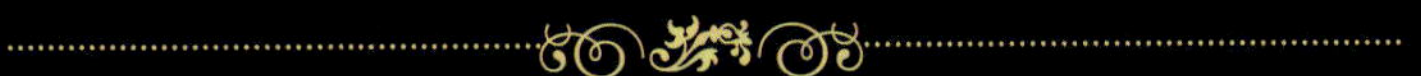

12-16 fresh daisy flower heads with petals attached
½ cup cosmetic almond oil, or the carrier oil of your choice
1 small (8-ounce) clean glass jar with a tight-fitting lid

Place the daisy heads into the jar. As you do, visualize filling the jar with healing light.

Pour the almond oil slowly over the daisies. Do your best to make sure all the flower heads are fully submerged. If necessary, add more oil until they are completely covered. Seal the jar and place it in a cool, dry place for two weeks.

After two weeks, strain the mixture through a fine mesh sieve into a glass measuring cup with a spout. Press down gently on the daisies with the back of a spoon to release every last drop of their golden goodness. Discard the daisies into your compost bin.

Wash, rinse, and thoroughly dry your jar. Pour in the finished oil. Label it and include the date you made it. Store the salve in the refrigerator, where it will keep for several weeks.

To use, apply a small amount of oil over minor aches, bruises, or dry patches of skin. Let each application be a small ritual of self-love—and thank the sweet daisies for their gift.

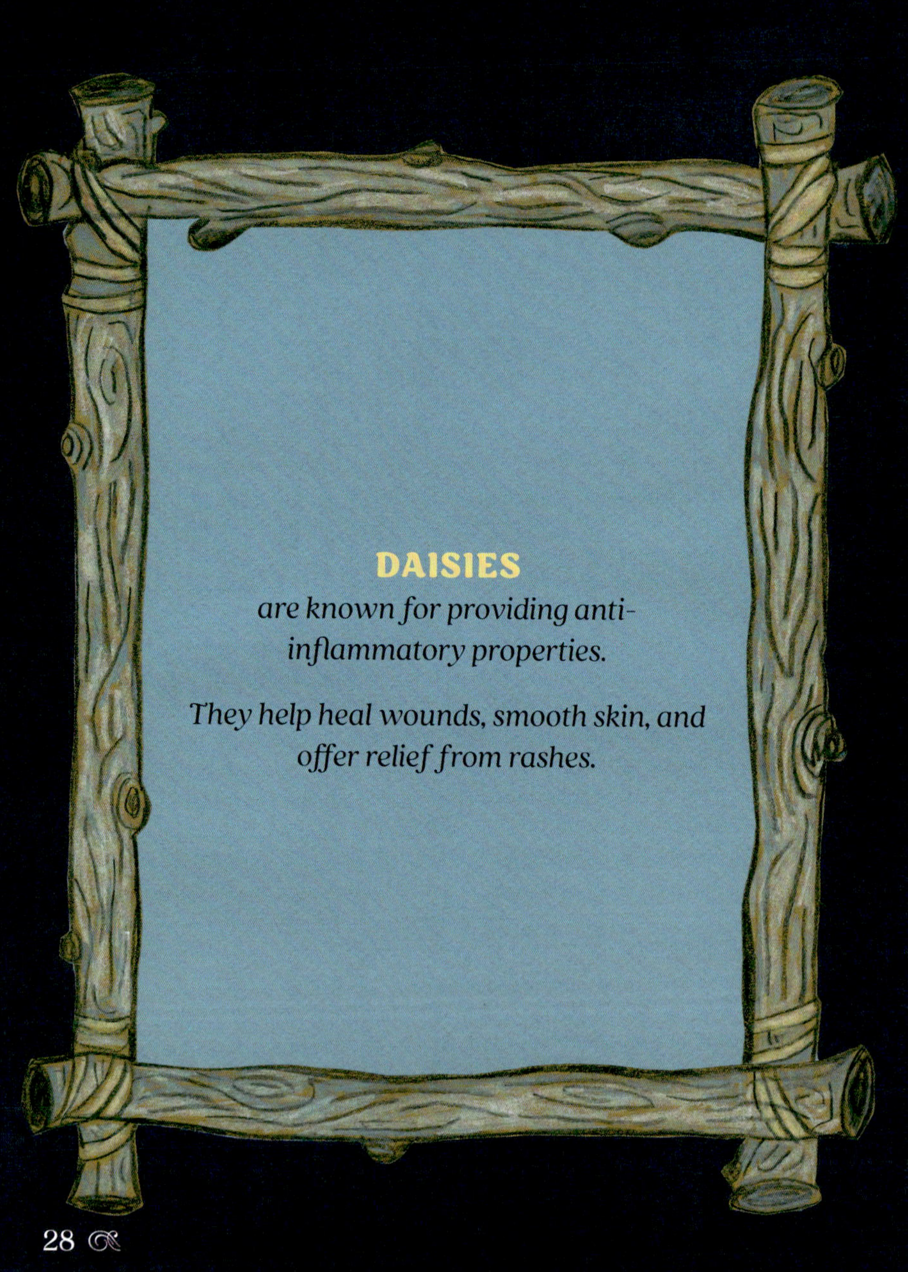

DAISIES

are known for providing anti-inflammatory properties.

They help heal wounds, smooth skin, and offer relief from rashes.

Did You Know?

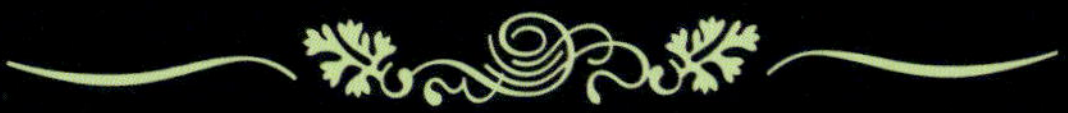

In medieval Europe, daisies were known as "bruisewort" for their powerful effect on bruises and wounds. Soldiers carried daisy poultices or used daisy infusions to treat injuries on the battlefield.

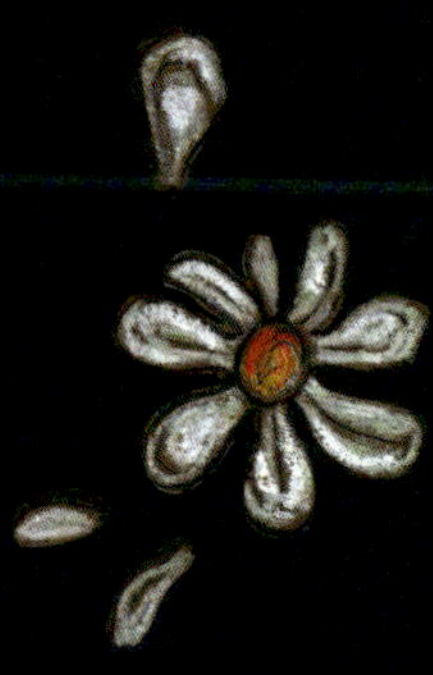

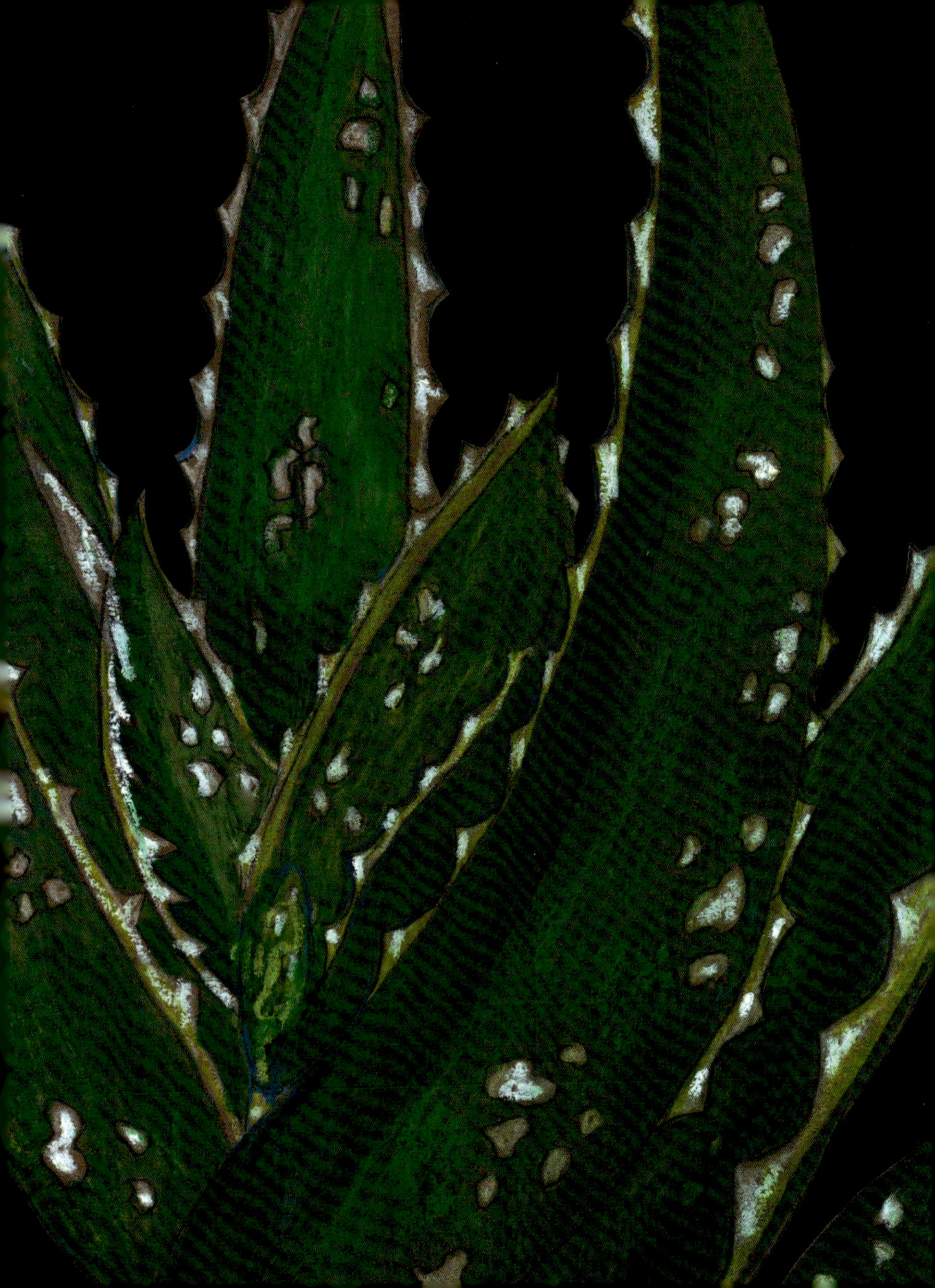

All's Well Aloe Elixir

(Makes about 2 applications)

To cool inflammation, nourish dry or sun-stressed skin, and bring your awareness back to your body with care and gratitude.

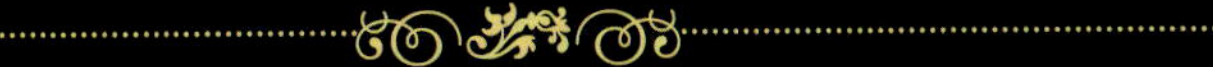

2 tablespoons fresh aloe vera gel
1 teaspoon coconut oil
2 drops lavender essential oil
1 teaspoon rose water

In a small glass bowl, stir together the aloe vera gel, coconut oil, lavender oil, and rose water. Stir slowly and mindfully, watching the textures blend.

Warm the mixture slightly by placing the bowl in your hands or setting it in a warm (not hot) water bath for a minute. Feel the energy of the ingredients activate.

Clean your skin gently and apply this elixir slowly and lovingly with special attention to areas affected by sunburn, dry skin, or soreness. Or simply apply it to your hands and chest to relieve stress.

After applying, sit or lie quietly for a few minutes. Let the aloe soak in. Let your breath be your balm.

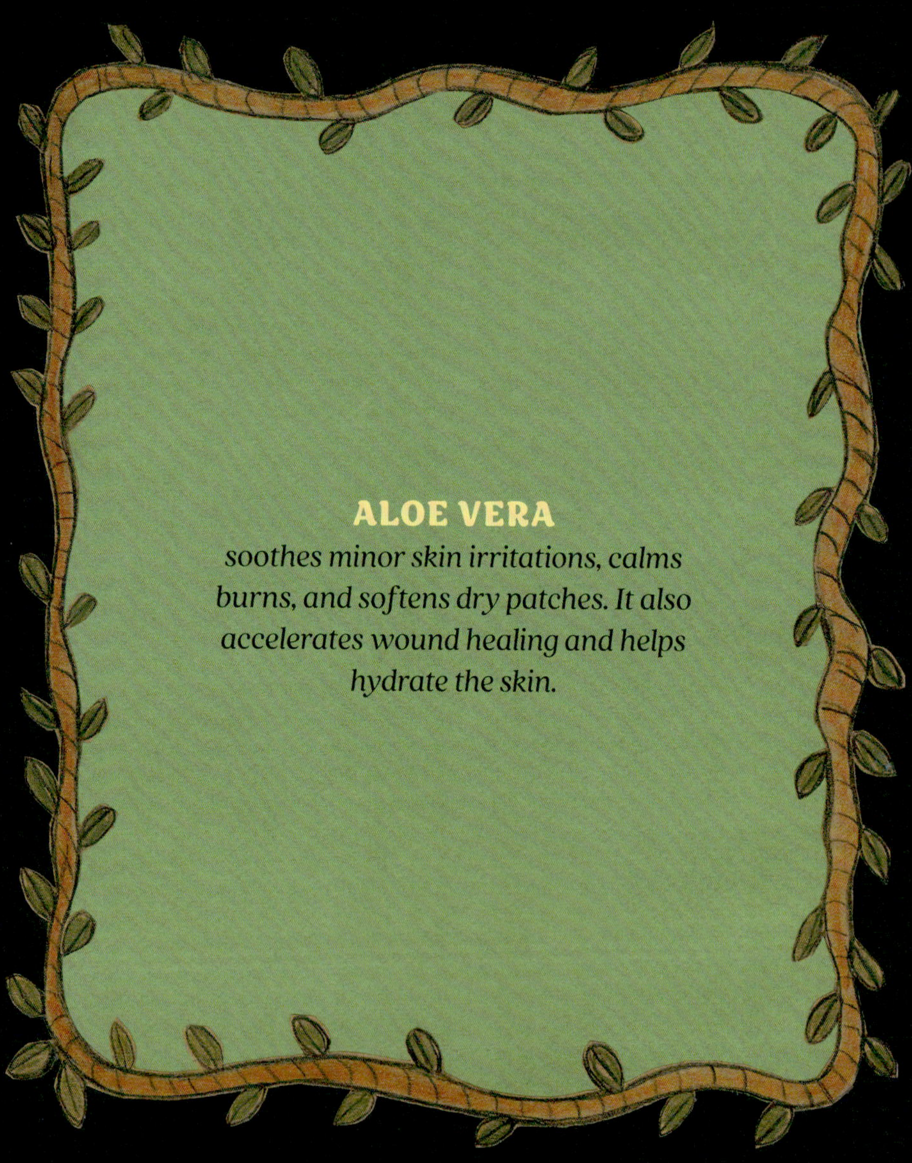

ALOE VERA

soothes minor skin irritations, calms burns, and softens dry patches. It also accelerates wound healing and helps hydrate the skin.

Did You Know?

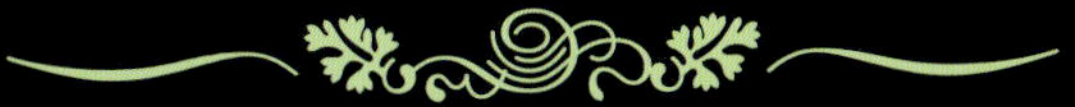

In ancient Egypt, aloe was said to have grown from the tears of Isis as she grieved the death of Osiris, giving it the power to heal the body and to soothe a mourning heart.

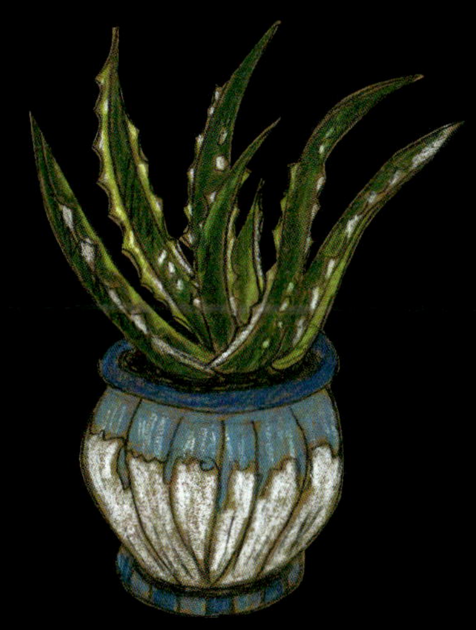

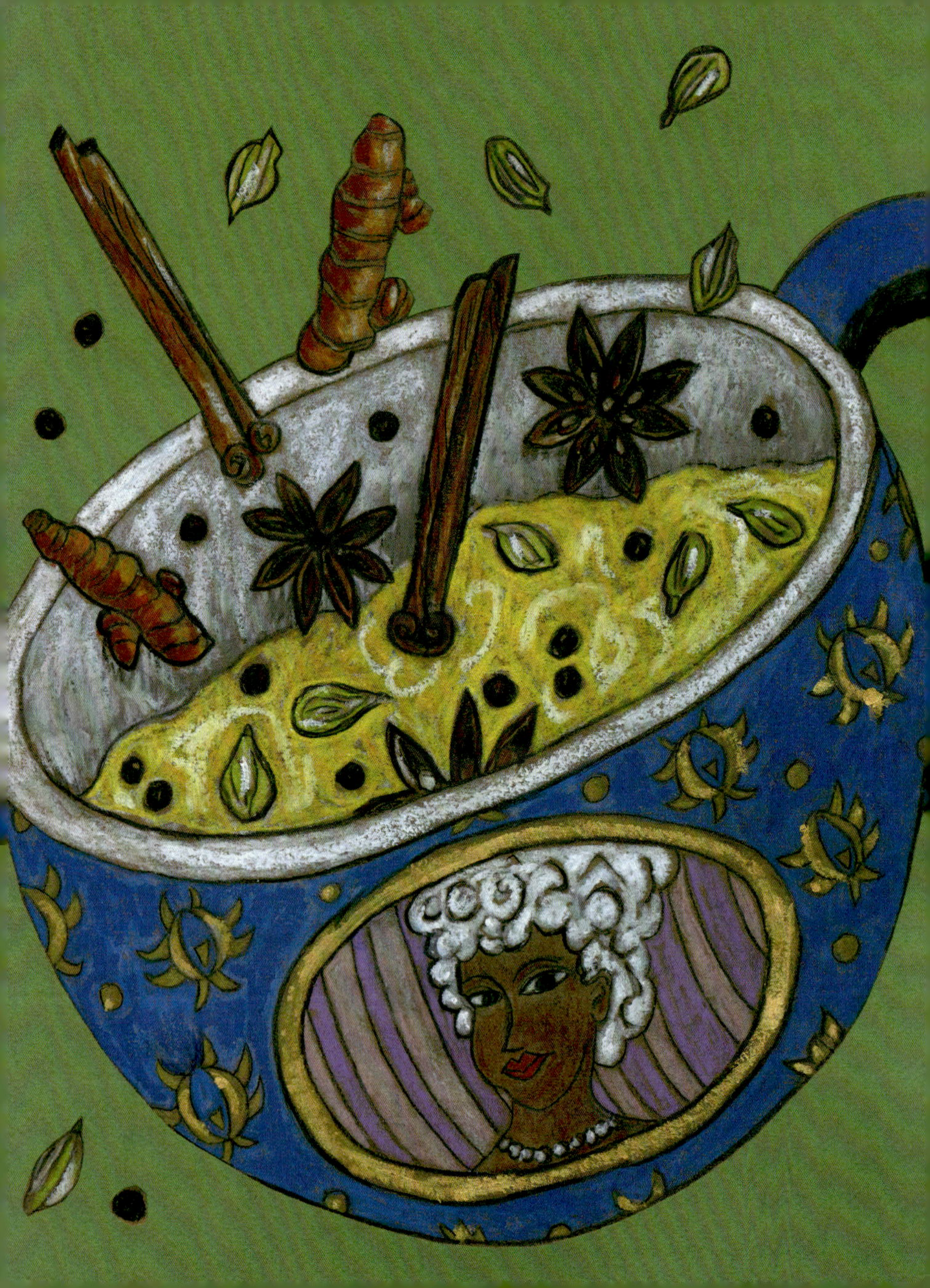

Golden Milk with Turmeric

(Serves 2)

This golden drink is more than nourishing—it's a cup of inner sunlight, brimming with ancient spices known to comfort the body, awaken the spirit, and invite mindful stillness.

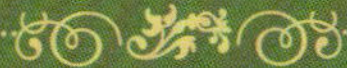

2 cups almond milk (or plant milk of your choice)
½ tablespoon grated fresh ginger
1 tablespoon fresh turmeric, peeled and grated
3-4 whole black peppercorns
3-4 cardamom pods, gently crushed
3-4 star anise pods
2 cinnamon sticks

Gently place all ingredients into a saucepan. As you do, reflect on the origin of each spice—the ancient roots of turmeric, the sacred bark of cinnamon, the protective power of pepper. Thank each one for its gift.

Bring the mixture to a gentle simmer over medium-high heat. Cover and let bubble softly for about 10 minutes.

Strain the golden mixture through a fine mesh sieve directly into mugs or teacups. Discard the spent spices into the compost bin. Imagine each cup is filled not just with golden milk, but with healing light.

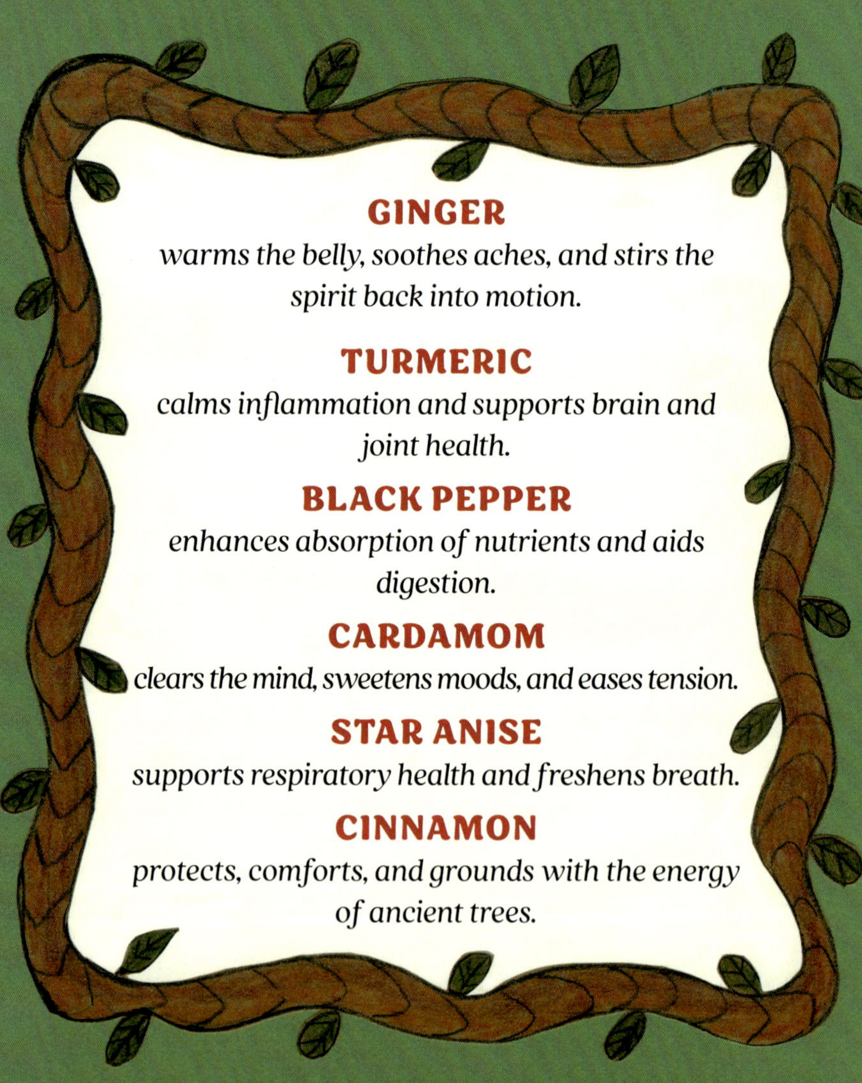

GINGER

warms the belly, soothes aches, and stirs the spirit back into motion.

TURMERIC

calms inflammation and supports brain and joint health.

BLACK PEPPER

enhances absorption of nutrients and aids digestion.

CARDAMOM

clears the mind, sweetens moods, and eases tension.

STAR ANISE

supports respiratory health and freshens breath.

CINNAMON

protects, comforts, and grounds with the energy of ancient trees.

Did You Know?

Golden milk, called haldi doodh in Hindi, comes directly from Ayurvedic medicine, an ancient Indian system dating back over 5,000 years. In Ayurveda, turmeric is revered as one of the most sacred of spices.

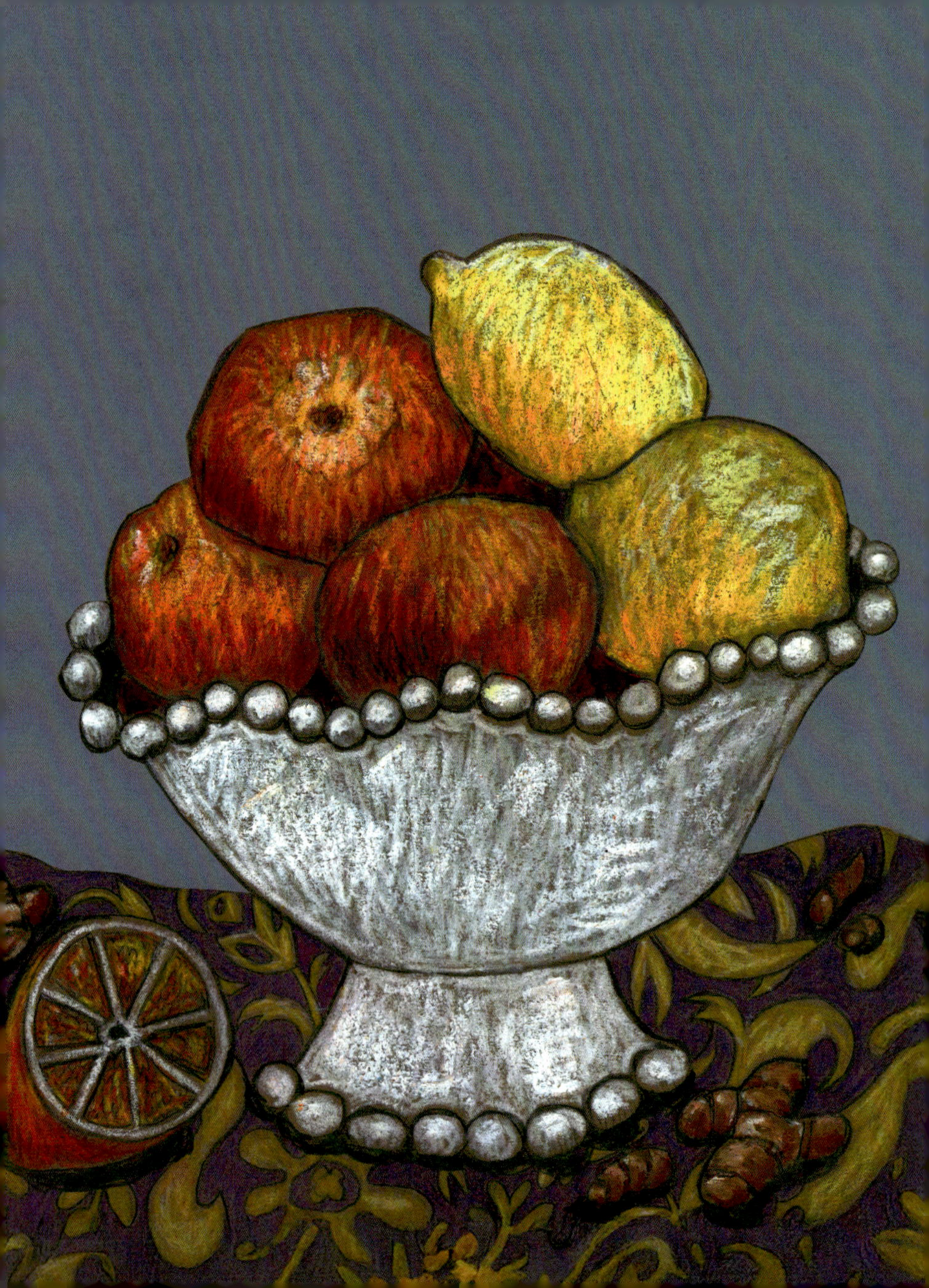

Blood Orange Tonic

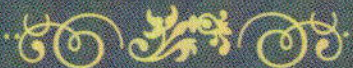

(Serves 2–3)

This bright, colorful tonic cleanses and invigorates from within,
reminding you that vitality begins with balance and nourishment.

3 blood oranges, washed and sliced into thin rounds
1 lemon, washed and sliced into thin rounds
2 teaspoons chopped fresh ginger
1 teaspoon ground turmeric
6 cups water

In a large pot, combine all ingredients. Bring mixture to a boil over high heat, then reduce to a gentle simmer. As the steam rises, take slow, deep breaths and let the scent clear your mind.

Let the liquid gently simmer for 5 to 10 minutes, allowing the ingredients to release their healing essences. Remove the pot from the heat and let it steep for 5 additional minutes. While it steeps, place a hand over your heart and silently set an intention for renewal or gratitude.

Strain through a fine mesh sieve into a pitcher or directly into mugs. Discard the solids into the compost bin. Add a slice of orange or lemon to your cup for an extra lift of aroma and beauty.

You may also refrigerate the tonic to enjoy as a chilled drink later.

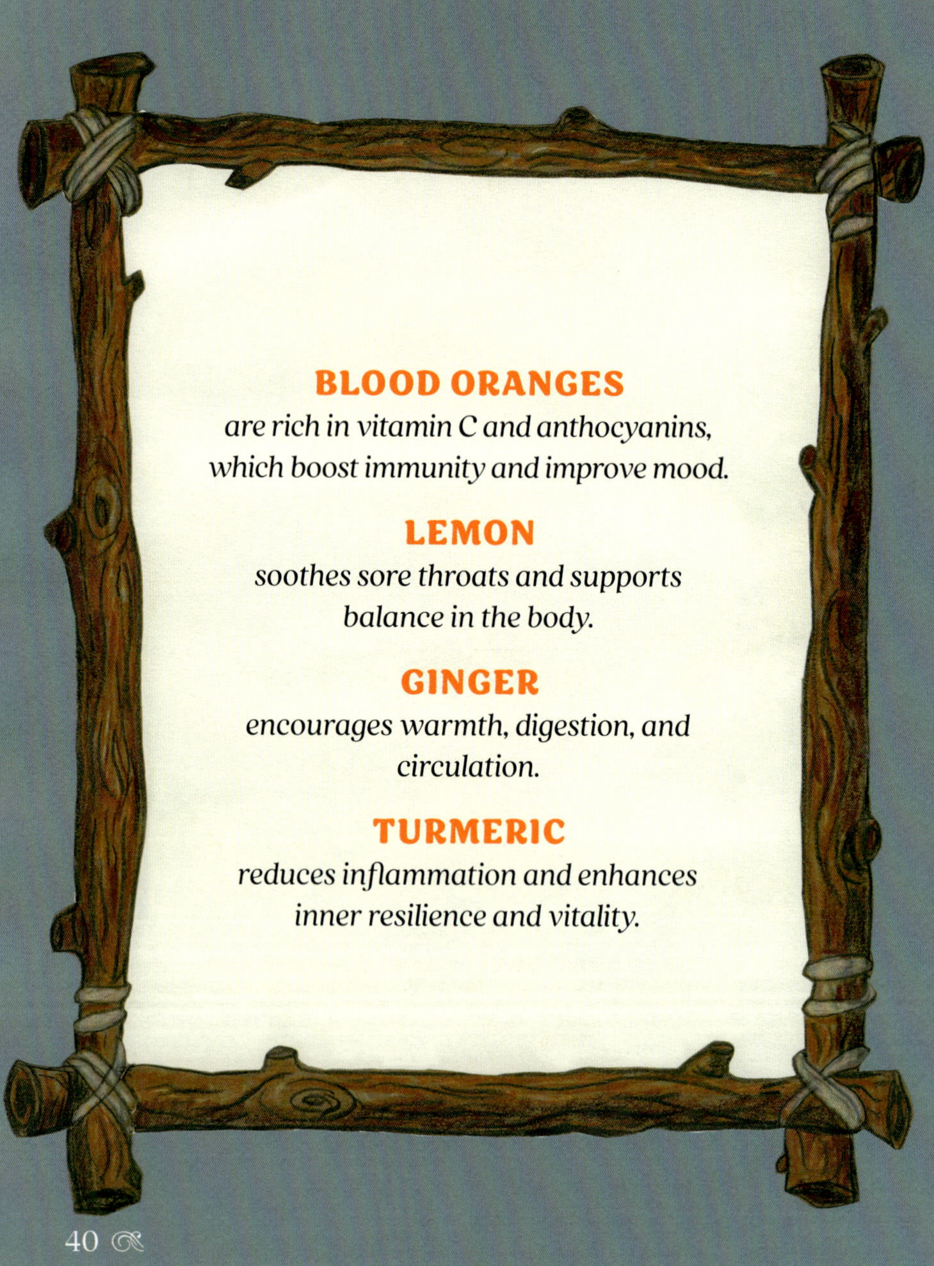

BLOOD ORANGES

*are rich in vitamin C and anthocyanins,
which boost immunity and improve mood.*

LEMON

*soothes sore throats and supports
balance in the body.*

GINGER

*encourages warmth, digestion, and
circulation.*

TURMERIC

*reduces inflammation and enhances
inner resilience and vitality.*

Did You Know?

According to Sicilian folklore, oranges were said to help people recover from heartbreak or sorrow, especially when paired with herbs such as rosemary or mint.

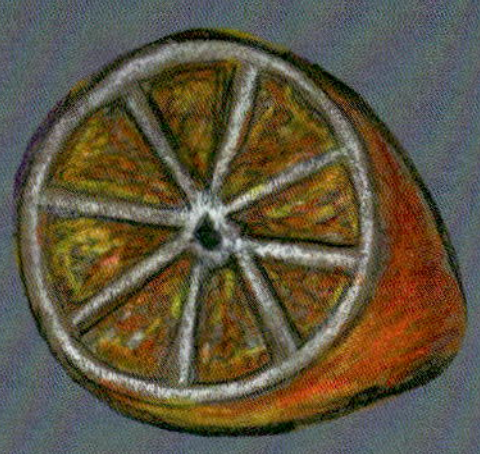

Carrot and Ginger Soup

(Serves 4)

**Carrot and ginger soup is not only delicious—
it's a vibrant bowl of warmth, comfort, and healing.**

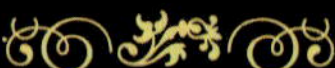

1 tablespoon olive oil
1 medium yellow onion, chopped
1 clove garlic, minced
3 tablespoons chopped fresh ginger
1 pound carrots, peeled and sliced
4 cups (32 ounces) vegetable broth
1 cup coconut milk
Salt and pepper to taste
Pumpkin seeds for garnish

Add the olive oil to a large saucepan, Dutch oven, or stock pot over medium-high heat. As it heats, watch for the shimmer that signals readiness.

Add the onion, garlic, and ginger. Stir slowly, letting their fragrance rise. As the onion turns translucent (about 5 minutes), imagine it easing your stress.

Add the carrots and vegetable broth and bring the mixture to a boil. Reduce the heat to a gentle simmer and cook, stirring occasionally to prevent scorching, for about 25 minutes.

Slowly stir in the coconut milk—creamy, cooling, nurturing. Watch the color shift to golden serenity.

Purée the soup until smooth. You can use an immersion blender directly in the pot, or you can use a food processor. If you choose the processor, wait for the soup to cool slightly (about 15 minutes) and blend it in small batches to avoid overflow.

Add salt and pepper to taste. Ladle the soup into bowls and top each serving with crunchy pumpkin seeds for texture and grounding.

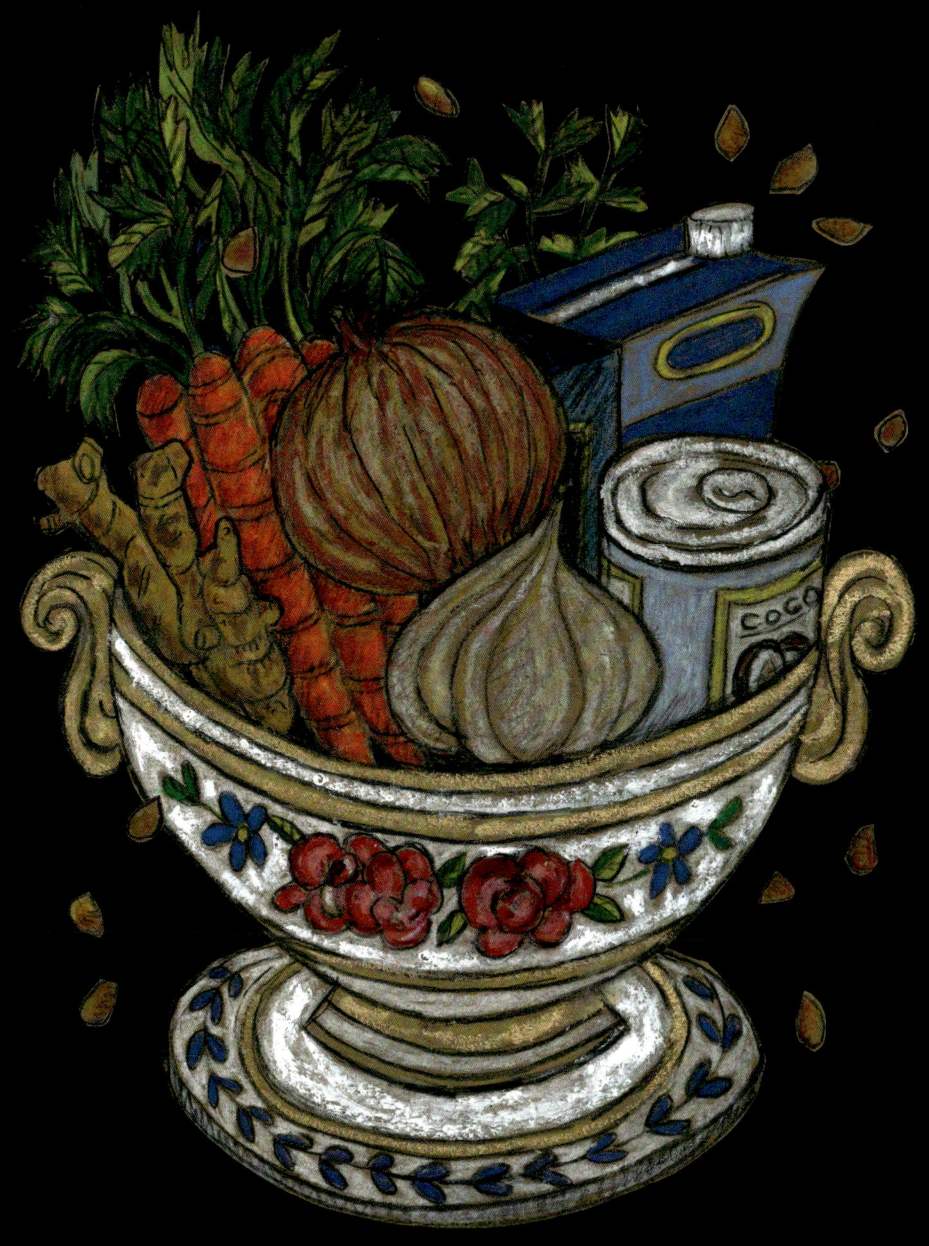

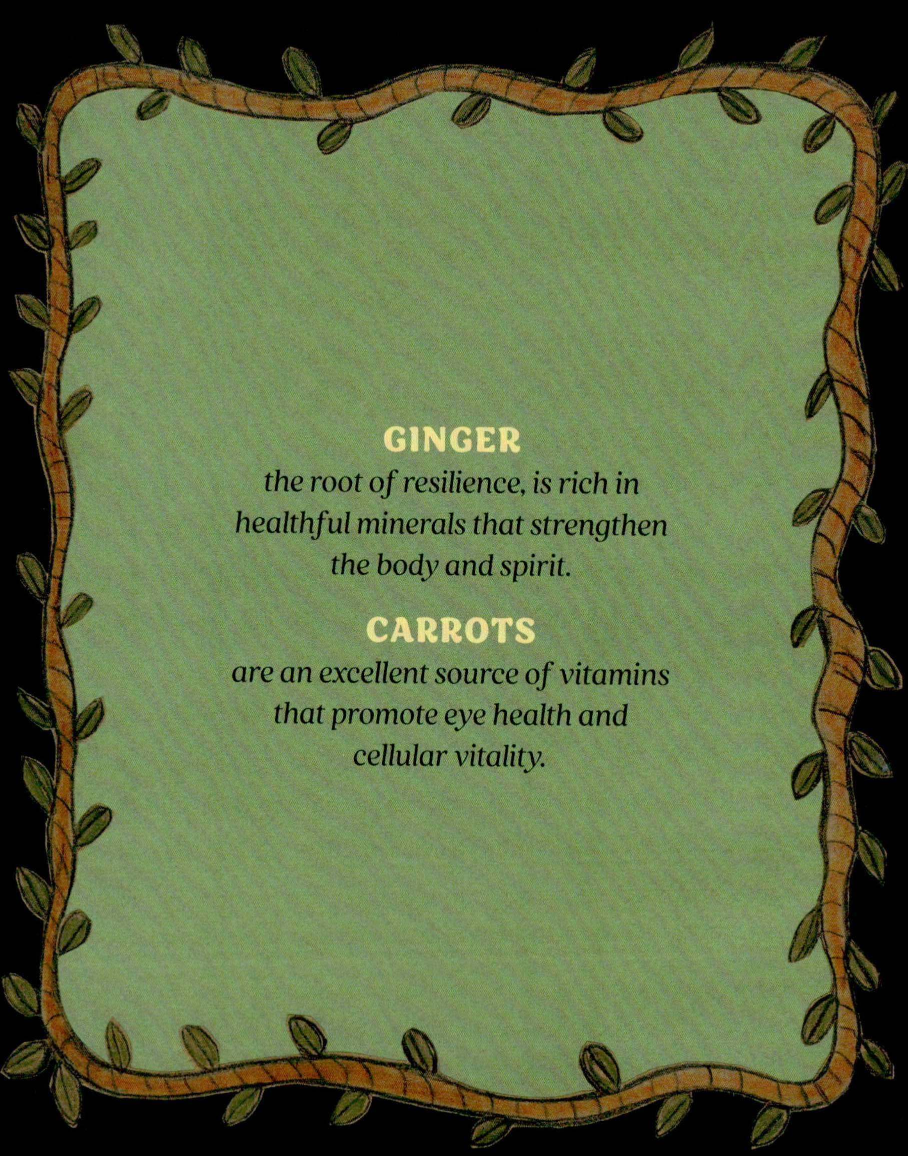

GINGER

the root of resilience, is rich in
healthful minerals that strengthen
the body and spirit.

CARROTS

are an excellent source of vitamins
that promote eye health and
cellular vitality.

Did You Know?

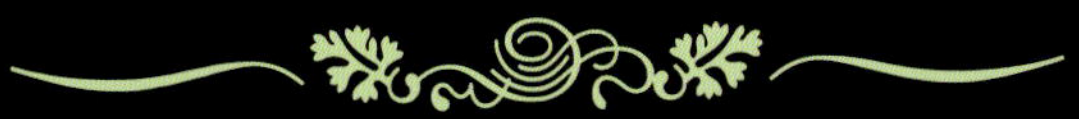

In ancient China and India, the carrot was revered as a sacred root, used by the legendary emperor Shennong for healing. In ancient Greece, the physician Dioscorides extolled the power of carrots to aid digestion and purify the blood.

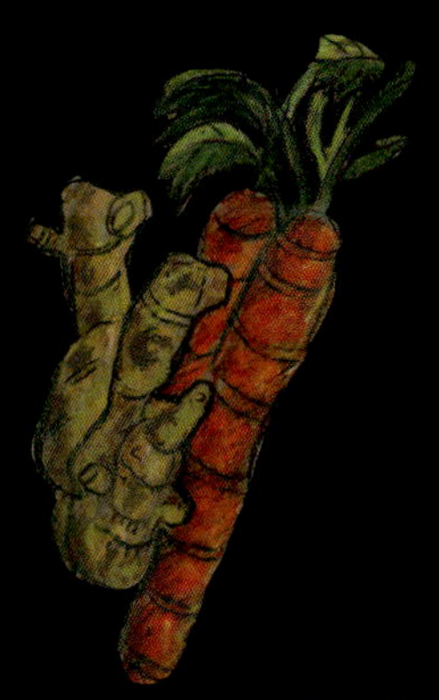

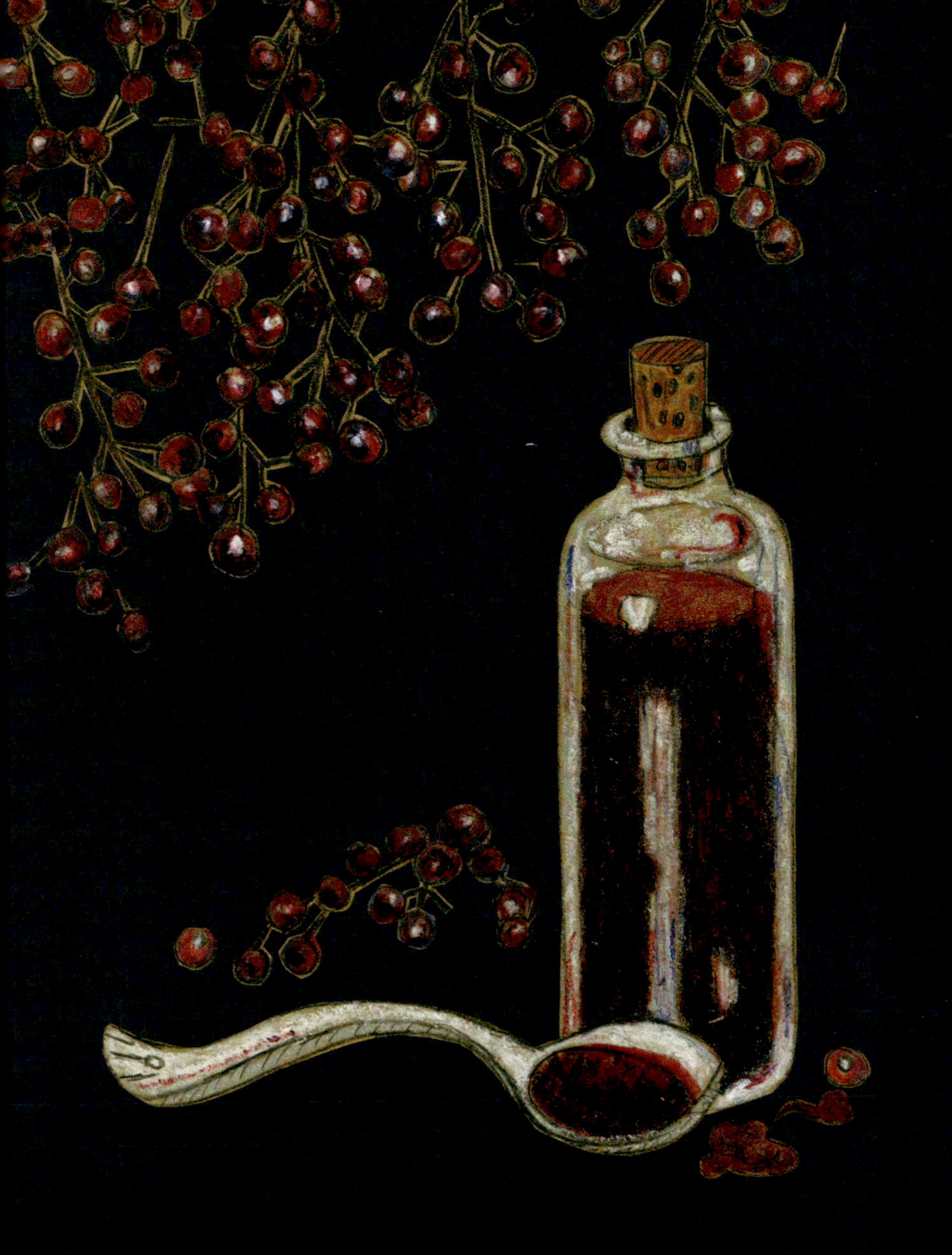

Elderberry Syrup

This elixir, crafted from the berries of the elder tree, has been lovingly used for generations to support wellness.

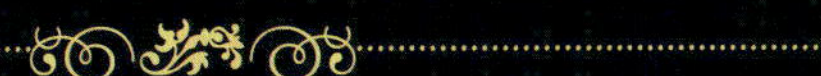

3 cups water
¾ cup dried elderberries
1 tablespoon grated fresh ginger
1 teaspoon dried cinnamon
1 teaspoon dried cloves
1 cup agave sweetener

In a large pot, combine water, elderberries, ginger, cinnamon, and cloves. Bring to a boil, then reduce heat to a gentle simmer. Simmer slowly for 20 to 25 minutes, or until the liquid is reduced by half. Breathe in the wonderful scent, setting your intention on healing.

Remove from heat and allow to cool.

Strain the mixture through a fine mesh sieve into a bowl, using the back of a wooden spoon to press all the goodness from the berries. Discard the spent solids into the compost bin.

Stir the agave into the mixture while focusing on warmth, sweetness, and wellness.

Taste a spoonful of the syrup, then store the rest in an airtight glass jar in the refrigerator. Your syrup will keep for up to two months. Enjoy 1 or 2 tablespoons a day, either by the spoonful or stirred into warm herbal tea, cool water, or a smoothie.

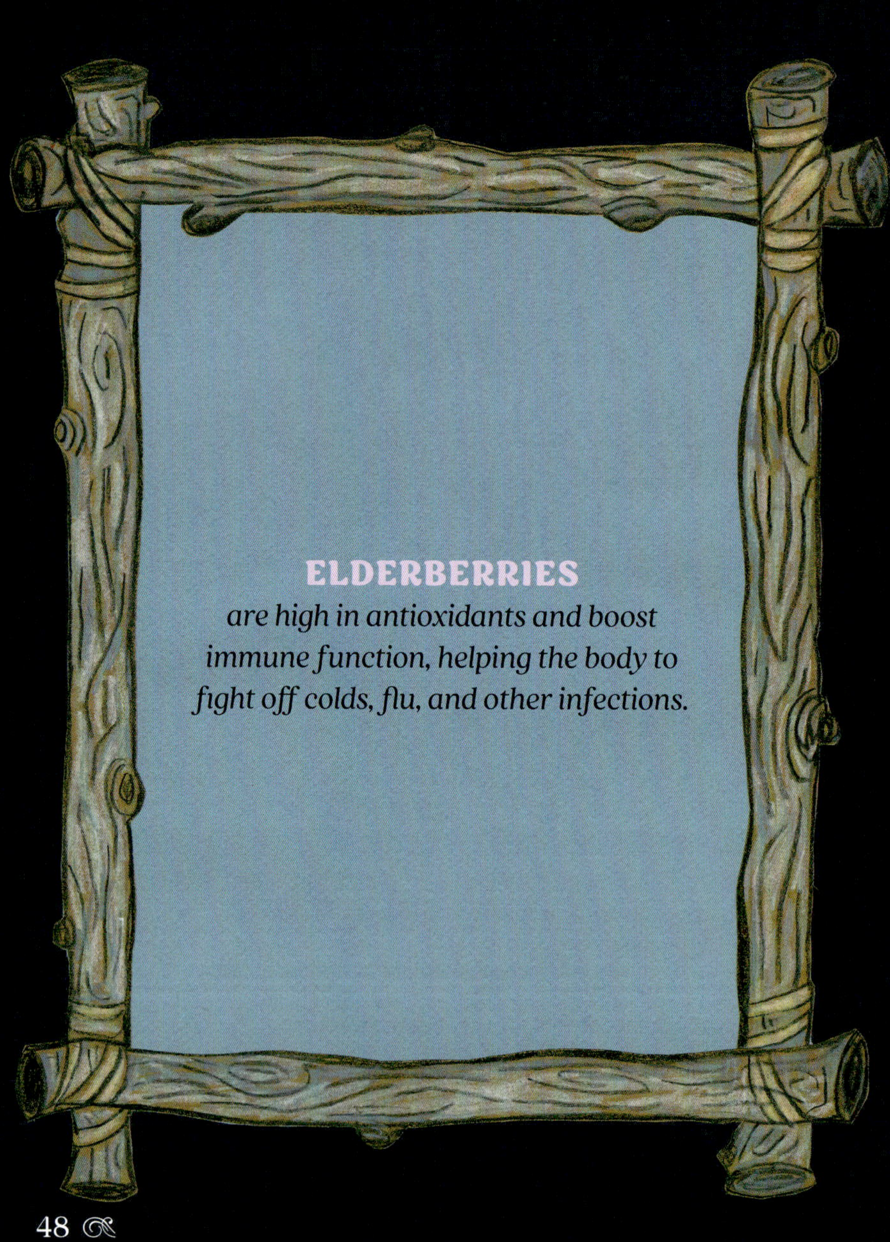

ELDERBERRIES
are high in antioxidants and boost
immune function, helping the body to
fight off colds, flu, and other infections.

Did You Know?

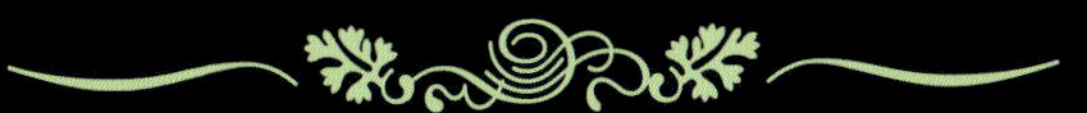

In Celtic lore, elderberry trees were grown near a home to keep illness at bay and banish bad spirits.

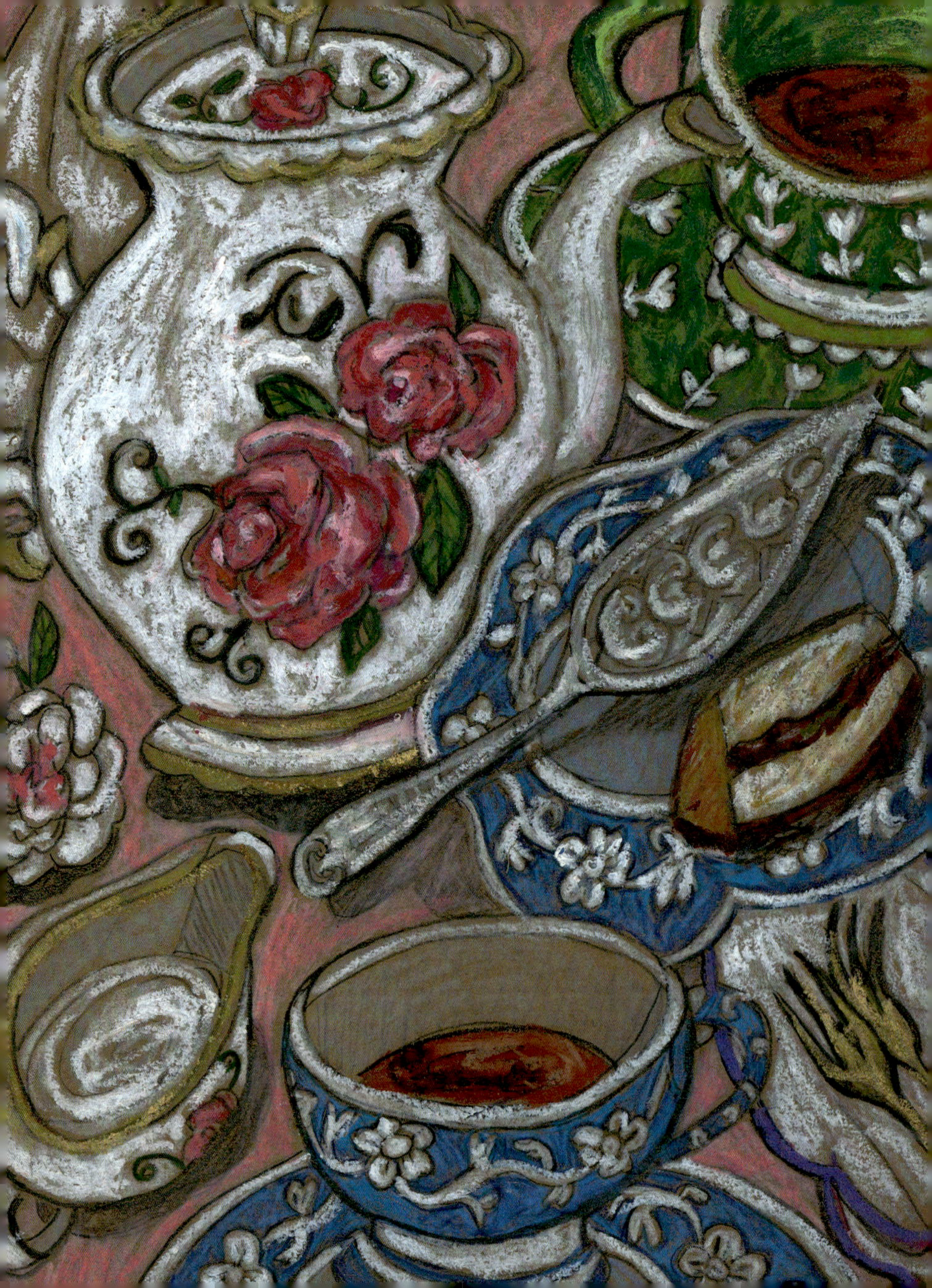

CHAPTER 2

HEAL YOUR LIFE

This chapter is all about creating harmony and finding nourishment, not just in food and drink but also in ritual, and, of course, nature. Plants are wonderful companions on this journey, reminding us that true well-being is more than just health—it is balance, protection, and joy.

Throughout history, people have turned to nature for medicine, good fortune, happiness, and renewal. Heather, beloved in Celtic folklore, was carried as a charm for protection and luck. Pomegranates, symbols of abundance and new beginnings, were celebrated in tales from Persephone's underworld story and in ancient fertility rites. These myths echo across time, reminding us that plants do more than just nourish the body. They help us shape our lives and fill them with intention.

Each recipe in this chapter is an act of self-care, infusing your life with self-love.

Here we begin with heather, a sweet wildflower known to bring luck to those who carry it. We have steeped it into a wonderful tea—*Malvina's Heather Tea for Protection and Luck*. Enjoy!

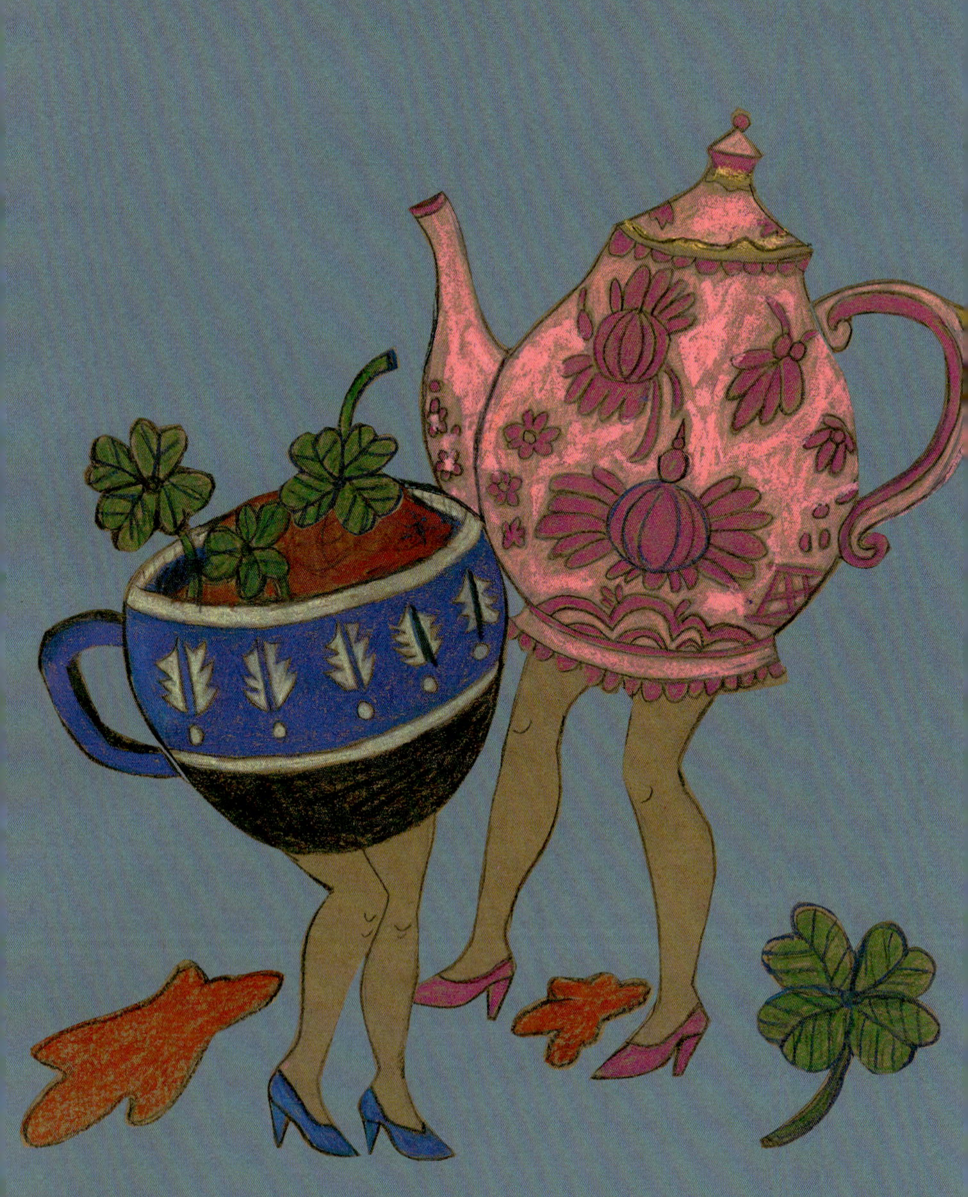

Malvina's Heather Tea
for Protection and Luck

(Serves 2)

Drink this tea for protection, luck, and peace.

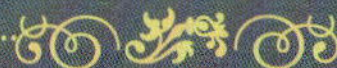

2 teaspoons dried heather flowers
2 teaspoons dried chamomile
2 teaspoons dried mint leaves
2 cups water

Combine the dried heather, chamomile, and mint in a bowl, noticing the subtle colors and aromas.

Bring water to a boil in a pot. As you wait, take a few deep breaths to center yourself and invite calm into the moment.

Add the herbal mixture to the simmering water and let it steep for about 5 to 7 minutes.

Strain the tea into 2 cups and deposit the spent herbs into your compost bin. Wrap your hands around your cup, noticing how the soothing heat relaxes any lingering tension in your body. Enjoy!

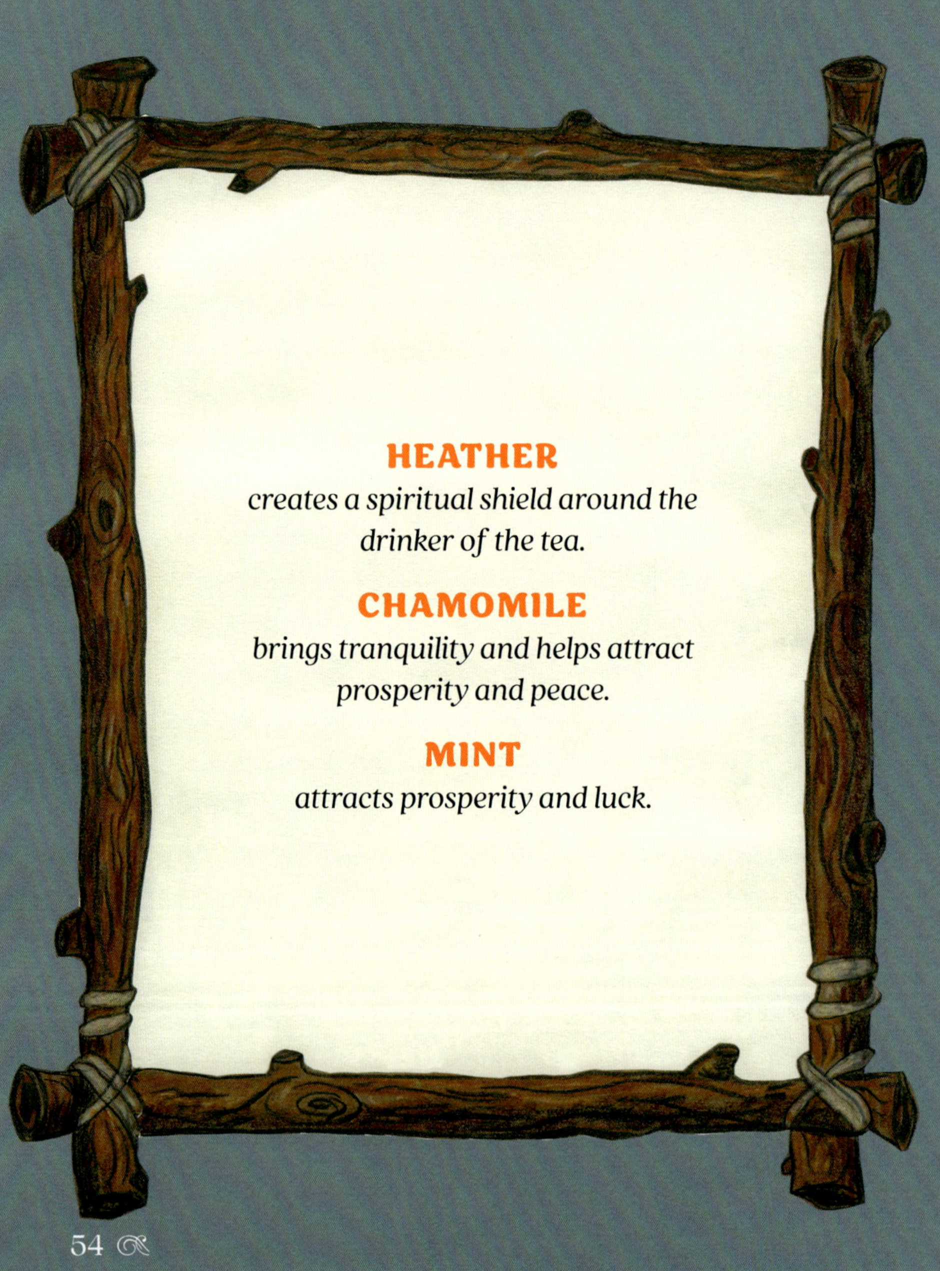

HEATHER

creates a spiritual shield around the
drinker of the tea.

CHAMOMILE

brings tranquility and helps attract
prosperity and peace.

MINT

attracts prosperity and luck.

Did You Know?

Malvina, the daughter of the Celtic bard Ossian, is a captivating figure in Scottish lore. After Malvina's lover, Oscar, was killed in battle, a messenger brought her a sprig of purple heather from his grave. Overcome with sadness, Malvina's tears turned the purple heather white. She declared that from then on, white heather would bring luck and protection to anyone who found it.

Note: The color of the heather used in your tea will bring luck and protection, be it purple or white.

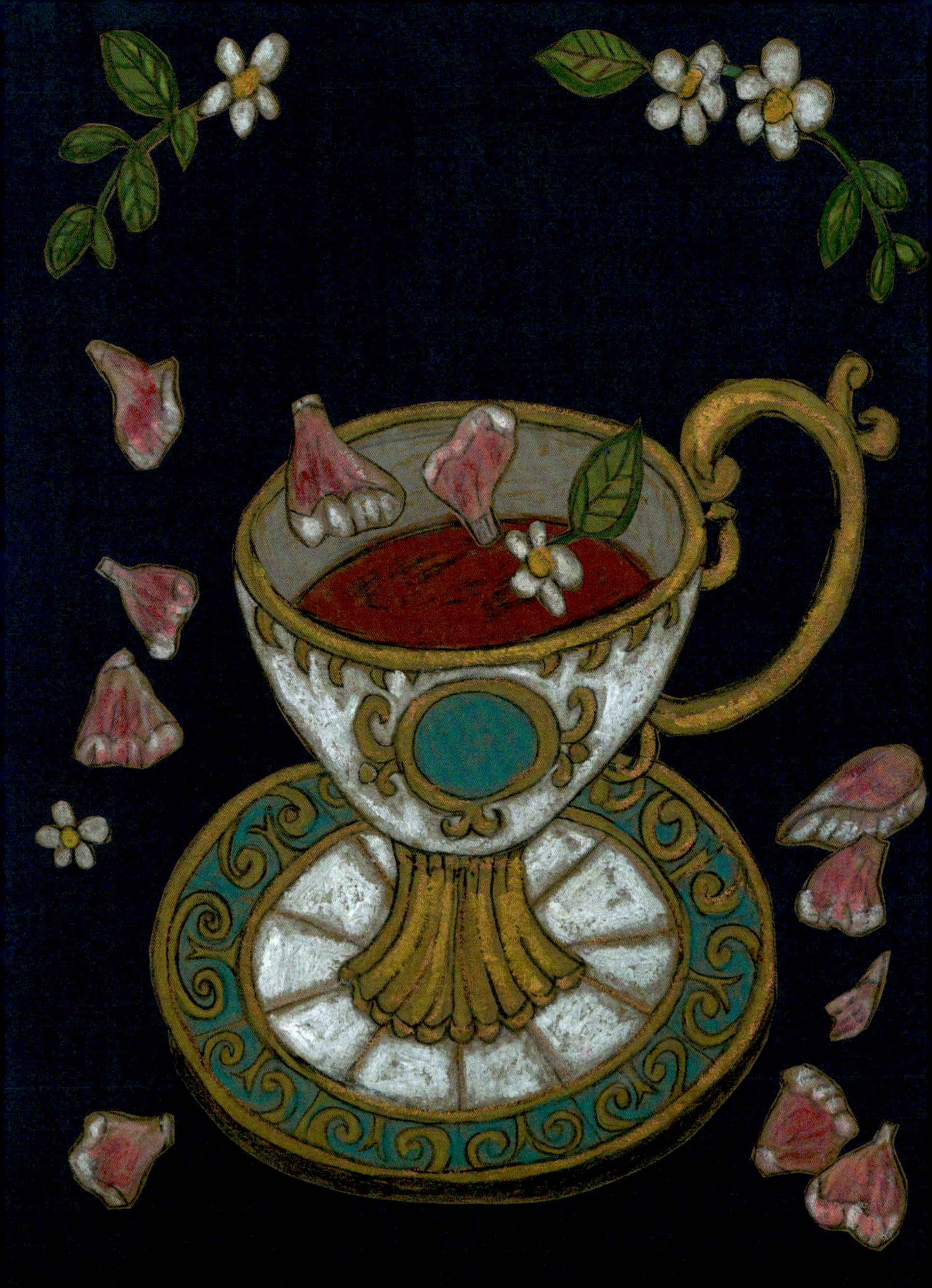

Euphrosyne's Happiness Tea

(Serves 2)

Sip this energizing and refreshing tea for an immediate sense of well-being!

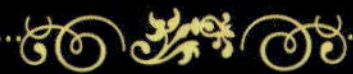

2 teaspoons black tea leaves
1 teaspoon dried chamomile flowers
1 teaspoon dried St. John's wort
1 teaspoon dried basil leaves
1 teaspoon dried rose petals
1 teaspoon dried orange peel
1 teaspoon dried peppermint leaves
2 cups water

Combine the black tea leaves, chamomile flowers, St. John's wort, basil leaves, rose petals, orange peel, and peppermint leaves in a bowl.

Bring water to a boil in a pot. As you wait, take a slow, mindful breath in and out, releasing any tension from your shoulders.

Once the water is boiling, reduce the heat to a simmer. Add the herbal mixture to the water. Let it simmer for about 10 to 15 minutes, allowing the flavors and beneficial properties to infuse. During this time, let the aromas of the steeping herbs soothe and ground you.

Strain the tea into your cups and place the used herbs in your compost bin. Serve and enjoy!

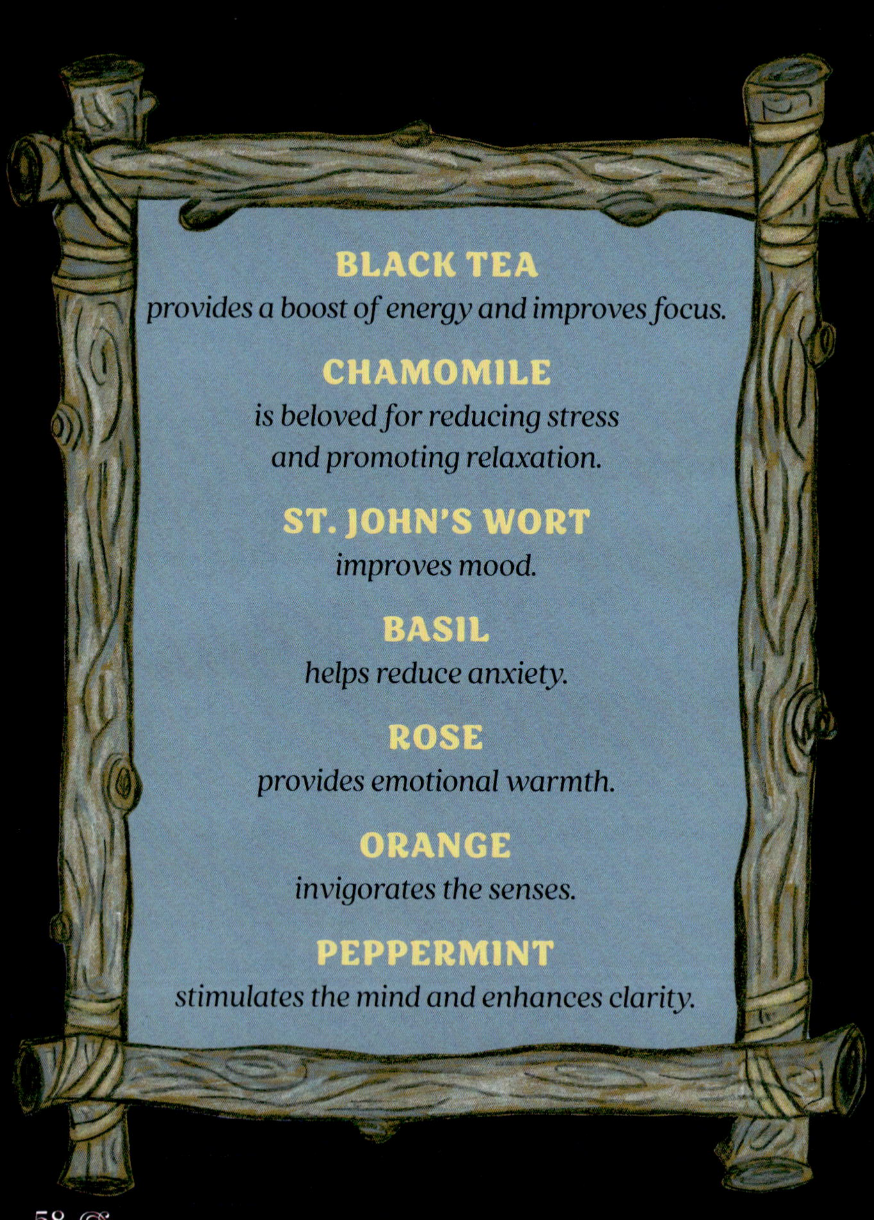

BLACK TEA
provides a boost of energy and improves focus.

CHAMOMILE
is beloved for reducing stress
and promoting relaxation.

ST. JOHN'S WORT
improves mood.

BASIL
helps reduce anxiety.

ROSE
provides emotional warmth.

ORANGE
invigorates the senses.

PEPPERMINT
stimulates the mind and enhances clarity.

Did You Know?

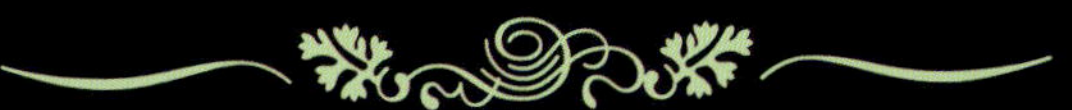

In Greek mythology, the Three Graces were goddesses of charm, beauty, nature, human creativity, and fertility. Euphrosyne, in particular, was the personification of joy and happiness. Along with her sisters Aglaea (splendor) and Thalia (good cheer), Euphrosyne was often depicted dancing, spreading happiness and good luck.

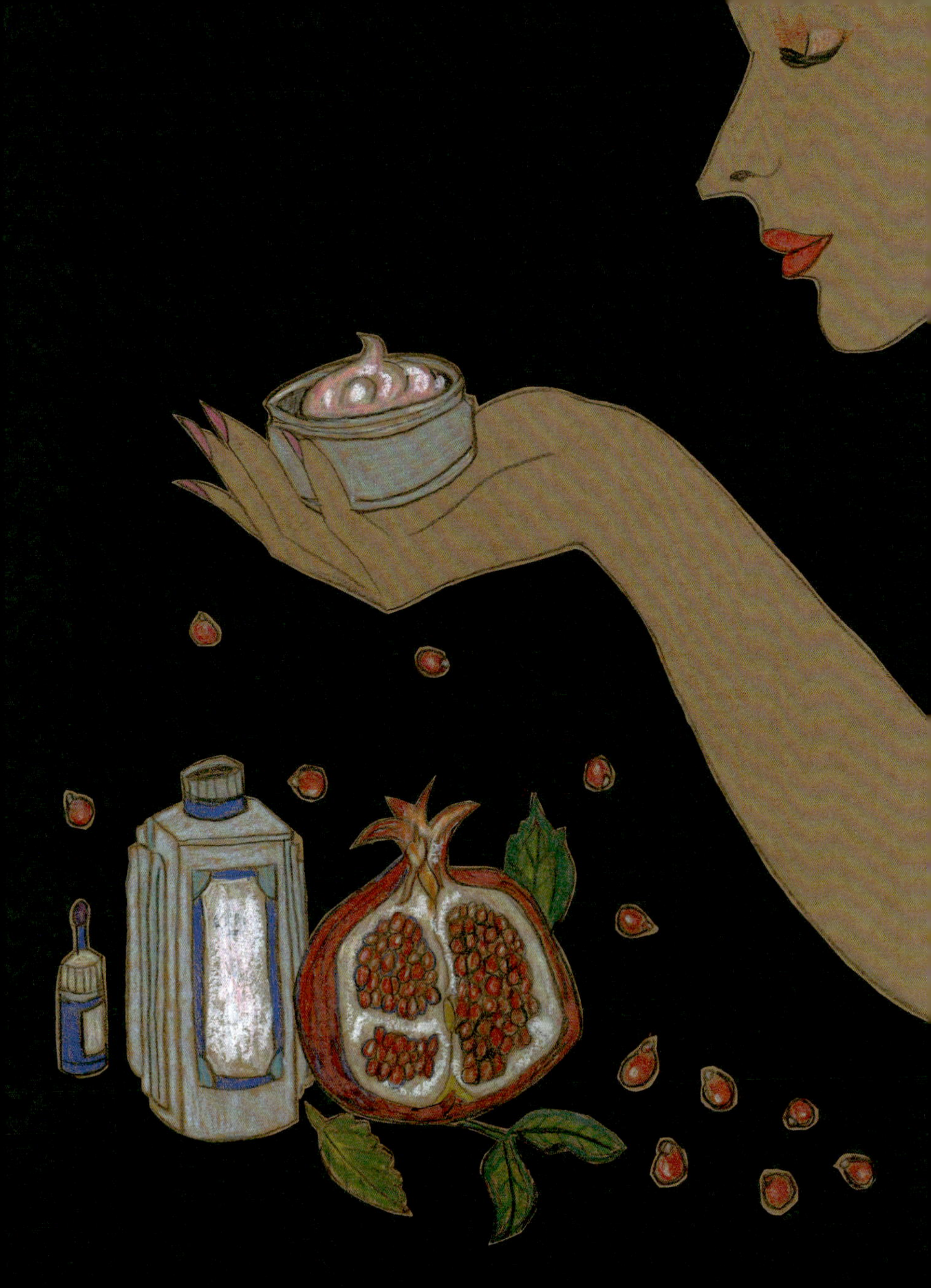

Pomegranate Lip Balm

(Makes 3–4 tins of lip balm)

This luxurious lip balm offers daily nourishment and protection while reminding you to slow down and honor small moments of self-care.

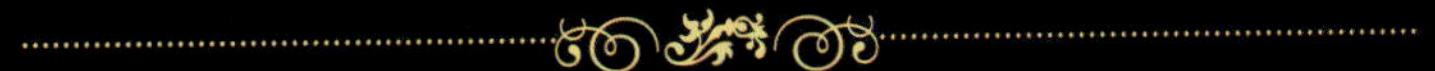

2 tablespoons coconut oil
2 tablespoons cocoa butter
1 tablespoon candelilla wax (a vegan alternative to beeswax)
1 tablespoon pomegranate seed oil
1 teaspoon maple syrup
2 drops peppermint essential oil
Lip balm containers or small tins

In a double boiler, combine the coconut oil, cocoa butter, and candelilla wax. Heat gently until melted, stirring occasionally. As the mixture melts, take a few slow breaths and notice the soothing aroma. Allow this small act to ground you in the present moment.

Once the wax mixture is melted, remove it from the heat and let it cool slightly, about 10 minutes. Stir in the pomegranate seed oil, peppermint essential oil, and maple syrup until mixture is smooth.

Use a small spoon to transfer the mixture into your lip balm containers or tins, taking care not to overfill. Allow the lip balm to cool and solidify completely at room temperature, which may take a couple of hours.

Once your lip balm is set, cap the containers and label them (remember to include the date you created your beautiful balm). Store in a cool, dry place, and use within 12 months.

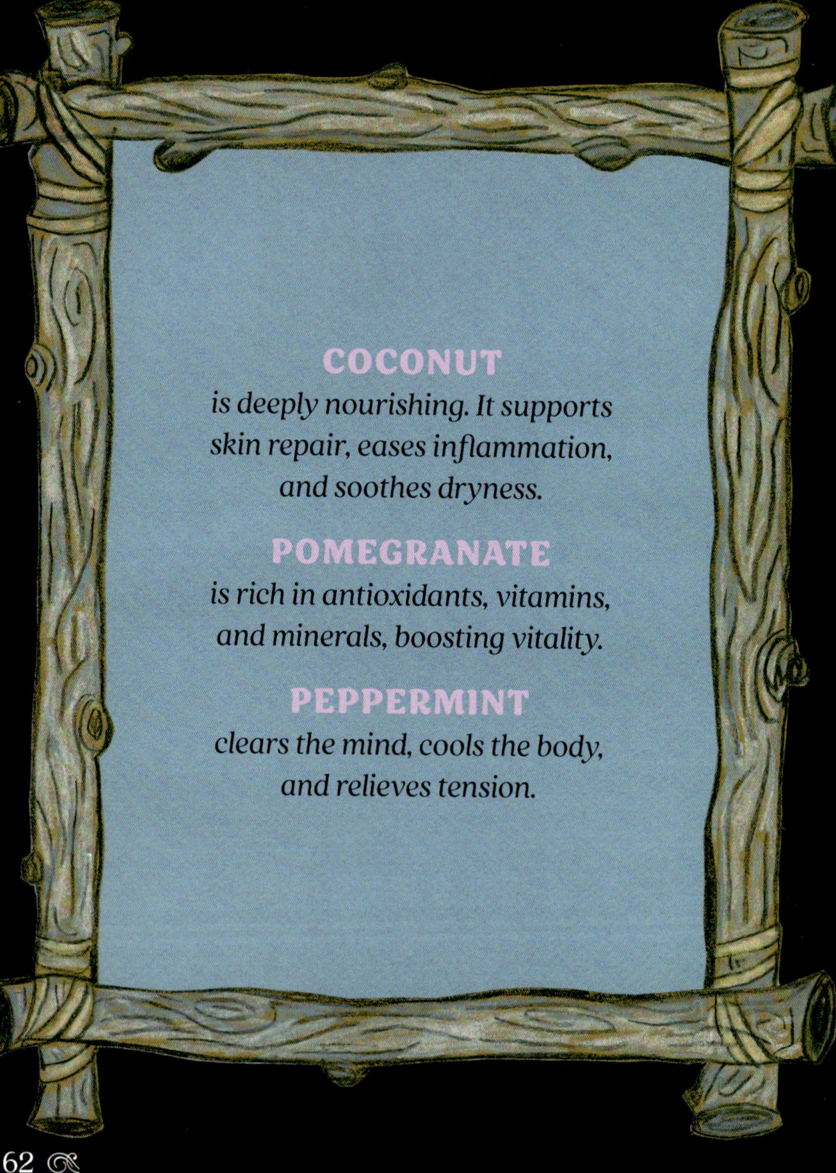

COCONUT

is deeply nourishing. It supports
skin repair, eases inflammation,
and soothes dryness.

POMEGRANATE

is rich in antioxidants, vitamins,
and minerals, boosting vitality.

PEPPERMINT

clears the mind, cools the body,
and relieves tension.

Did You Know?

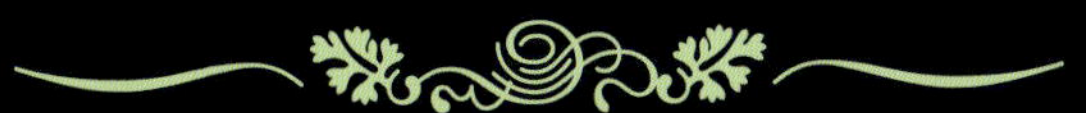

In Greek mythology, the pomegranate plays a central role in the story of Persephone and Demeter. When Hades abducted Persephone to the underworld, Demeter, goddess of the harvest, fell into a deep depression, causing all life on Earth to suffer. Eventually, a deal was struck that allowed Persephone to return to the surface, but because she had eaten pomegranate seeds in the underworld, she had to spend part of each year down there with Hades.

Though some see this as a tale of loss, the pomegranate ultimately brought healing by creating the cycle of the seasons, teaching humans about renewal and the promise of rebirth after hardship.

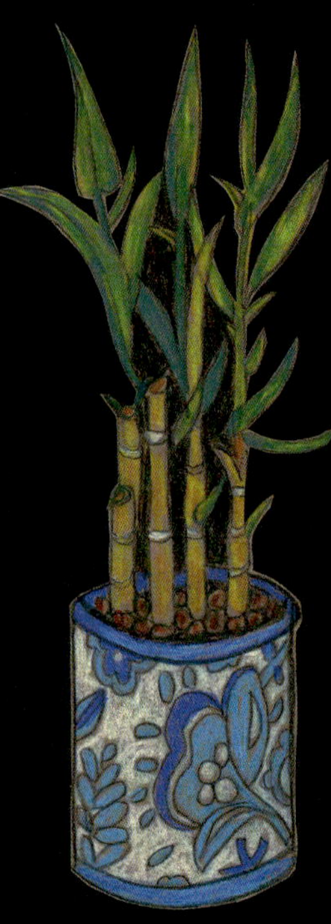

Lucky Houseplants for the Home

(6 potted plants of any size)

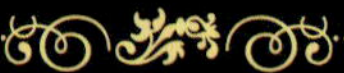

Bringing plants into your home is more than decoration—it is an act of creating wellness in your living space. Plants purify the air and calm the nervous system. Many plants have a reputation for luck or protection, making them allies not only for health but for harmony and good fortune.

Note: Some houseplants can be toxic to pets, so be sure to check with your veterinarian before bringing new plants into your home.

ALOE VERA

Known as the "plant of immortality" in ancient Egypt, the aloe vera plant attracts healing energy and helps refresh the air in your home. Place your aloe in a sunny window and harvest its healing gel to soothe sunburns and protect the skin.

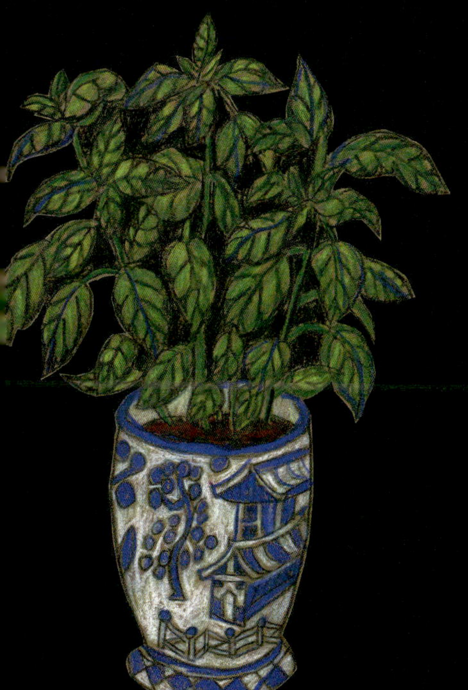

BASIL

More than a culinary herb, basil is a plant of prosperity and protection in Mediterranean and Indian traditions. Its scent uplifts your mood.

ROSEMARY

This aromatic herb helps with memory and clear thinking. Keeping rosemary in your home helps ward off stagnant energy. Each day, rub the leaves of your rosemary plant between your fingers and breathe its scent deeply.

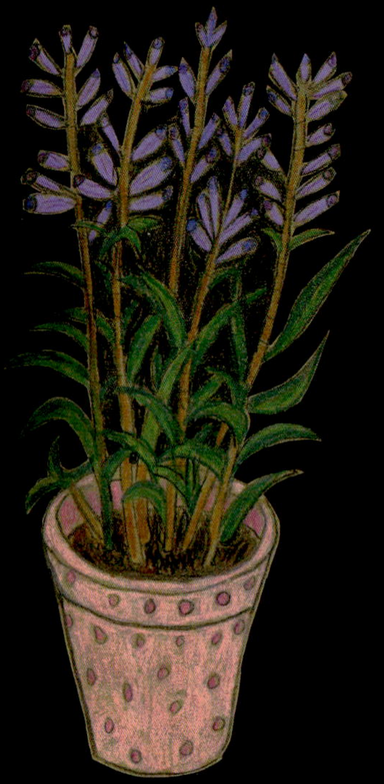

LAVENDER

A beloved plant for calm and sleep, lavender in a sunny indoor spot brings relaxation into your home. It also attracts luck in love and peace.

LUCKY BAMBOO

A classic plant in feng shui traditions, lucky bamboo attracts good fortune and resilience. Easy to care for, it thrives in water or soil and grows quickly.

JADE PLANT

Often called the "money plant," jade attracts abundance, growth, and harmony.

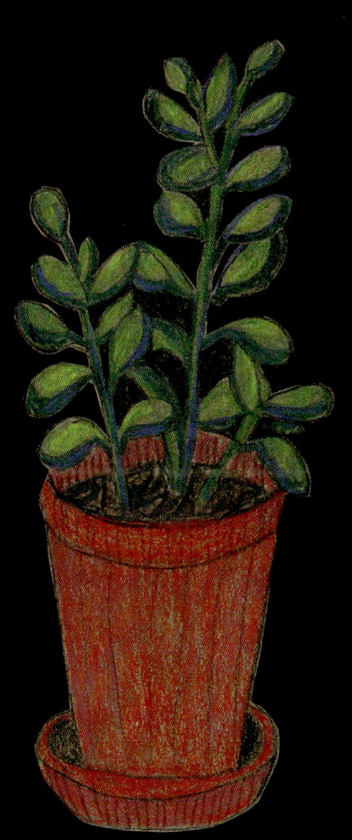

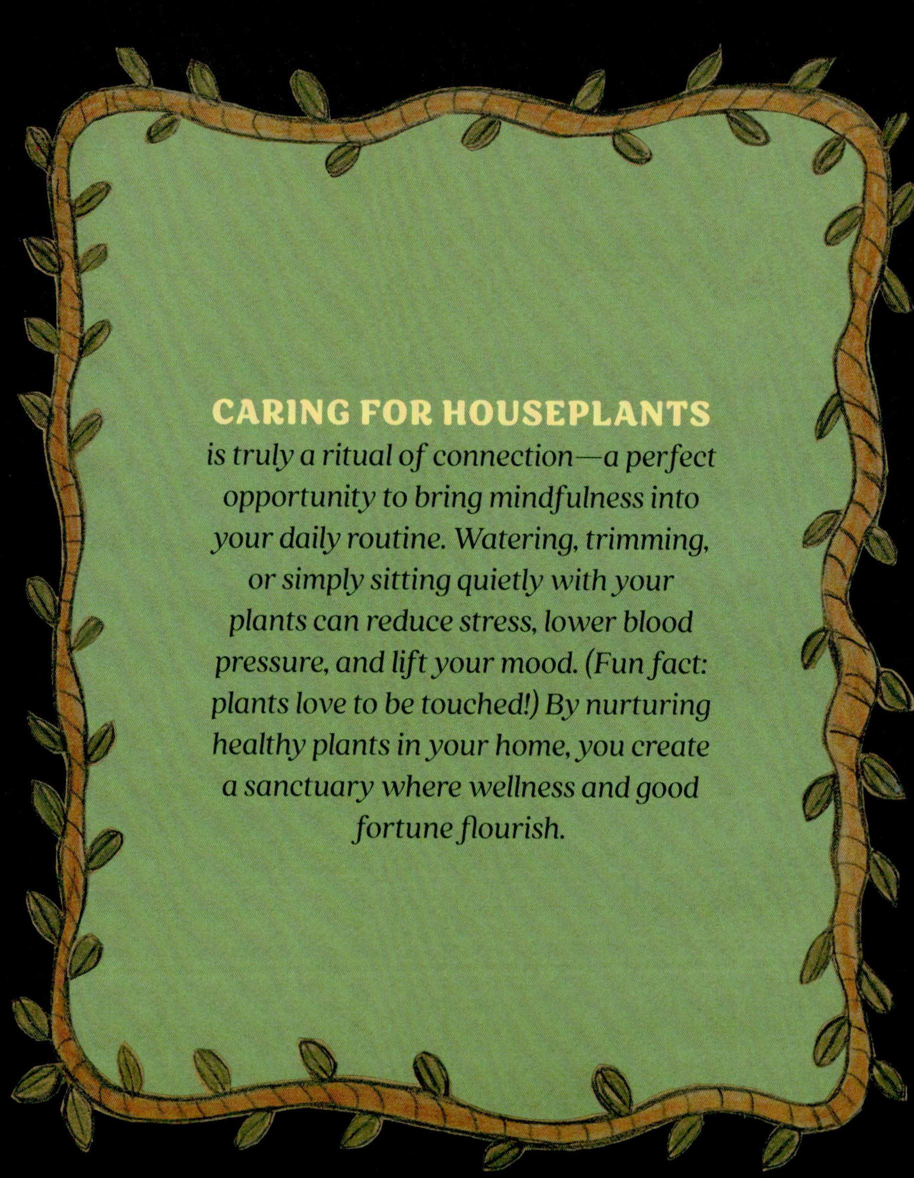

CARING FOR HOUSEPLANTS

is truly a ritual of connection—a perfect opportunity to bring mindfulness into your daily routine. Watering, trimming, or simply sitting quietly with your plants can reduce stress, lower blood pressure, and lift your mood. (Fun fact: plants love to be touched!) By nurturing healthy plants in your home, you create a sanctuary where wellness and good fortune flourish.

Did You Know?

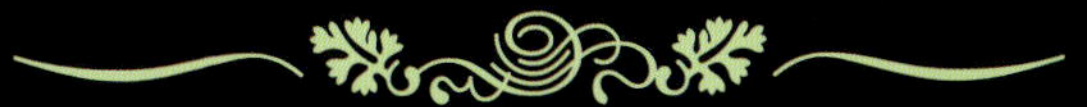

A plant may be called "lucky" when it attracts prosperity, love, or protection. Plants are considered "healthy" when they offer benefits like refreshing indoor air, producing oxygen, or emitting soothing fragrances.

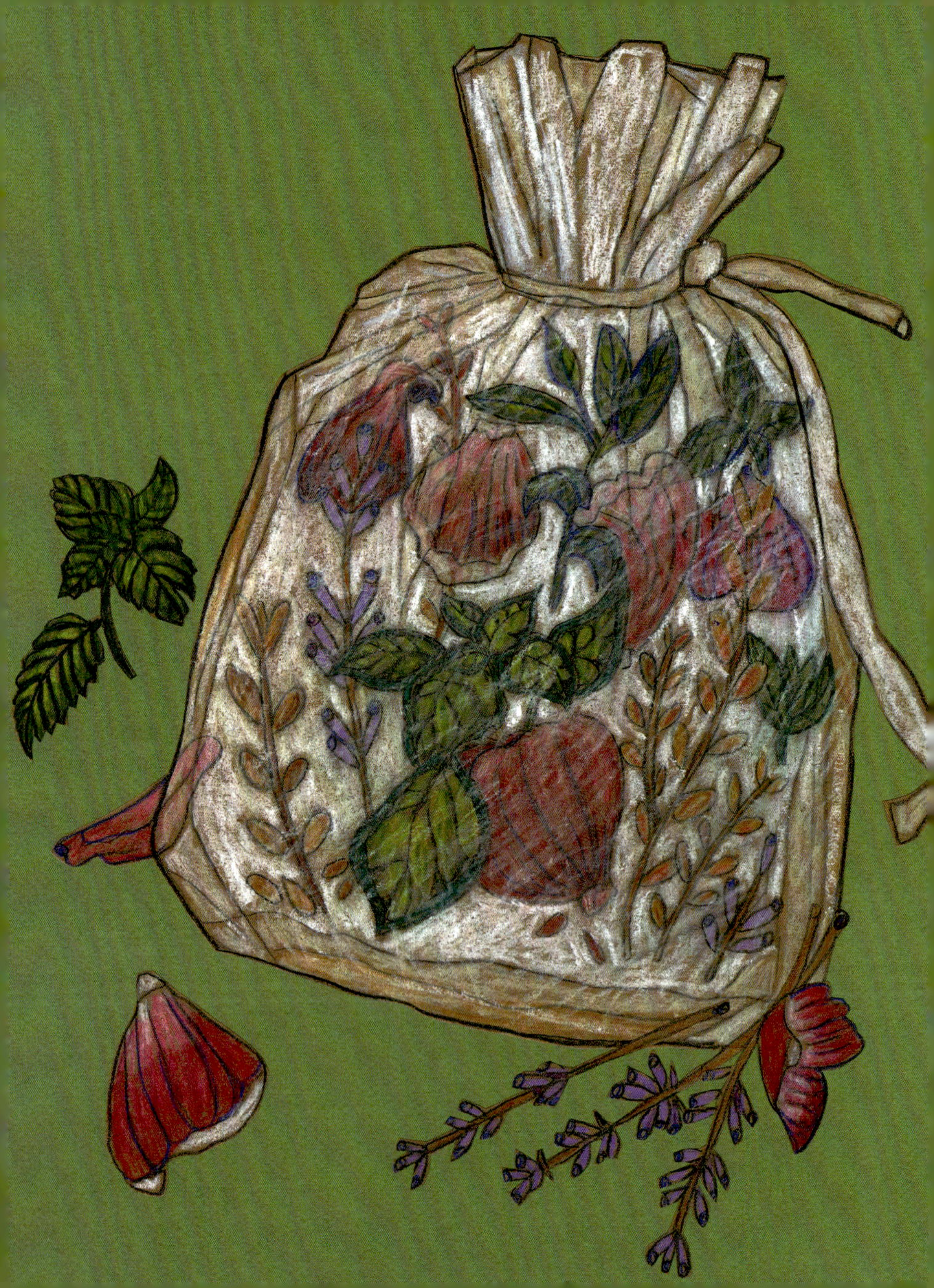

Rejuvenation Sachet

(Makes 1 sachet)

This sachet promotes balance, joy, and emotional rejuvenation through the energies of its aromatic herbs.

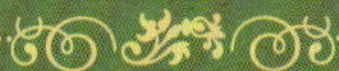

1 tablespoon dried heather
1 tablespoon dried rose petals
1 teaspoon dried mint leaves
1 teaspoon dried basil leaves
1 teaspoon dried lavender buds
Small cotton or muslin sachet bag with drawstring

Combine the heather, rose petals, mint, basil, and lavender in a bowl. As you mix, take a slow breath in and out, setting an intention for joy and balance in your life. Pause here to smile gently to lift your mood and release stress.

Spoon the mixture into a sachet bag and tie it securely. Hold the sachet in your hands for a moment and visualize light and warmth surrounding you.

Place the sachet in a drawer or under your pillow, or carry it in your bag to invite luck, protection, and wellness as you move through the world.

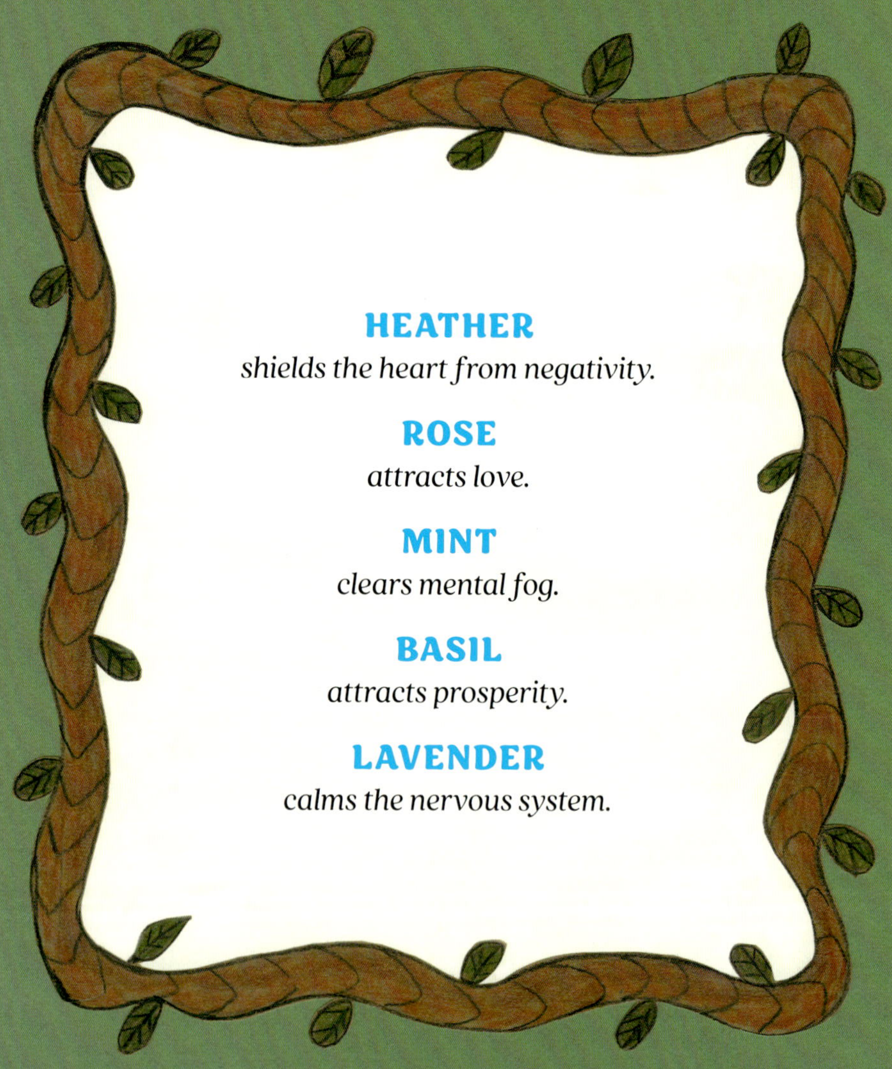

HEATHER

shields the heart from negativity.

ROSE

attracts love.

MINT

clears mental fog.

BASIL

attracts prosperity.

LAVENDER

calms the nervous system.

Did You Know?

In medieval Europe, travelers and soldiers often carried small sachets filled with protective herbs like mint, lavender, and heather. Knights kept sachets inside their armor to guard them from plague and poison.

Watermelon and Basil Granita

(Serves 4)

This invigorating granita will help hydrate the body, cool the spirit, and offer a refreshing reminder to savor life's simple pleasures.

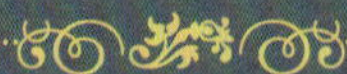

4 cups cubed seedless watermelon
½ cup fresh basil leaves
¼ cup sugar
1 tablespoon lime juice
Pinch of salt

In a food processor, blend all ingredients until smooth. As you watch the ingredients transform, take a moment to notice the vibrant colors and fresh aroma—let these remind you of the simple joys of nourishing your body.

Strain the mixture through a fine mesh sieve. Discard the solids into your compost bin.

Pour the mixture into an 8 × 8-inch metal baking pan. Place it in the freezer.

Check the granita after 1 hour. When the edges start to freeze, scrape through the mixture with a fork to break up any ice crystals. As you scrape, breathe deeply and imagine you are also breaking up any tension within yourself. Return the granita to the freezer.

Every 30 minutes for the next 3 to 4 hours, scrape through the granita. Eventually you will create a light, grainy, crushed-ice texture.

Scoop the finished granita into serving bowls. Garnish with extra basil leaves or slices of lime if desired and serve.

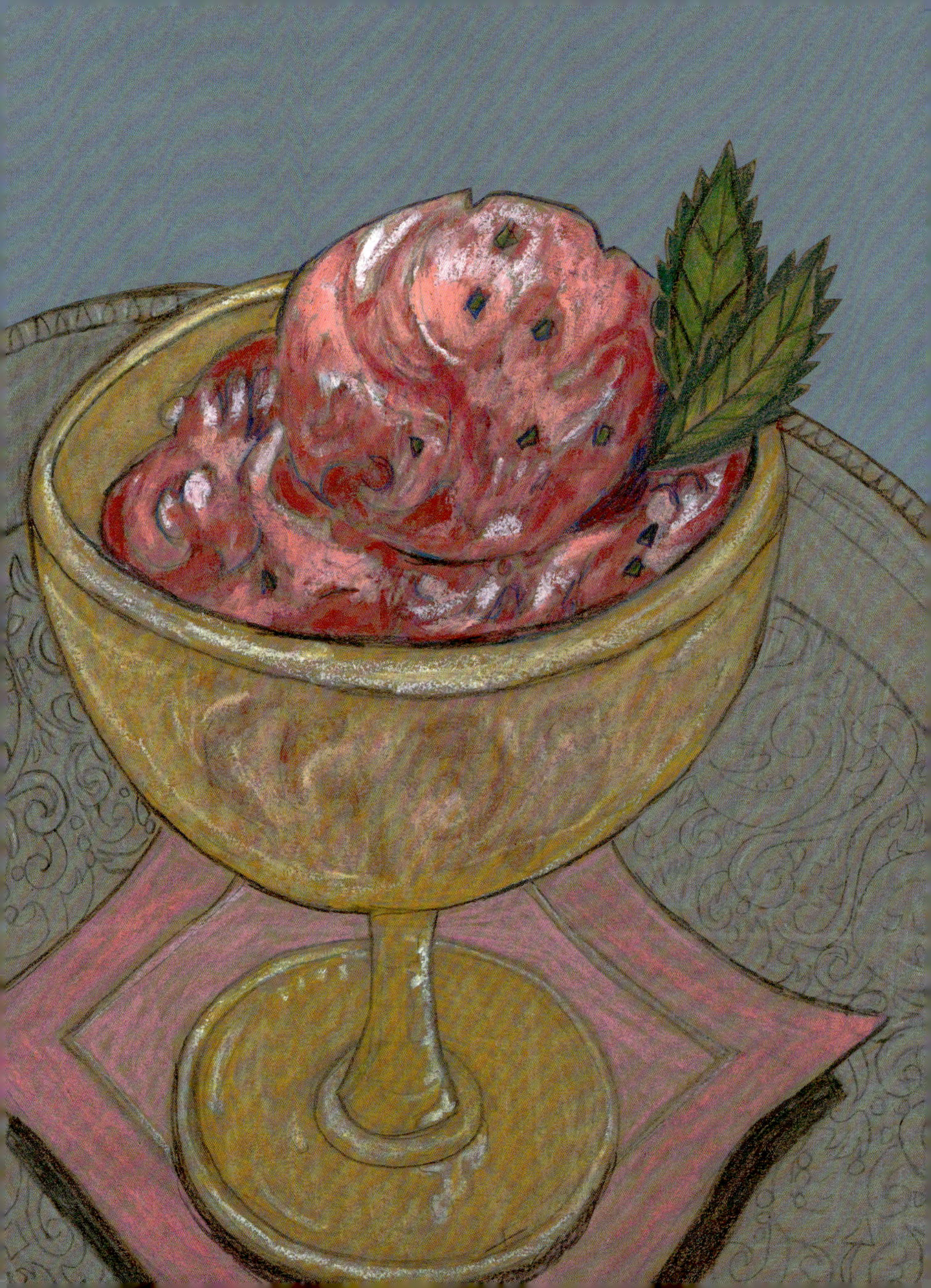

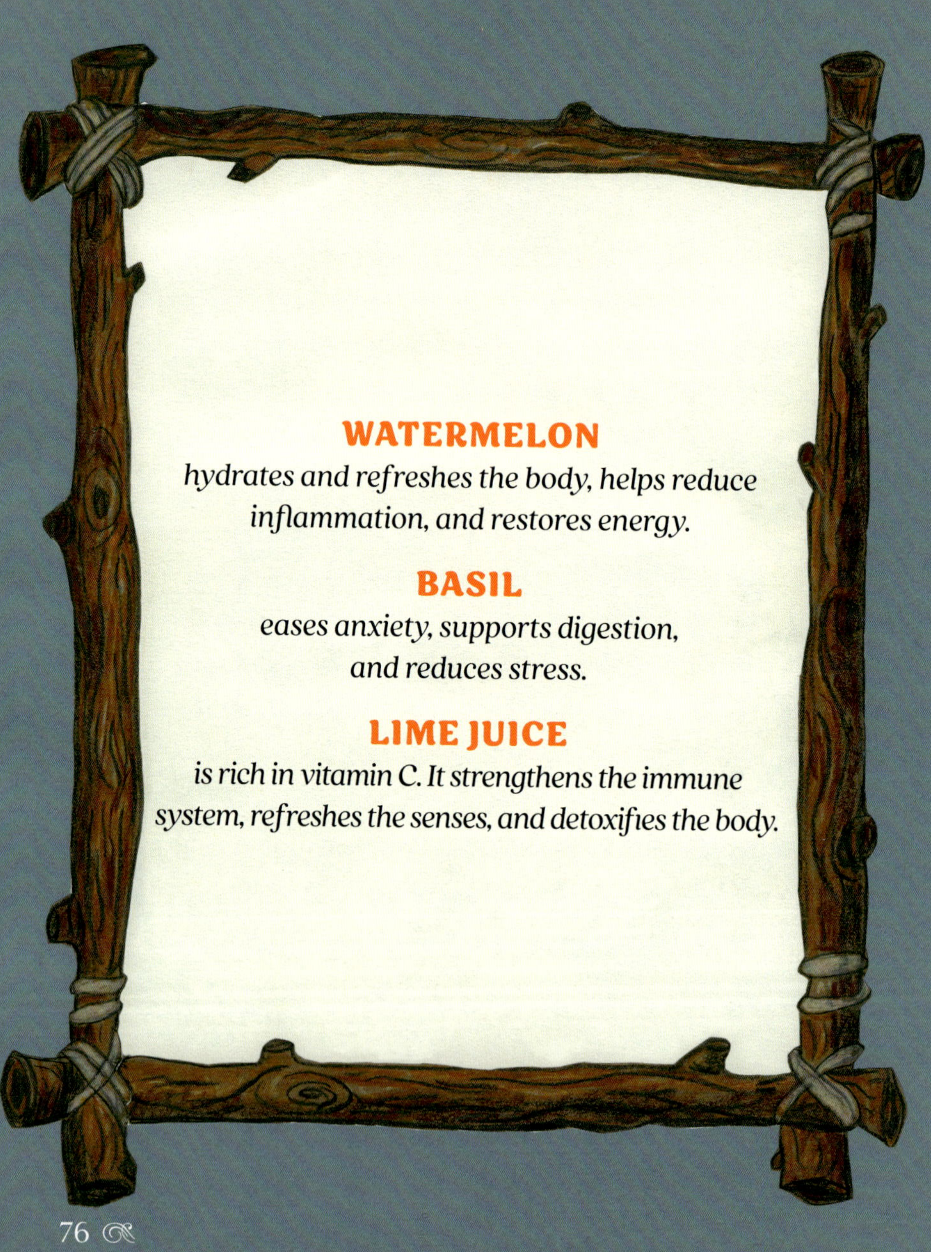

WATERMELON
hydrates and refreshes the body, helps reduce inflammation, and restores energy.

BASIL
eases anxiety, supports digestion, and reduces stress.

LIME JUICE
is rich in vitamin C. It strengthens the immune system, refreshes the senses, and detoxifies the body.

Did You Know?

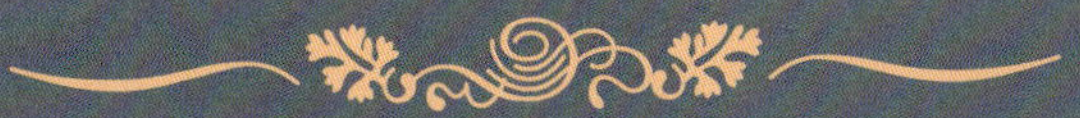

In ancient Egypt, watermelon was placed in tombs to nourish the dead and to give them strength on their journey to the afterlife. In Italian folklore, basil is cherished as a plant of love and reconciliation. Young women were advised to place a pot of basil on their windowsill to show they were available to potential suitors.

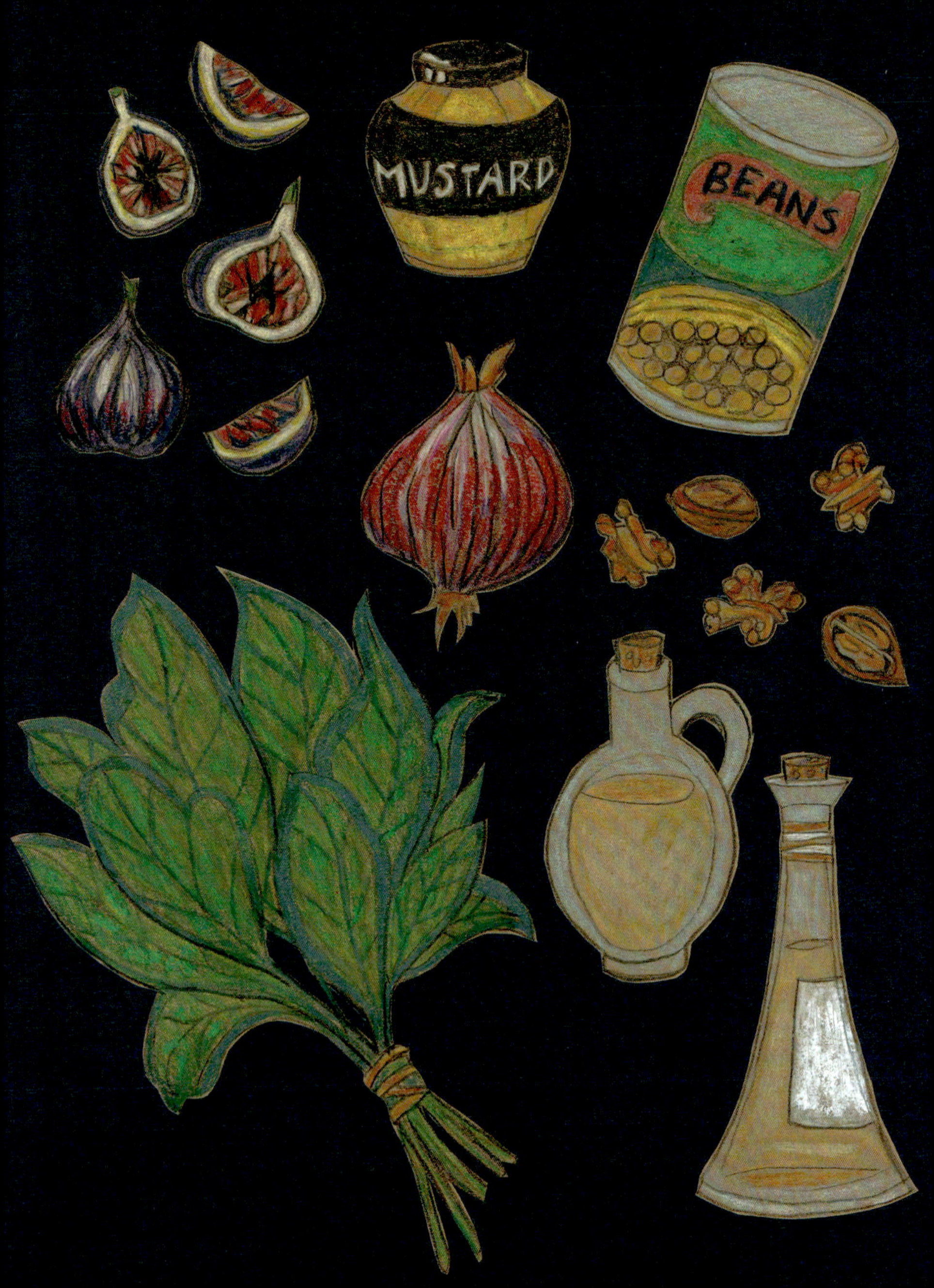

MUSTARD
BEANS

Spinach, Fig, and Walnut Salad with Aquafaba and Miso Dressing

(Serves 4)

This refreshing salad is enhanced by its rich dressing. The key ingredient, aquafaba—the liquid strained from canned chickpeas—has a magical ability to transform into a light, airy froth, giving the dressing a delightful, creamy texture.

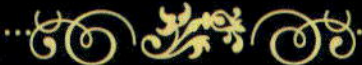

¼ cup aquafaba
2 tablespoons apple cider vinegar
1 tablespoon white miso paste
1 tablespoon Dijon mustard
1 tablespoon maple syrup
1 teaspoon fresh lemon juice
⅓ cup olive oil
Salt and pepper to taste
4 cups fresh spinach, washed and dried
1 cup fresh figs, cut into quarters
½ cup chopped and toasted walnuts
½ small red onion, thinly sliced
Sea salt and black pepper to taste

In a food processor, blend the aquafaba, apple cider vinegar, miso paste, Dijon mustard, maple syrup, and lemon juice until smooth. With the motor running, add the olive oil through the processor's feed tube until the dressing is emulsified. Season with salt and pepper to taste. Set aside.

In a large salad bowl, toss the fresh spinach, quartered figs, toasted walnuts, and sliced red onion. Drizzle the dressing over the salad, sprinkle with salt and pepper, and toss gently to combine. Before enjoying your salad, take a deep breath and inhale its fresh, earthy aroma to awaken your senses and invite mindfulness into your meal.

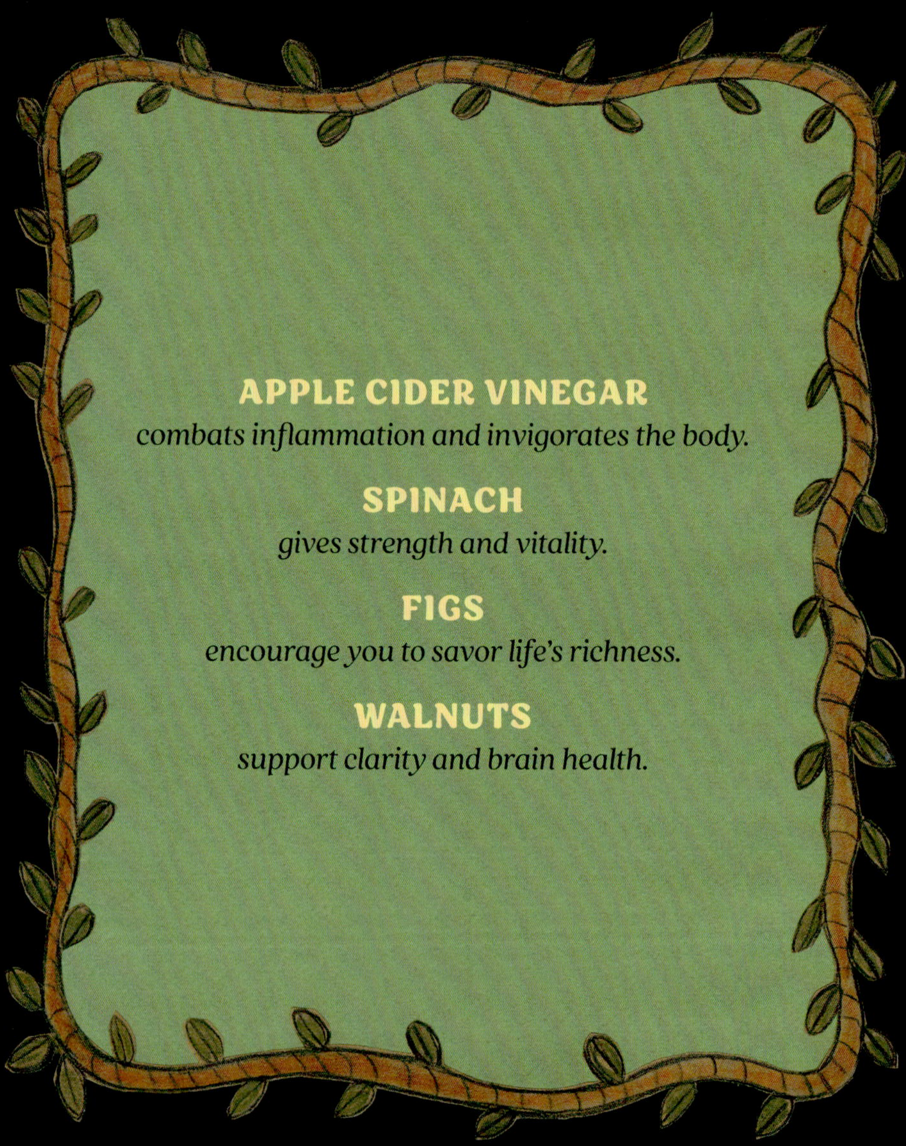

APPLE CIDER VINEGAR
combats inflammation and invigorates the body.

SPINACH
gives strength and vitality.

FIGS
encourage you to savor life's richness.

WALNUTS
support clarity and brain health.

Did You Know?

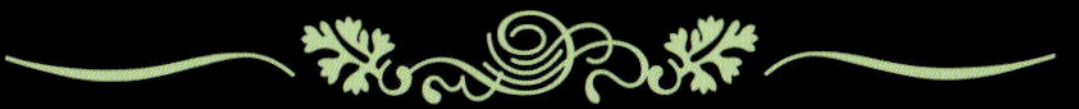

Pliny the Elder praised figs for a long life, and in Greek mythology the fig tree was a gift from Dionysus and represented recovery after hardship. Walnuts were loved for providing wisdom and healing in both Roman and Celtic traditions. Hippocrates himself prescribed vinegar for health. And in American pop culture, Popeye the Sailor Man made spinach famous as a food that instantly restored energy and resilience.

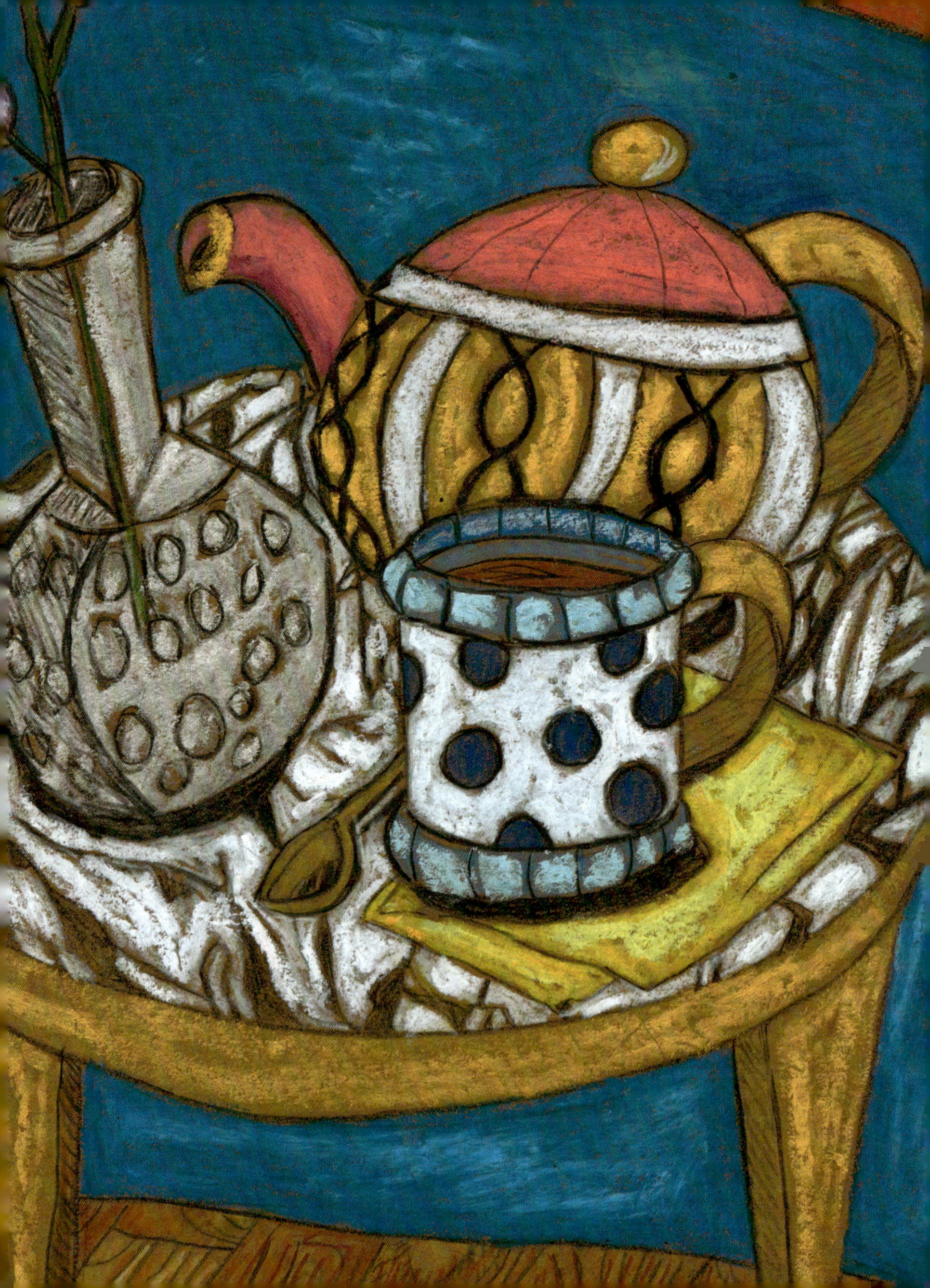

HEAL YOUR HOME

Home should be more than walls and windows—it is the sanctuary that holds your spirit. Here, our goal is to fill it with warmth, balance, and care, turning ordinary spaces into places of renewal.

Through the ages, people have turned to nature to bless and protect their homes. In this chapter, you'll find teas to soothe the air, sachets to invite calm, natural cleaners to refresh your space, and recipes to link body and home in wellness. Each small act—boiling water, lighting a candle, tying a sachet—becomes a mindful ritual to bring you peace.

Let's begin with a pot of *Home Sweet Home Lavender Tea*, a gentle brew that fills the air with calm and invites serenity.

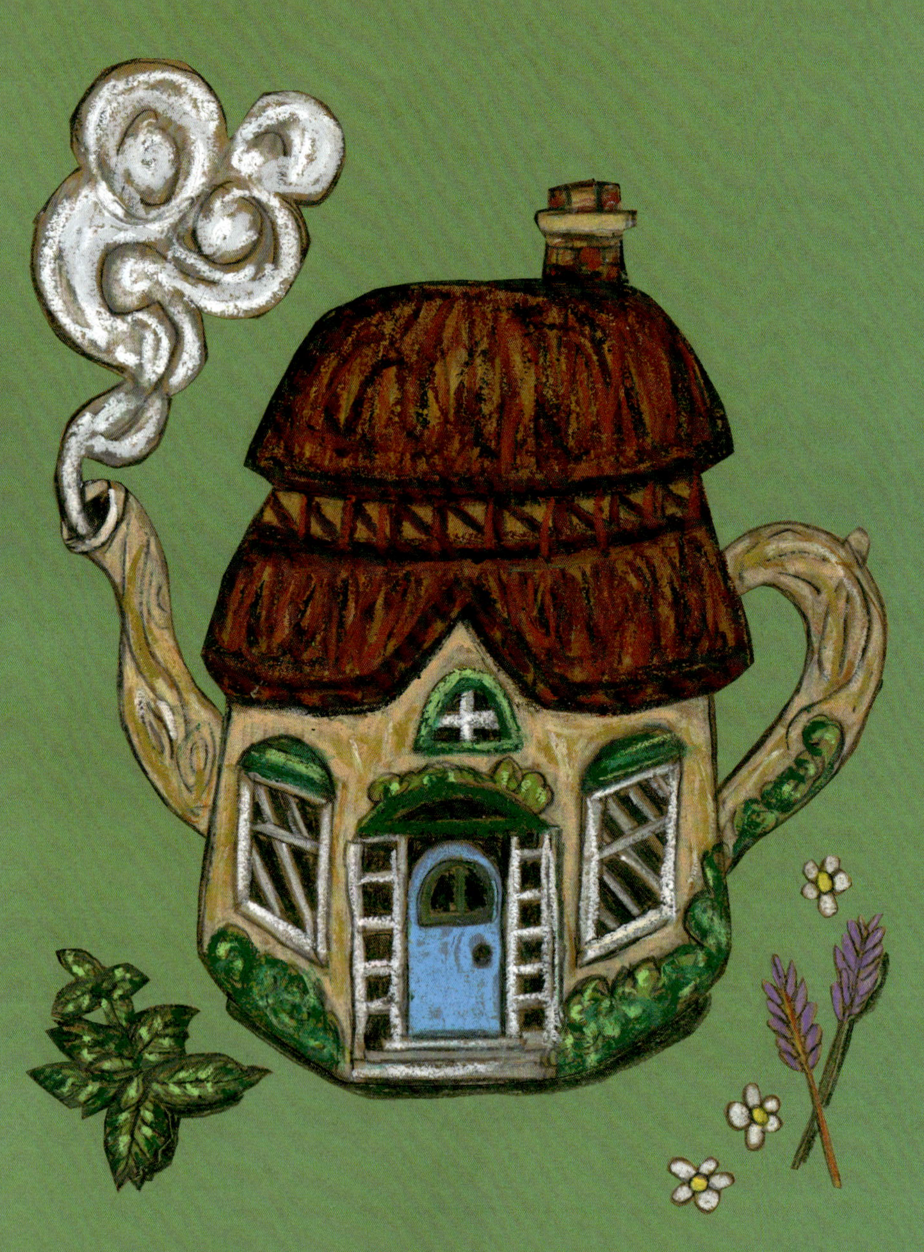

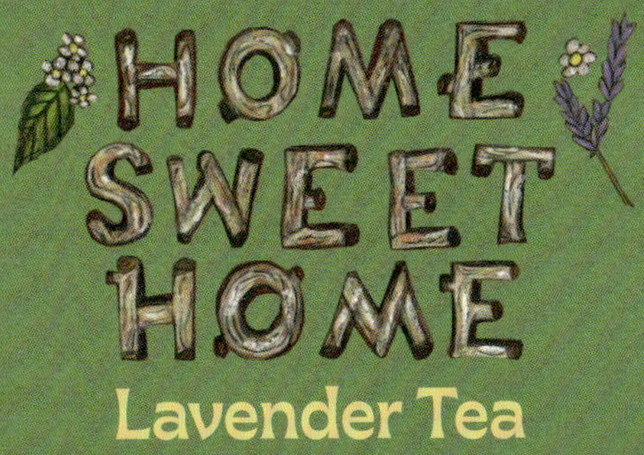

Lavender Tea

(Serves 2)

Let the act of making this calming, aromatic, deeply delicious tea become an act of mindfulness.

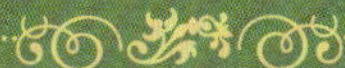

2 cups water
1 tablespoon dried lavender buds
1 teaspoon dried chamomile flowers
1 teaspoon dried peppermint leaves
1 teaspoon dried lemon balm leaves
1 teaspoon dried thyme leaves

Combine the lavender buds, chamomile flowers, peppermint leaves, lemon balm leaves, and thyme leaves in a bowl. As you measure and mix, breathe deeply. Let the scent of each herb invite you into a calm space.

Boil water. As you wait, take a quiet moment for yourself to stretch your body or simply zone out!

Place 1 tablespoon of the herbal mixture in a teapot or tea infuser. Pour the boiling water over the herbs and cover. Let the tea steep for 5 to 7 minutes. Place your hands around the vessel. Feel the warmth and notice the beautiful aroma the tea lends to your home.

Strain the tea into a cup and toss the soaked herbs into the compost bin.

Add a slice of lemon to your tea if you desire. Let it float gently, like a tiny sun in your cup.

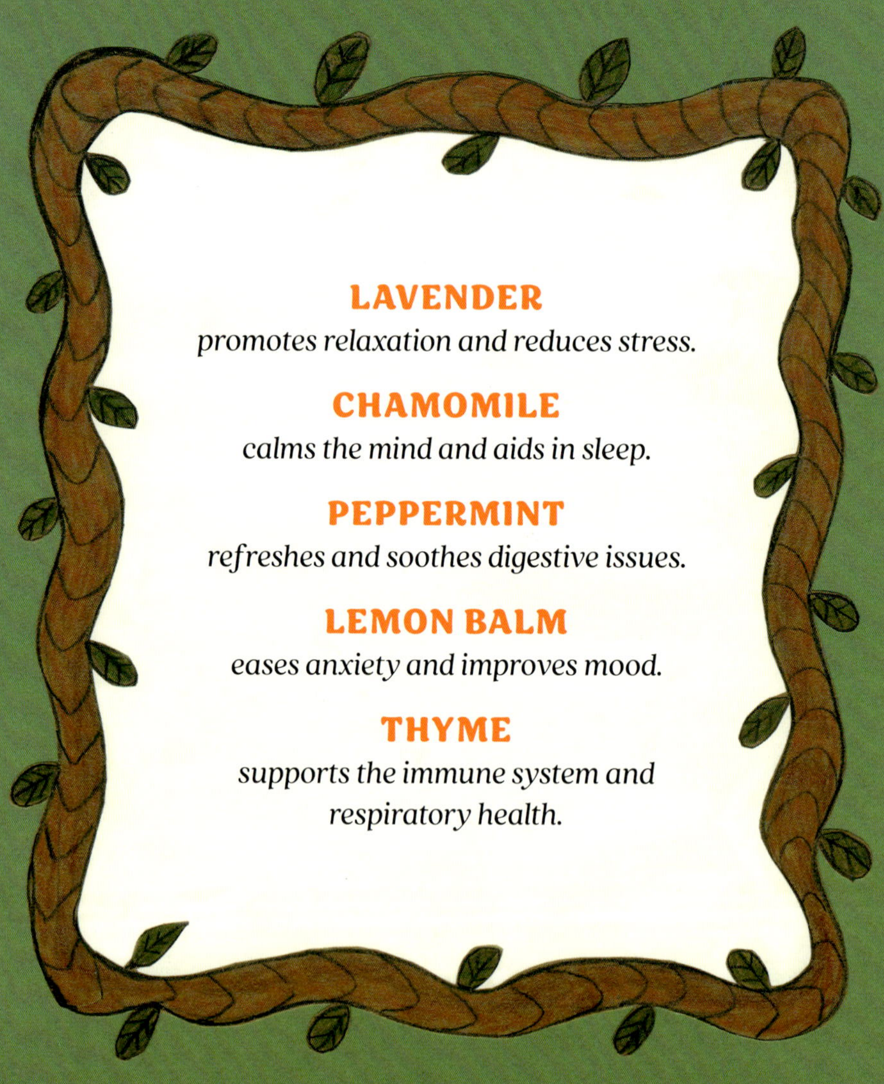

LAVENDER

promotes relaxation and reduces stress.

CHAMOMILE

calms the mind and aids in sleep.

PEPPERMINT

refreshes and soothes digestive issues.

LEMON BALM

eases anxiety and improves mood.

THYME

supports the immune system and
respiratory health.

Did You Know?

Ancient Egyptians used lavender oil in embalming, and the ancient Greeks benefited from its medicinal properties. Roman soldiers carried lavender to war with them to dress their wounds.

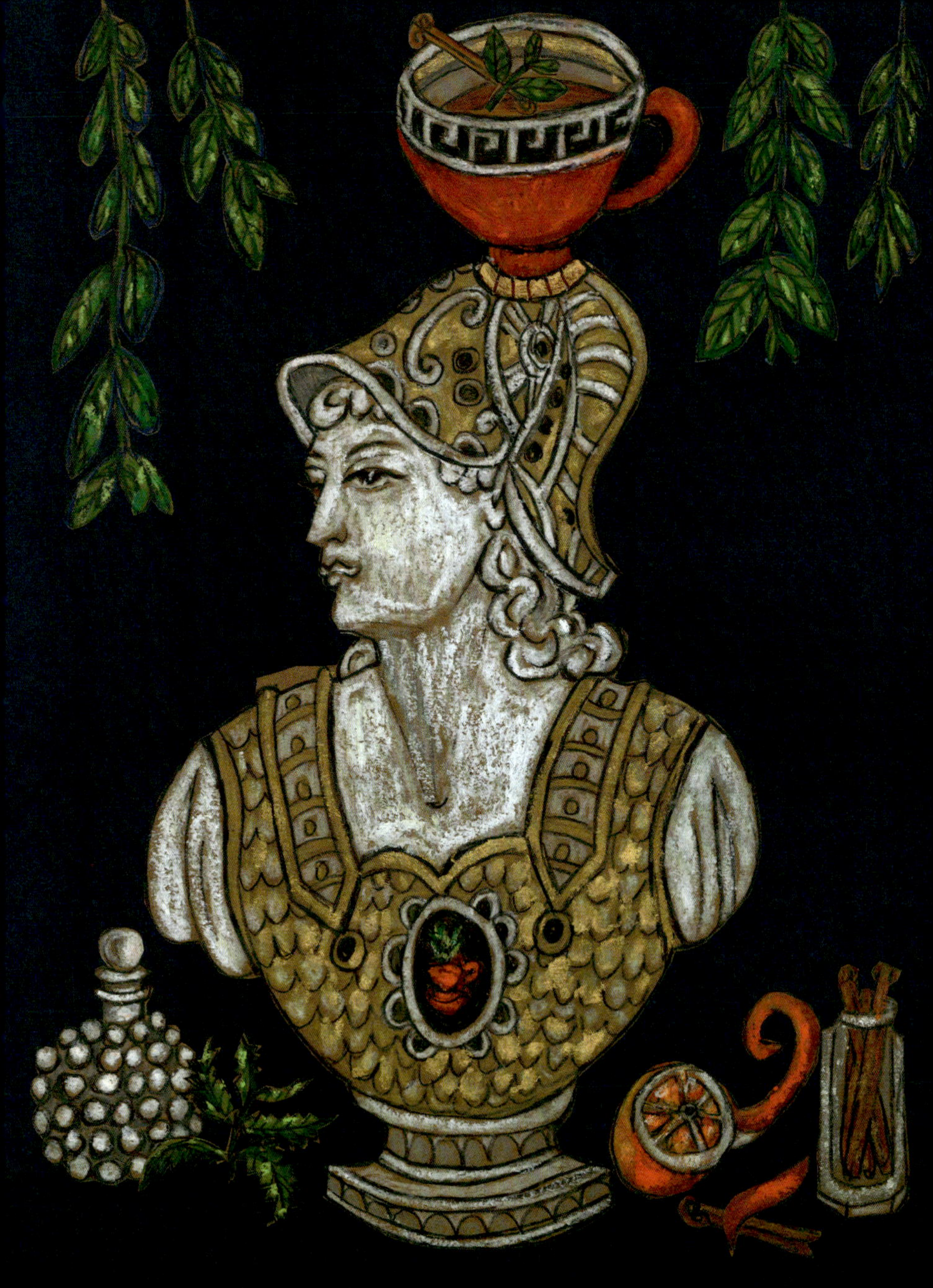

Athena's Brave Heart Tea

(Serves 2)

**A warming, fortifying tea to summon your inner courage
and clarity—one mindful sip at a time.**

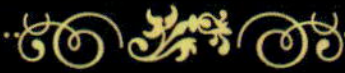

1 tablespoon dried ginger root
1 teaspoon dried cinnamon bark
1 teaspoon dried nettle leaves
1 teaspoon dried basil leaves
1 teaspoon dried orange peel
2 cups water

In a quiet space, combine the dried ginger root, cinnamon bark, nettle leaves, basil leaves, and orange peel in a bowl. As you mix, take a deep breath in through the nose and exhale slowly through the mouth.

Bring water to a boil. As the water heats, close your eyes and visualize Athena's shield, a glowing symbol of protection and wisdom, rising before you.

Add the herbal mixture to a teapot or tea infuser. Slowly pour the water over the herbs. Cover and allow the tea to steep for 7 to 10 minutes. As it steeps, place your hands around the vessel and feel the warmth radiate. Inhale the fragrant steam and anchor your breath in the present moment.

Strain the tea into a red teacup and toss the used herbs into your compost bin. Red symbolizes vitality, bravery, and life-force energy—let the color uplift and energize your spirit. Drink and savor the warmth and the power each herb imparts. Let this moment be your sacred pause.

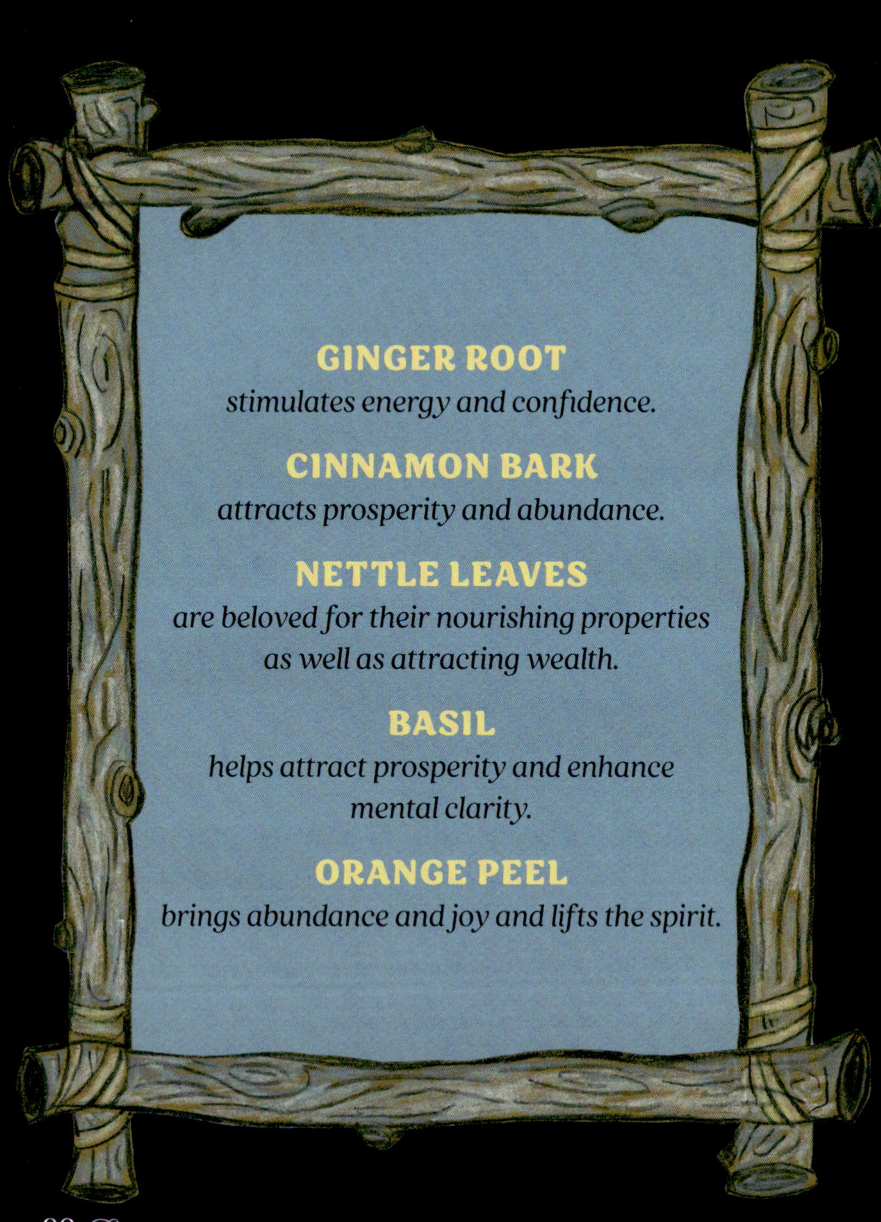

GINGER ROOT
stimulates energy and confidence.

CINNAMON BARK
attracts prosperity and abundance.

NETTLE LEAVES
are beloved for their nourishing properties
as well as attracting wealth.

BASIL
helps attract prosperity and enhance
mental clarity.

ORANGE PEEL
brings abundance and joy and lifts the spirit.

Did You Know?

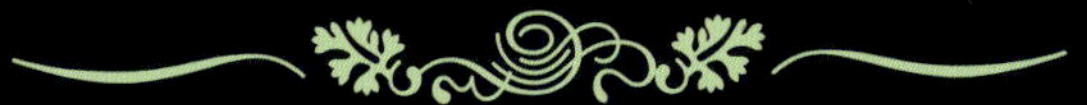

In Greek mythology, Athena is the goddess of wisdom, courage, and strategic warfare. The daughter of Zeus, she was respected for her intellect, fairness, and rationality. She was born fully grown and armored, and came from Zeus's forehead, which symbolized her emergence from the mind of the King of the Gods.

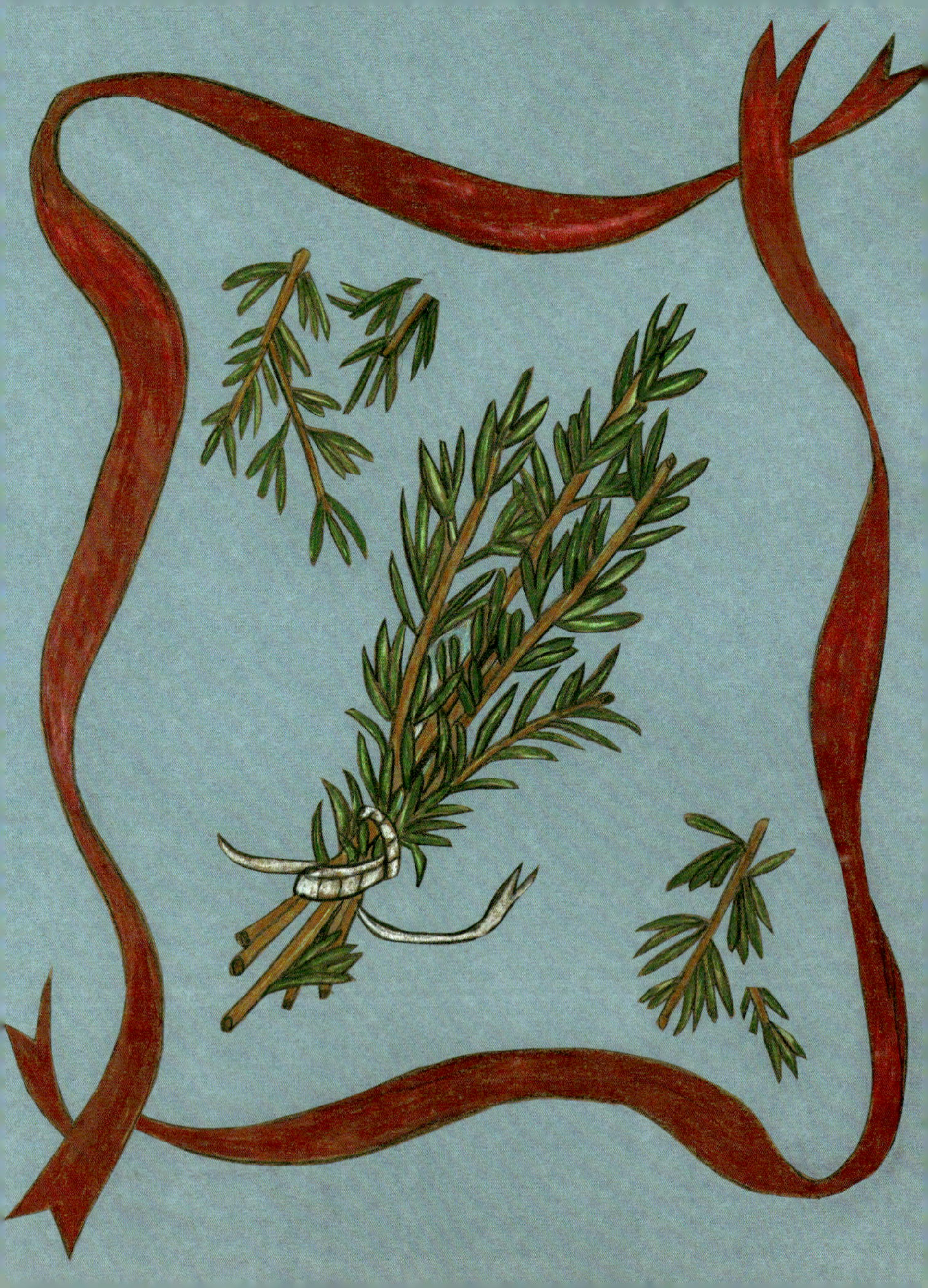

Home Protection Sachet

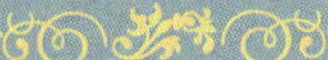

(Makes 1 sachet)

A calming and mindful project to attract peace and safety into your home.

1 tablespoon dried rosemary
1 teaspoon dried lavender
Pinch of black salt or sea salt
1 small clear quartz crystal
1 small muslin sachet bag with drawstring

Hold the rosemary in your hands. Breathe in its fresh, earthy scent. Add it to your sachet bag.

Add the lavender. As you sprinkle it in, enjoy how the scent calms you.

Add the salt. Appreciate the emotional balance it represents.

Add the crystal. Admire its beauty.

Pull the drawstring to close the sachet bag. Place it under your pillow before bed, or, during moments of stress, grasp it in your hands to reconnect with the powerful ingredients. Refresh the herbs every few weeks.

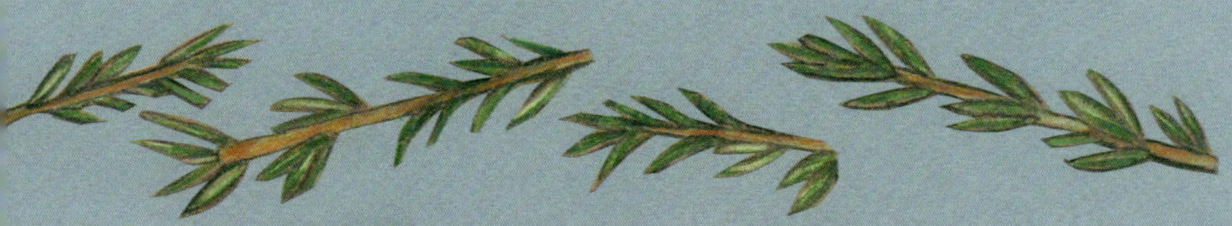

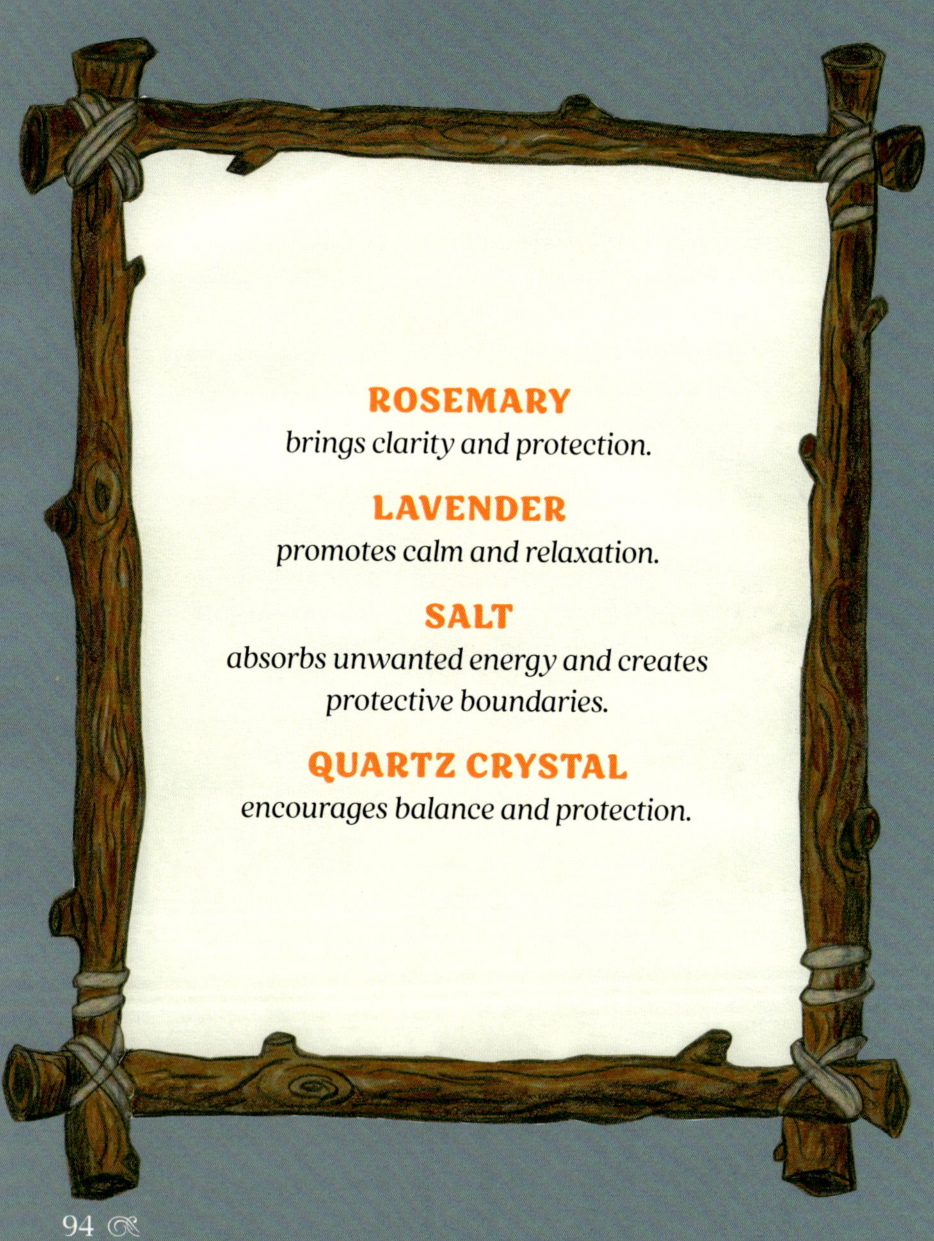

ROSEMARY
brings clarity and protection.

LAVENDER
promotes calm and relaxation.

SALT
absorbs unwanted energy and creates
protective boundaries.

QUARTZ CRYSTAL
encourages balance and protection.

Did You Know?

During medieval times, rosemary
was burned in homes and hospitals to
perfume the air, protect against illness,
and offer spiritual clarity.

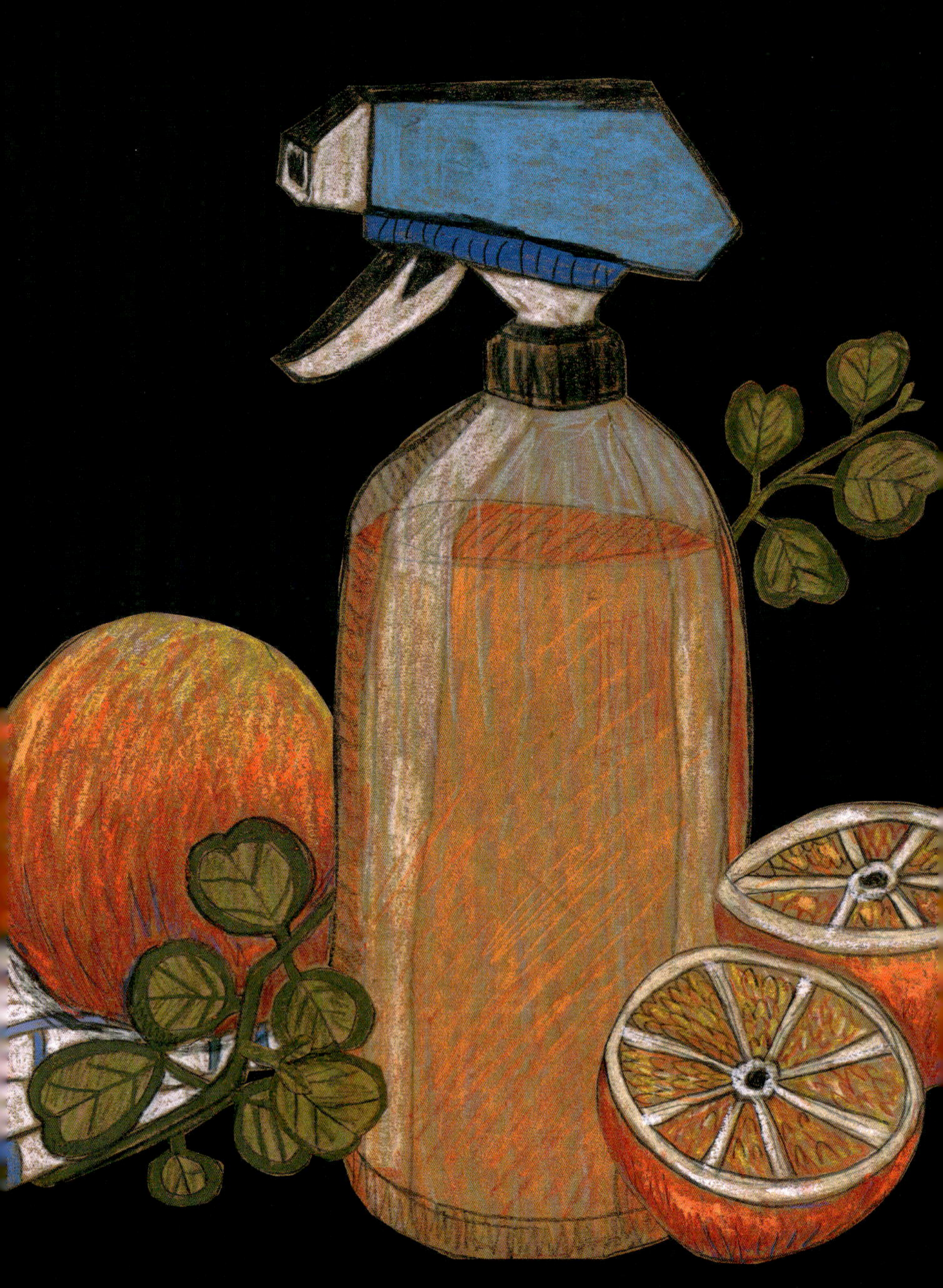

Orange and Eucalyptus Cleaning Spray

(Makes one 16-ounce bottle)

When your cleaning products smell like a grove of citrus and forest leaves, cleaning the home becomes a calming, sensory experience. Use this wonderful product to clean your kitchen, floors, and bathrooms.

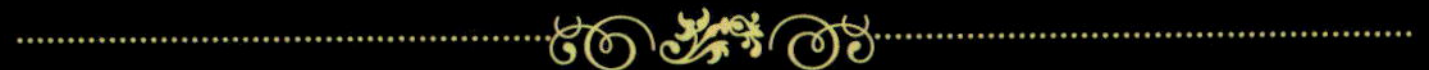

1 teaspoon orange essential oil
20 drops eucalyptus essential oil
½ cup clear, flavorless alcohol (120 proof vodka or
90% isopropyl alcohol)
12 ounces white vinegar

Add all ingredients to a 16-ounce glass spray bottle. Screw on the spray top to secure.

Shake the bottle for a few moments to thoroughly mix the ingredients. As you shake, take slow, steady breaths and imagine you are not only cleaning your home, but refreshing your spirit as well.

Store the spray bottle in a cool, dry place, away from direct sunlight, to preserve its potency and effectiveness.

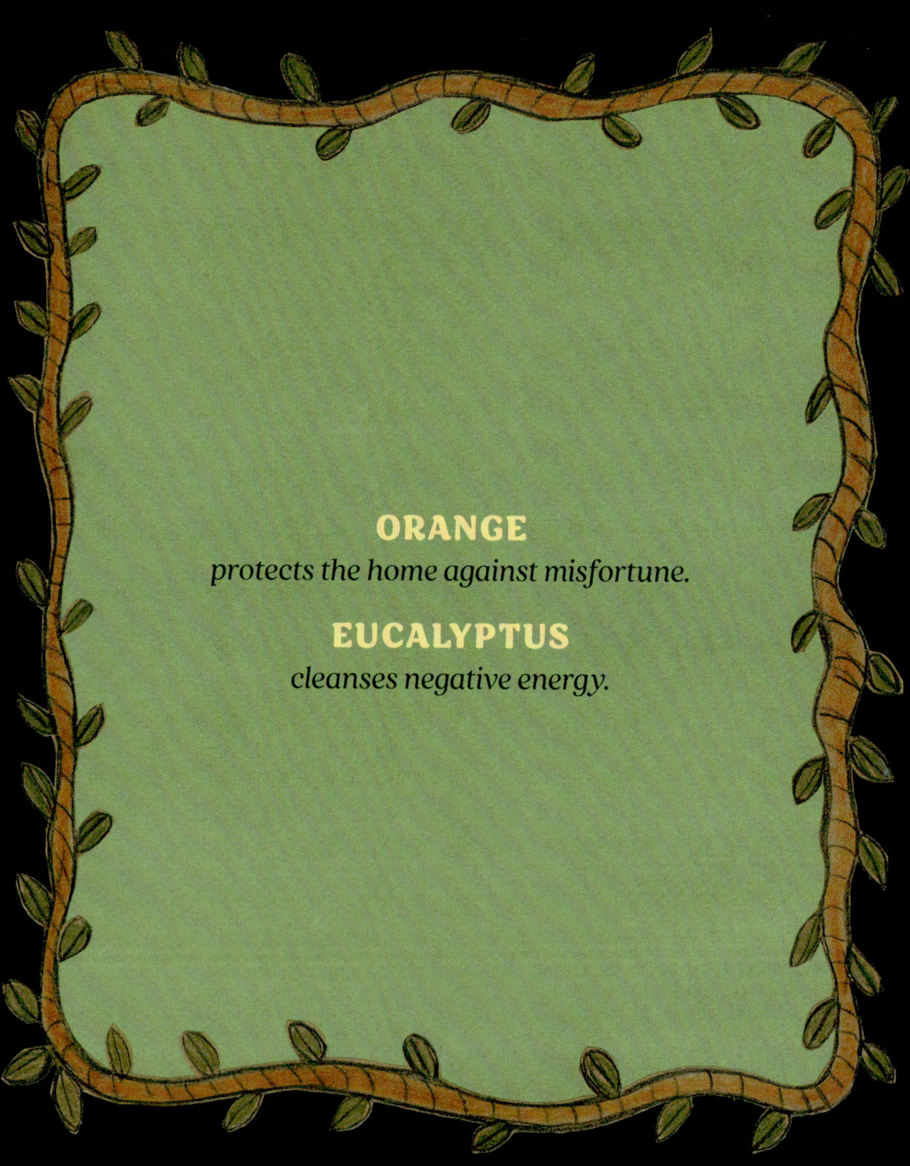

ORANGE
protects the home against misfortune.

EUCALYPTUS
cleanses negative energy.

Did You Know?

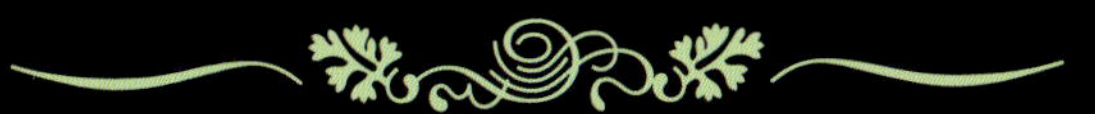

There are many advantages of using natural cleaners such as this orange and eucalyptus spray.

Commercial chemical cleaners often contain harsh ingredients like ammonia, bleach, and synthetic fragrances, which can cause respiratory irritation or allergic reactions.

Rosemary, Lavender, and Sage Cleansing Stick

(Makes 1 cleansing bundle)

This cleansing stick is designed to clear bad energy out of your home or workspace. Enjoy its gorgeous earthy scent!

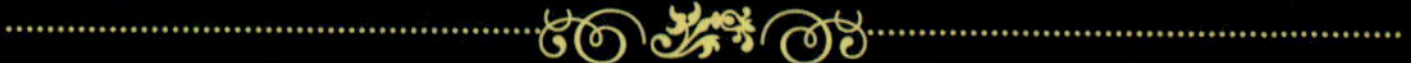

5 sprigs fresh rosemary (about 6 inches each)
5 sprigs fresh lavender (about 6 inches each)
3 sprigs fresh white sage (about 6 inches each)
Cotton twine (about 24 to 36 inches)

Gather the herbs together and trim if necessary to create even lengths. Tie them together at one end with the cotton twine, then, holding them tightly, wrap the twine around the sprigs, spiraling upward and then back down again to create a stick shape. As you bind them together, take a deep breath and set an intention for refreshed energy.

Hang the bundle in a cool, airy place for 1 to 2 weeks until dry.

Once the herbs are thoroughly dry, light the tip and, just after it catches, blow out the flame. Let the herbs smolder and the smoke rise. Slowly waft the smoke around your space, especially in doorways, corners, or anywhere that feels heavy or stagnant.

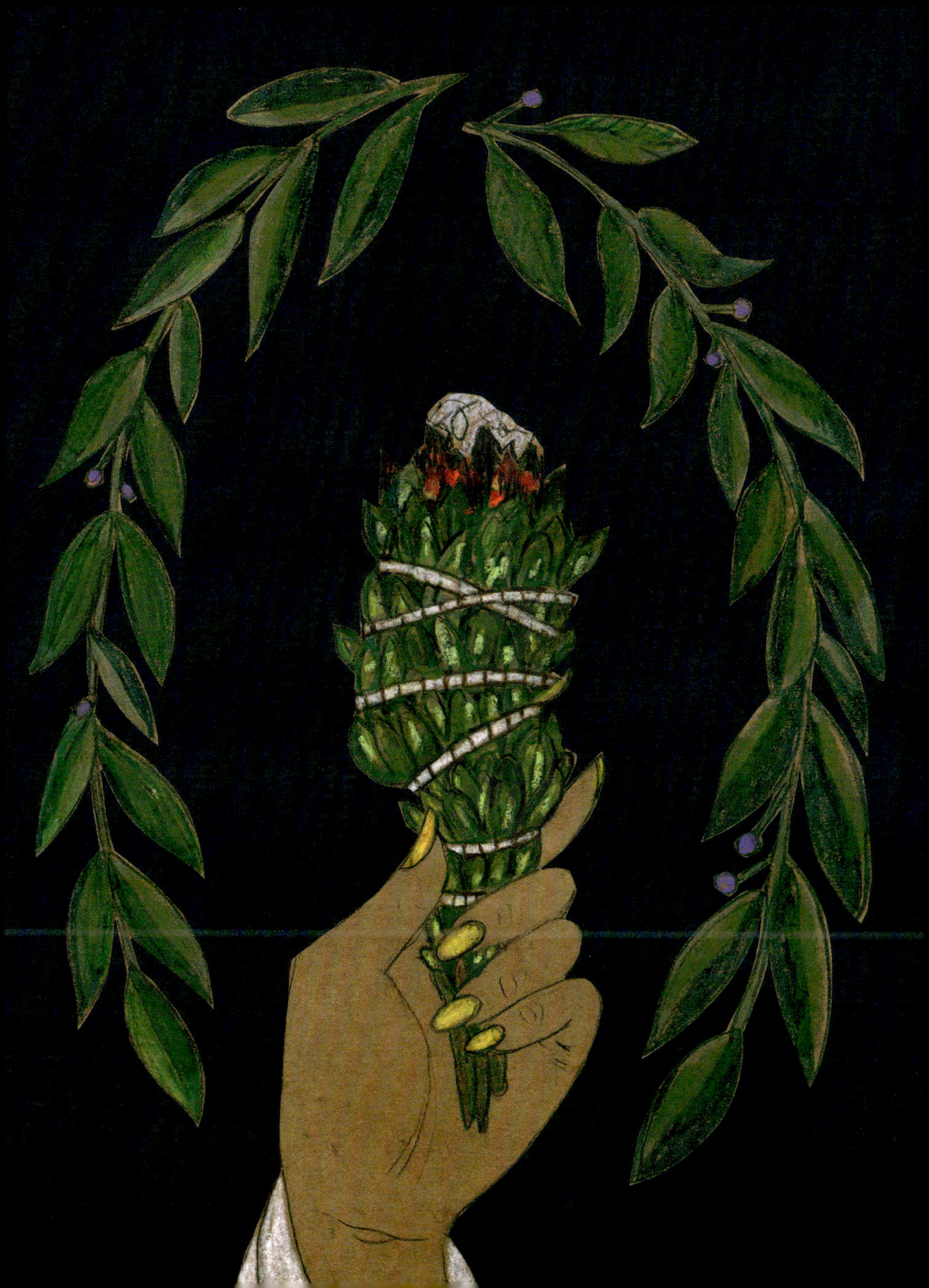

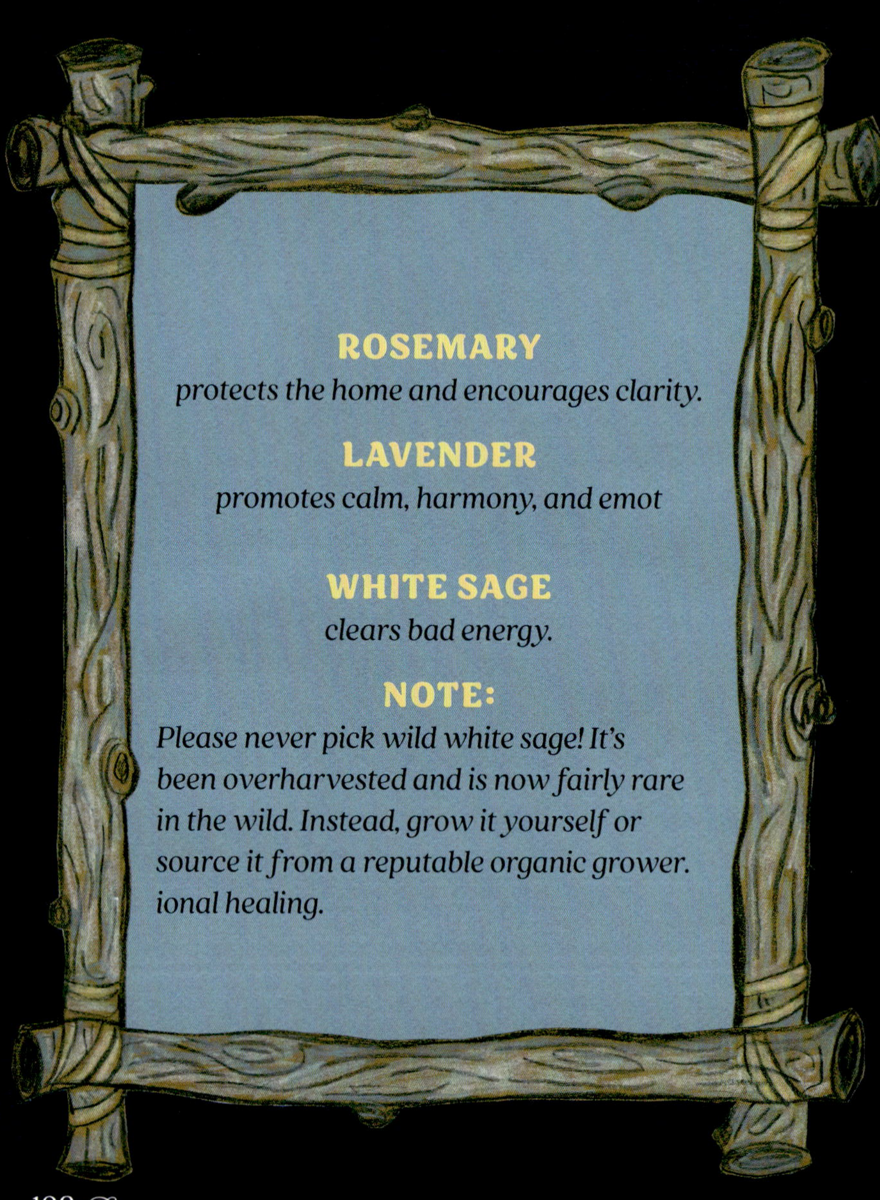

ROSEMARY

protects the home and encourages clarity.

LAVENDER

promotes calm, harmony, and emot

WHITE SAGE

clears bad energy.

NOTE:

Please never pick wild white sage! It's been overharvested and is now fairly rare in the wild. Instead, grow it yourself or source it from a reputable organic grower. ional healing.

Did You Know?

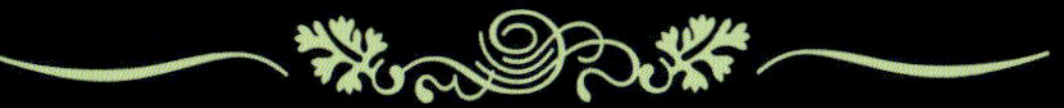

The burning of sage bundles (smudge sticks) has roots in the ceremonies of many Indigenous communities in North America. Smudging rituals purify spaces, ward off negative energy, and invite spiritual protection.

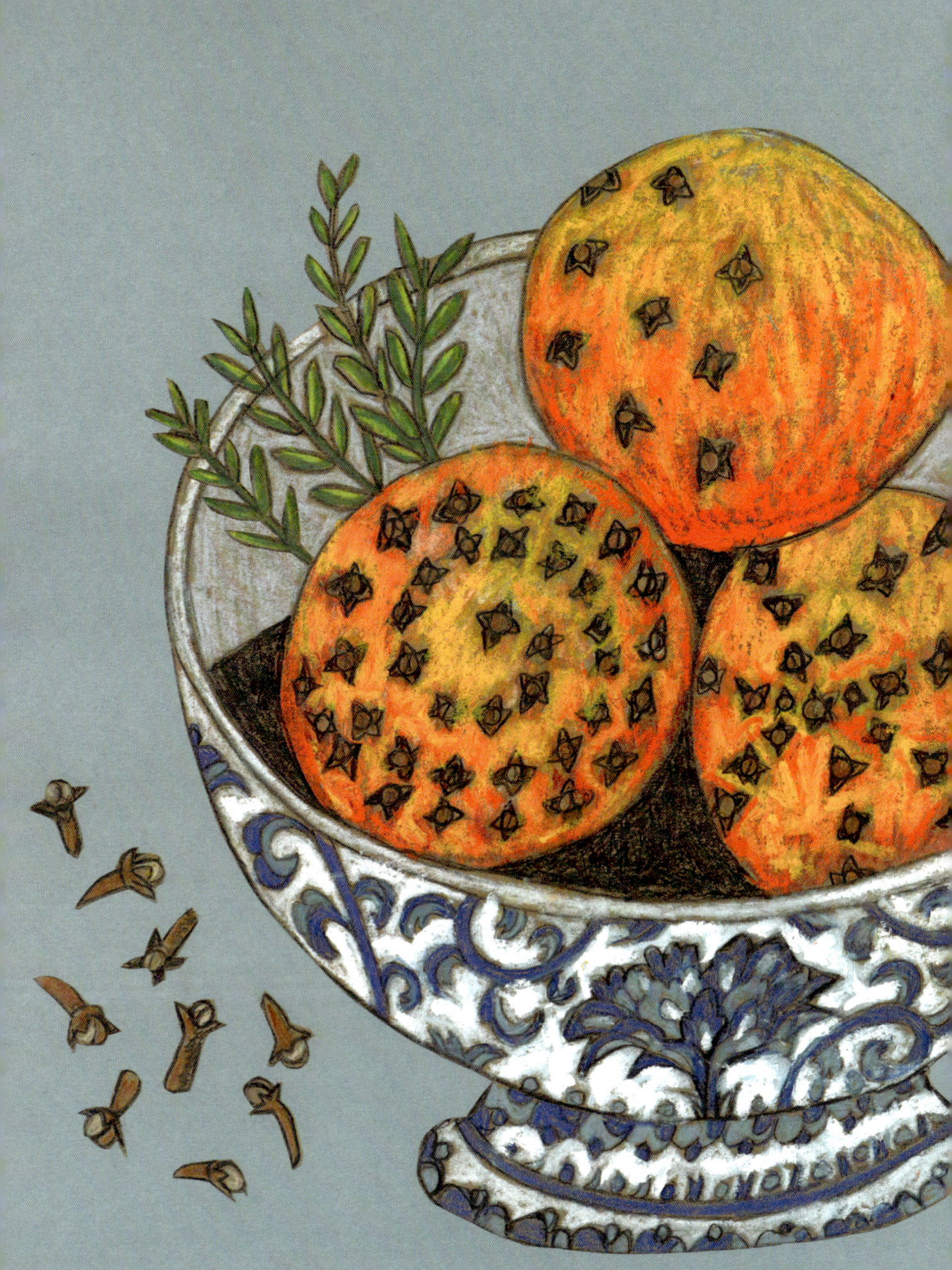

Refreshing Pomander Balls

(Makes 2)

Not only do these pomander balls bring a lovely scent to your indoor space, they also protect it from negative energy!

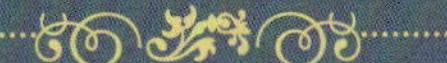

2 firm oranges, any variety
¼ cup whole cloves

Wash the oranges thoroughly. As you wash, take a slow breath and imagine you are rinsing away any tension from your day, leaving only freshness and clarity.

Pat the oranges dry with a clean towel. Using a wooden skewer, gently poke holes into the surface of each orange, creating spaces to receive the cloves.

Carefully insert cloves into the holes you've created. Feel free to be creative with your designs; arrange the cloves in patterns such as diamonds, circles, or spirals for a visually appealing look. As you press in each clove, pause for a moment of gratitude, letting the warm scent remind you to be present and centered.

As the oranges dry, they will release a delicate, spicy, floral fragrance to perfume your home, welcoming positive energy.

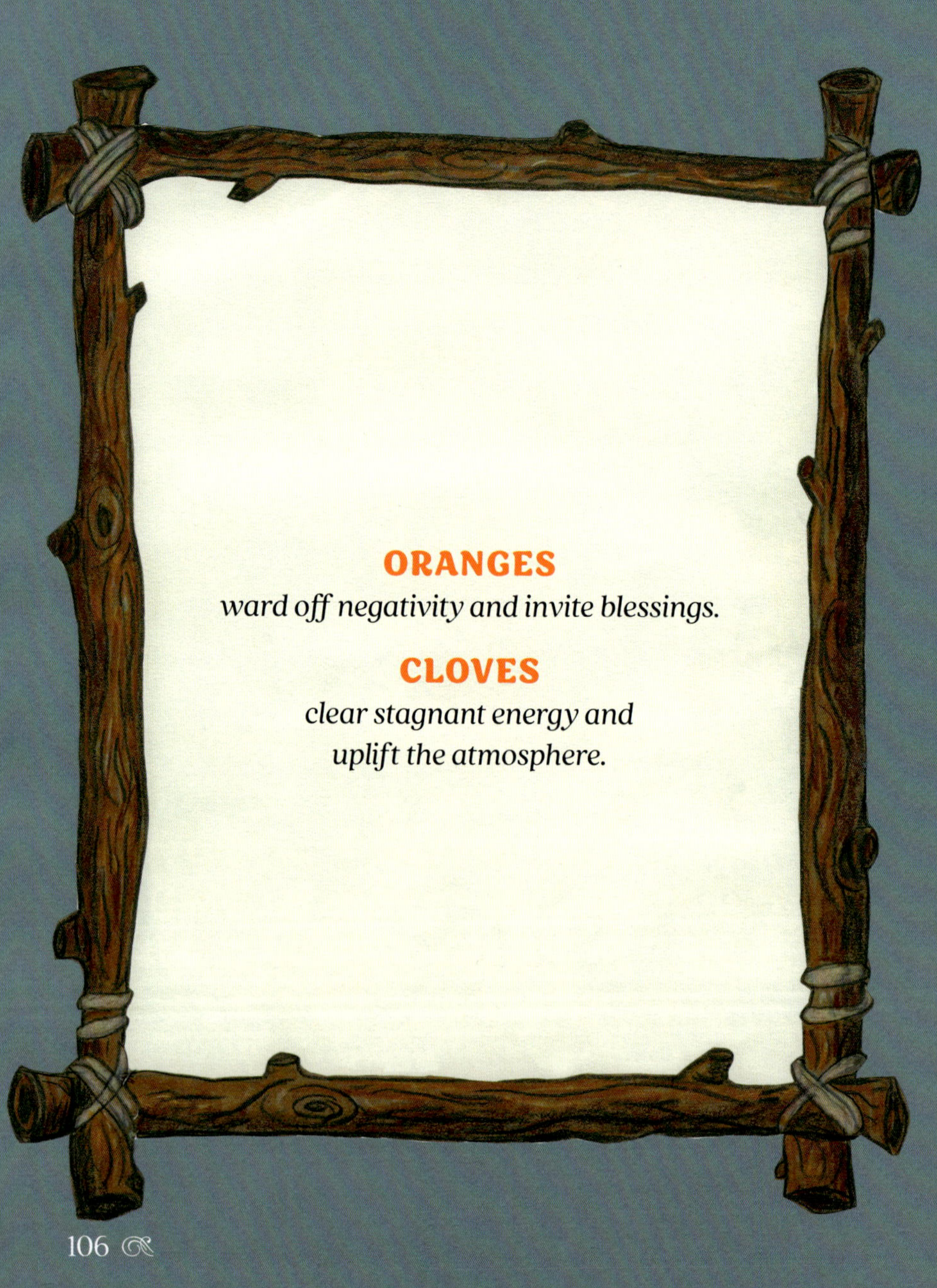

ORANGES

ward off negativity and invite blessings.

CLOVES

*clear stagnant energy and
uplift the atmosphere.*

Did You Know?

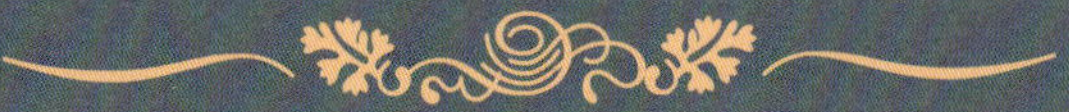

Medieval herbalists used pomanders to ward off illness. Pomanders were used during the Black Death to cover up and purify "bad air."

Cinnamon and Clove Vintage Teacup Candles

(Makes 2 candles)

Transform your mismatched and vintage teacups into delightful candles!

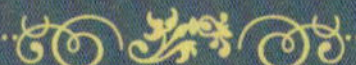

Microwave-safe container for melting wax
1-2 cups soy wax, depending on the size of the teacups
10-15 drops cinnamon essential oil
10-15 drops clove essential oil
Pouring pitcher or container with a spout
2 candle wicks with candle wick holders
2 vintage teacups
10-12 amber crystal chips or beads

Add wax to the microwave safe container. Heat wax in 30-second intervals until fully melted, stirring in between each interval.

Once the wax is melted, allow it to cool slightly. Add cinnamon oil and clove oil to the melted wax. Stir well to combine. Transfer wax mixture to a pouring pitcher.

Secure a candle wick in the center of each teacup using the wick holder. Make sure it's straight and centered.

Carefully pour the melted wax into each teacup. As you pour the wax, take a slow, deep breath and focus on the beautiful candles you're creating. Sprinkle amber crystals on the surface before the wax hardens to create a beautiful decorative finish.

Allow the candles to cool and harden completely at room temperature. This may take a few hours.

When the candles are fully set, trim the wicks to about ¼ inch above the wax surface. Enjoy your wonderful teacup candles!

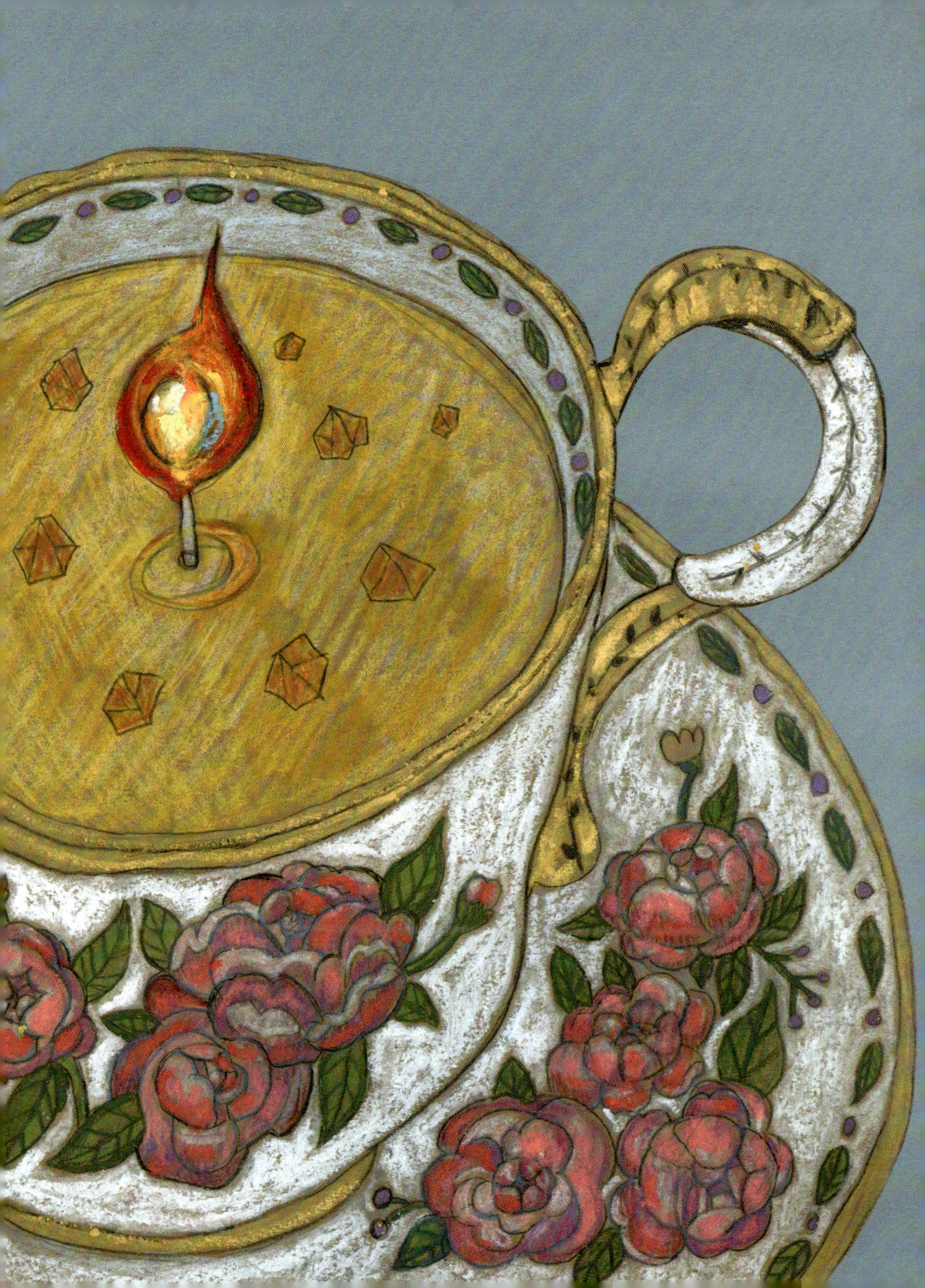

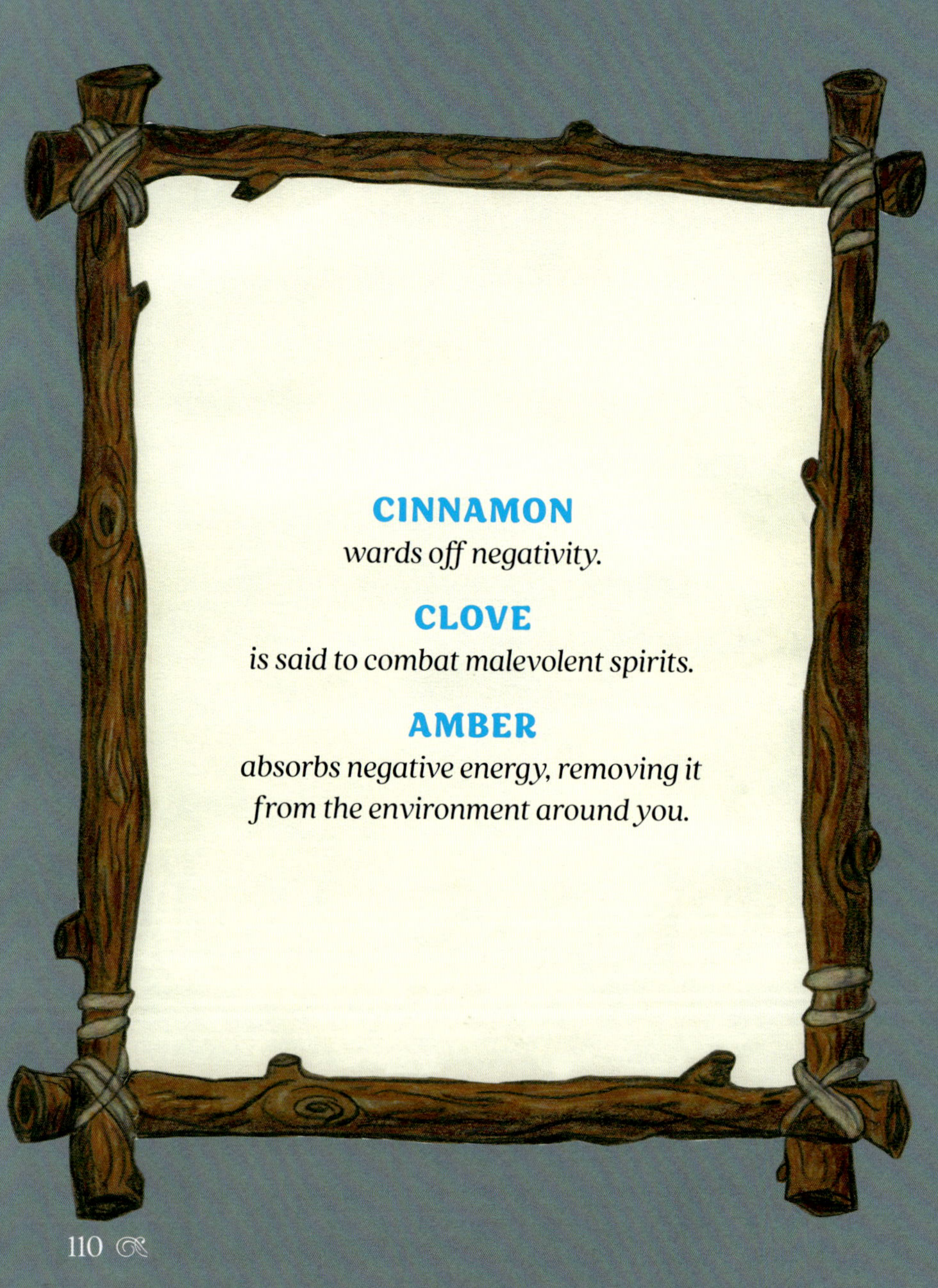

CINNAMON

wards off negativity.

CLOVE

is said to combat malevolent spirits.

AMBER

*absorbs negative energy, removing it
from the environment around you.*

Did You Know?

The act of lighting a candle calls upon a higher power to protect against harm. The flicker of flame is a reminder that even in darkness, one small light can keep fear at bay.

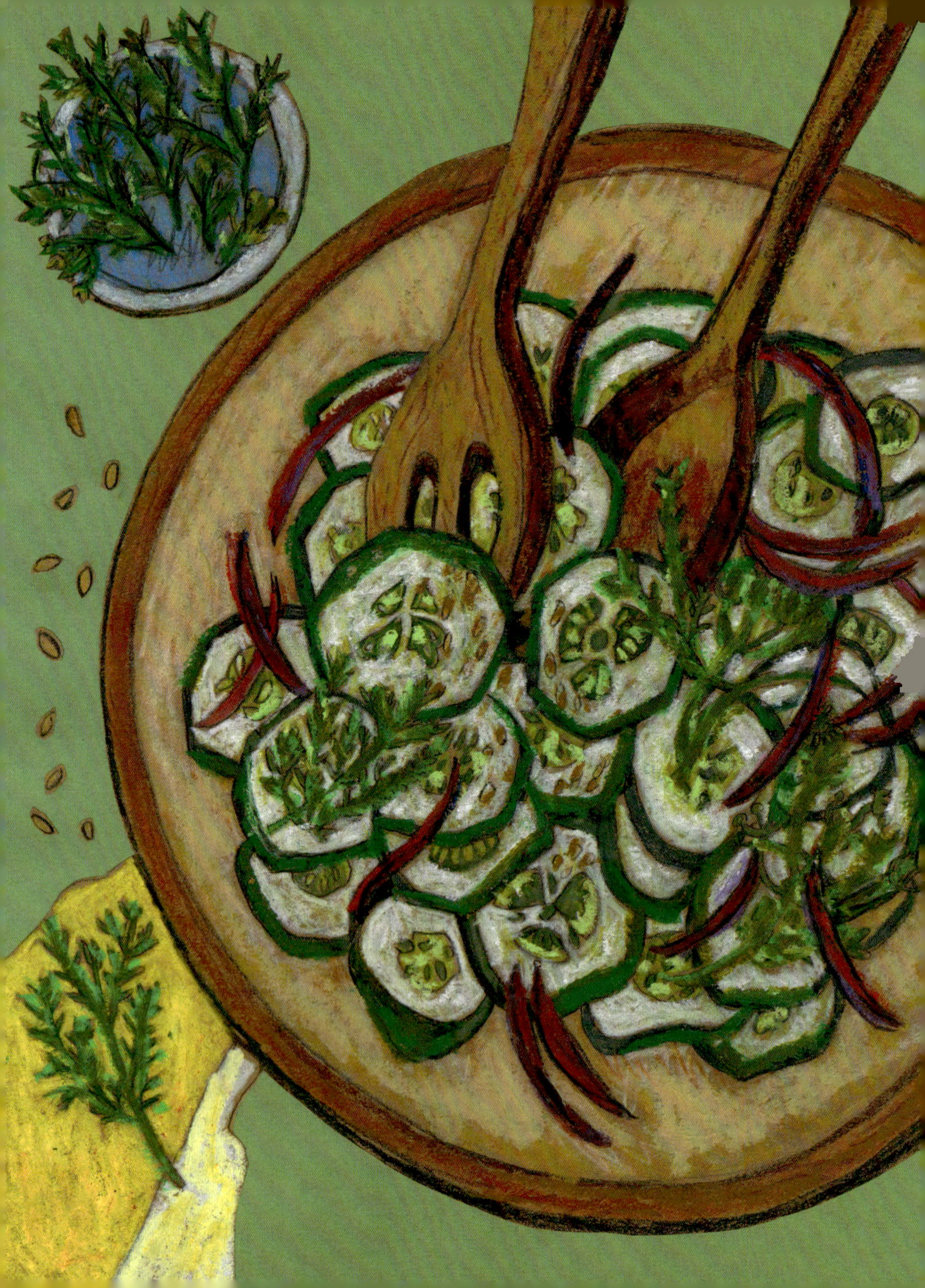

Cucumber Salad with Red Onion, Dill, and Flaxseeds

(Serves 4 as a side dish)

Together, these ingredients bring protection, harmony, and renewal—
qualities that nourish the body when eaten but also the spirit
of the home itself.

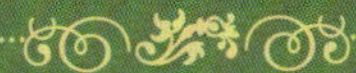

2 large cucumbers, thinly sliced
½ medium red onion, thinly sliced
3 tablespoons olive oil
2 tablespoons white wine vinegar or apple cider vinegar
1 teaspoon maple syrup (optional, for sweetness)
Salt and pepper to taste
2 tablespoons fresh dill, chopped
2 tablespoons flaxseeds

Add the cucumbers to a large bowl. Breathe slowly and notice the crisp freshness of the vegetables, letting their fresh scent bring you into the present moment. Add the red onion.

In a small bowl, whisk together the olive oil, vinegar, maple syrup (if using), salt, and pepper until well combined.

Drizzle the dressing over the cucumber and onion mixture. Add the chopped dill and flaxseeds and toss everything gently to coat.

For the best flavor, cover the salad and let it chill in the refrigerator for 20–30 minutes. Toss again just before serving. Enjoy your refreshing salad!

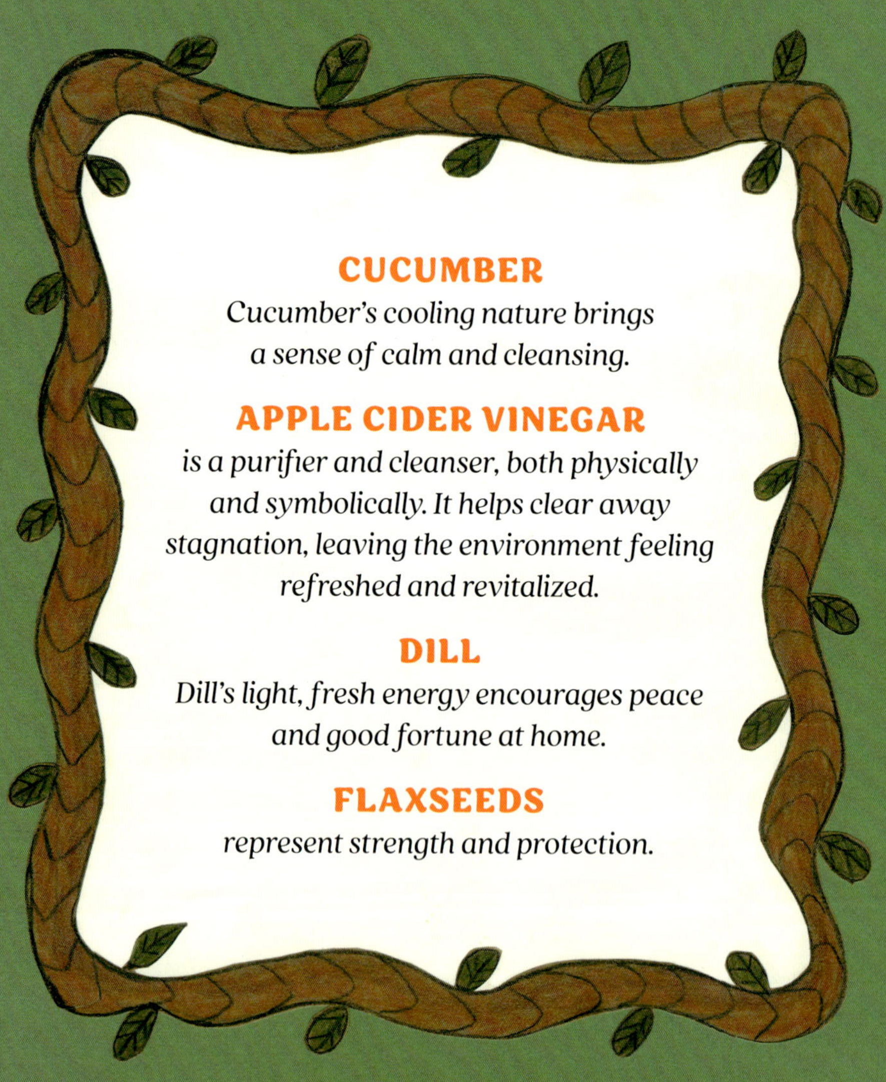

CUCUMBER

Cucumber's cooling nature brings
a sense of calm and cleansing.

APPLE CIDER VINEGAR

is a purifier and cleanser, both physically
and symbolically. It helps clear away
stagnation, leaving the environment feeling
refreshed and revitalized.

DILL

Dill's light, fresh energy encourages peace
and good fortune at home.

FLAXSEEDS

represent strength and protection.

Did You Know?

Placing cucumber peels in entryways can soak up bad energy or bad luck. Also, in many cultures, dill is kept in the home to ward off negativity. Red onions historically were used to protect the home from illness and bad luck by hanging them in doorways or windows, where they absorbed and dispelled harmful forces in the air. Flaxseeds have long been symbols of domestic harmony and abundance, blessing the home with peace.

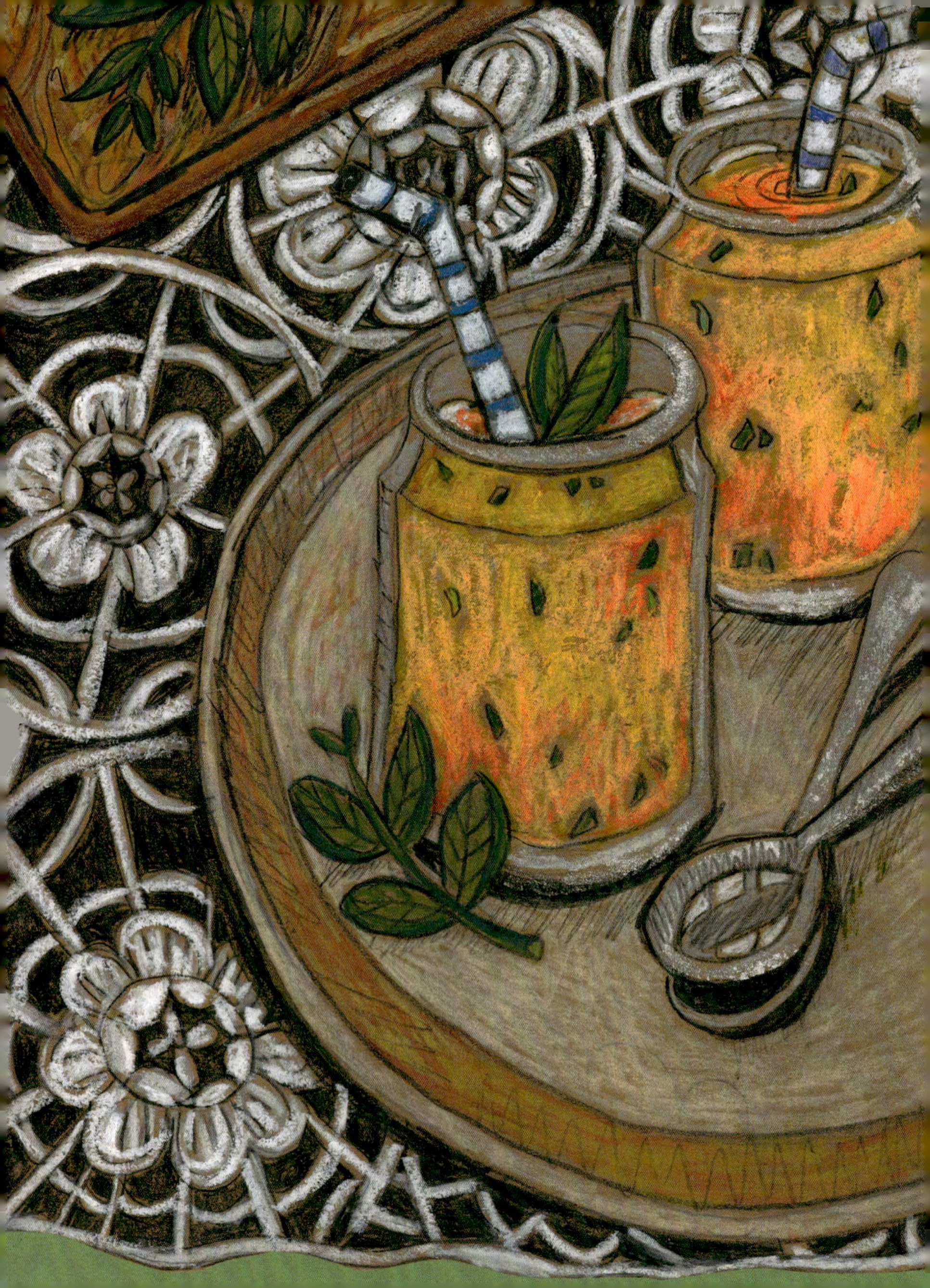

Protective Mint and Mango Smoothie

(Serves 2)

In this smoothie, mint and mango together invite uplifting,
protective energy into your home.

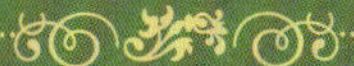

10 fresh mint leaves, plus 2 sprigs for garnish
2 fresh mangoes, or 1½ cups frozen mango cubes
1½ cups coconut milk, chilled
1 tablespoon agave sweetener (optional,
    you can adjust to your taste)
1 teaspoon fresh lime juice
Ice cubes (optional, for a colder smoothie)

Rinse mint leaves. If using fresh mangoes, peel, pit, and chop into 1-inch cubes. As you prepare the herbs and fruit, pause to notice their colors and fragrances, letting them remind you of nature's freshness and vitality.

In a blender, combine the mint leaves, mangoes, chilled coconut milk, agave (if using), and lime juice. Add a few ice cubes, if using.

Blend on high speed until the mixture is smooth and creamy, ensuring all ingredients are well incorporated. As the blender whirs, take a slow breath and set an intention for renewal and protection, imagining these qualities blending into your drink.

Pour the smoothie into 2 serving glasses. Garnish each glass with a sprig of mint.

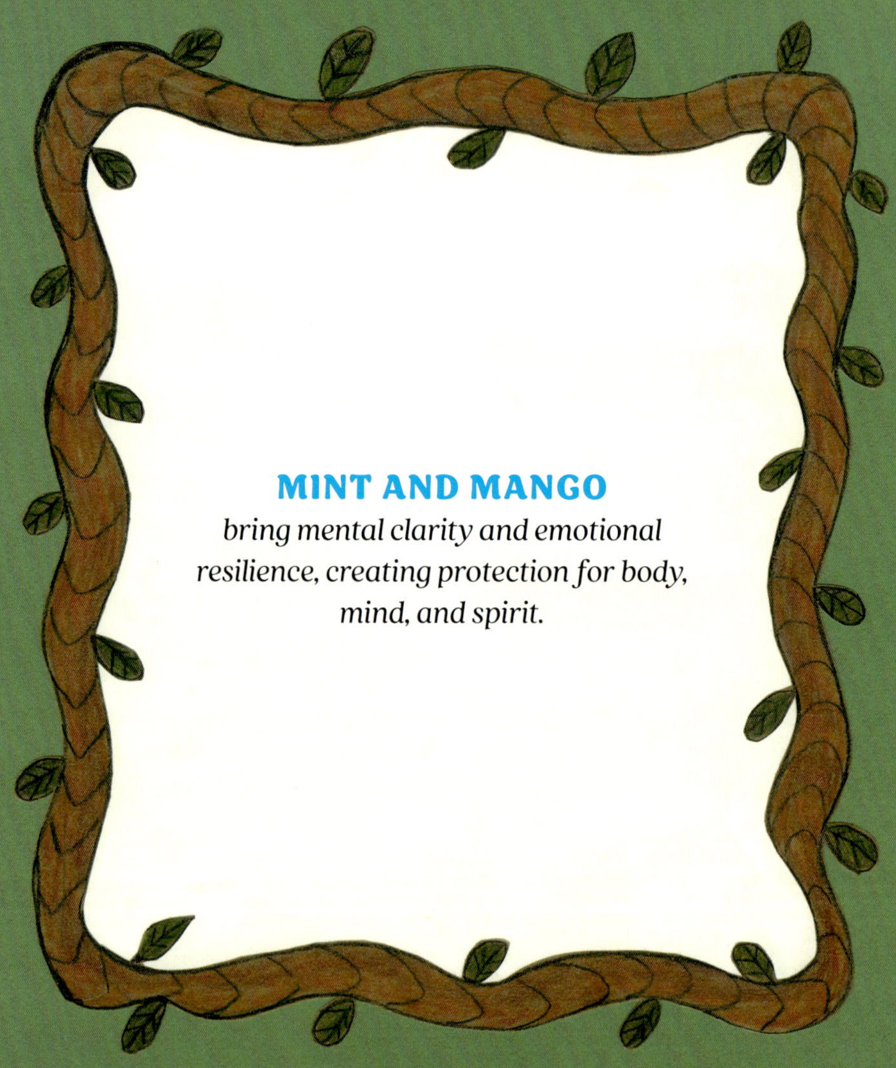

MINT AND MANGO

bring mental clarity and emotional
resilience, creating protection for body,
mind, and spirit.

Did You Know?

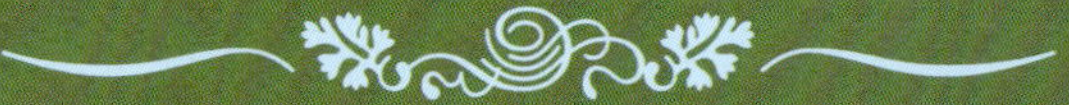

Mint can be used in protective sachets, threshold spells, and teas to guard against evil spirits. Hung at the door or held in one's pockets, mint acts as a protective charm for travelers.

Mango leaves are used to purify the home and ward off negative mojo.

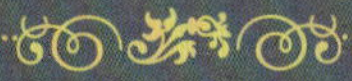

BONUS:
THE PROTECTIVE CAT!

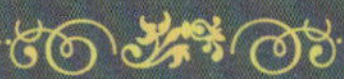

We wanted to give a special shout-out to our feline home protectors, because we love them so much! Have you ever noticed a statue of a waving white cat in the window of a Japanese business? That cat statue, known as Maneki-neko (literally "beckoning cat"), is an adorable symbol of luck, protection, and prosperity. With one paw raised in a welcoming gesture, the cat is placed near doorways or shop entrances to draw in good fortune. Traditionally, a raised left paw is to attract customers, while the right paw attracts wealth.

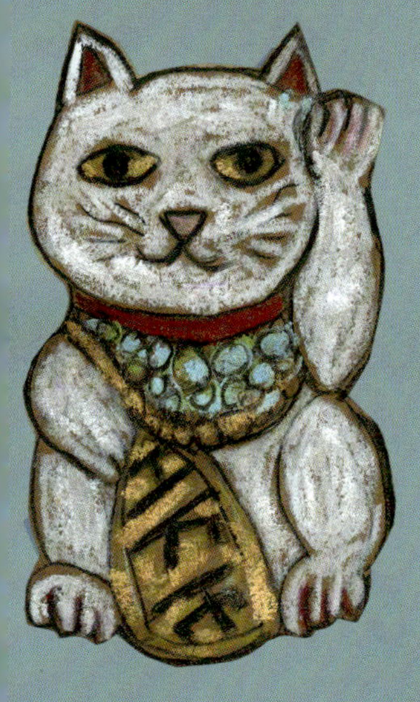

Around the world, cats have long been regarded as protectors of the home. They are known to sense unseen spirits, guard against evil, and maintain energetic harmony. Their quiet vigilance and acute ability to detect subtle shifts in energy make them natural guardians of your home or business.

Always give your cats love, affection, food, and lots of treats! We can't imagine our homes without them.

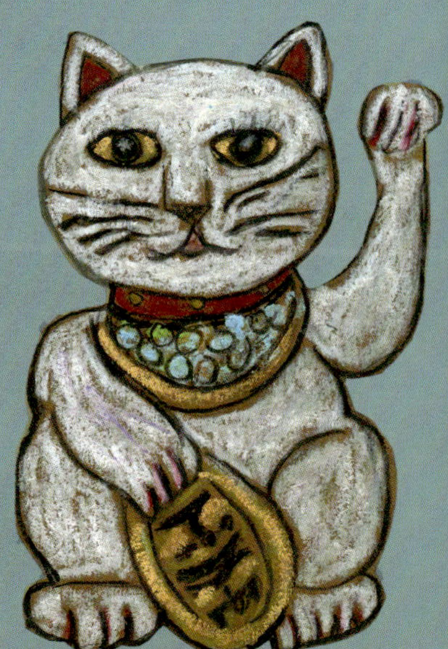

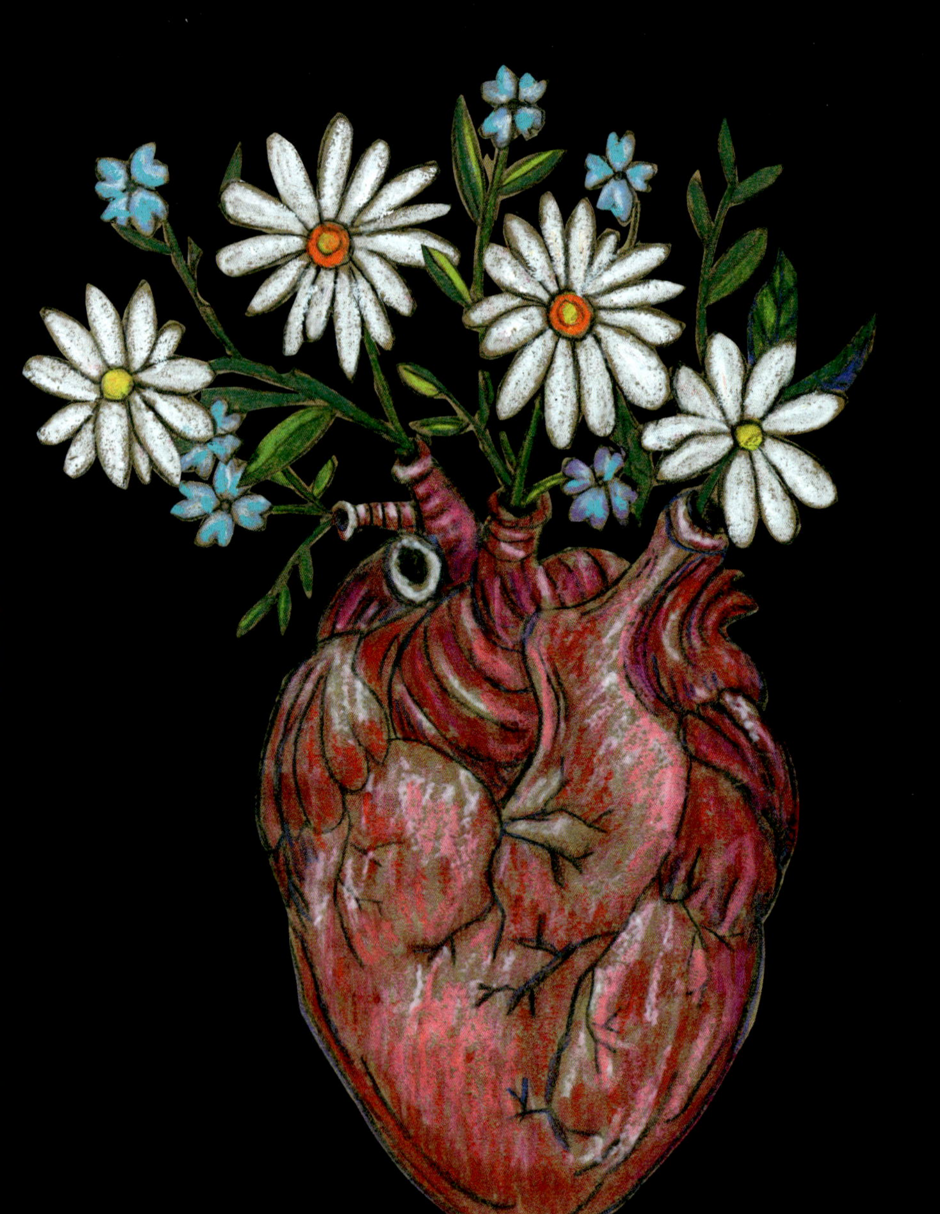

CHAPTER 4

HEAL YOUR HEART

The heart is more than a muscle—it is the holder of love, courage, sorrow, and joy. And plants, our ever-wise allies, remind us that true strength blooms from softness.

Throughout time, lovers have carried rose petals for devotion, warriors held hawthorn for bravery, and poets honored herbs that eased grief. Here you'll find teas, tonics, and creations to comfort, awaken, and strengthen the heart.

Before you begin any recipe or project, place your hand over your heart and take three deep breaths, inviting warmth and gratitude. As you create, welcome whatever feelings arise and remember that healing flows from acceptance.

We begin with *Orpheus's Heartbreak Helper Tea*, a renewing blend of rose, hawthorn, and passionflower to remind you that even in loss, the love you had will always remain in your heart.

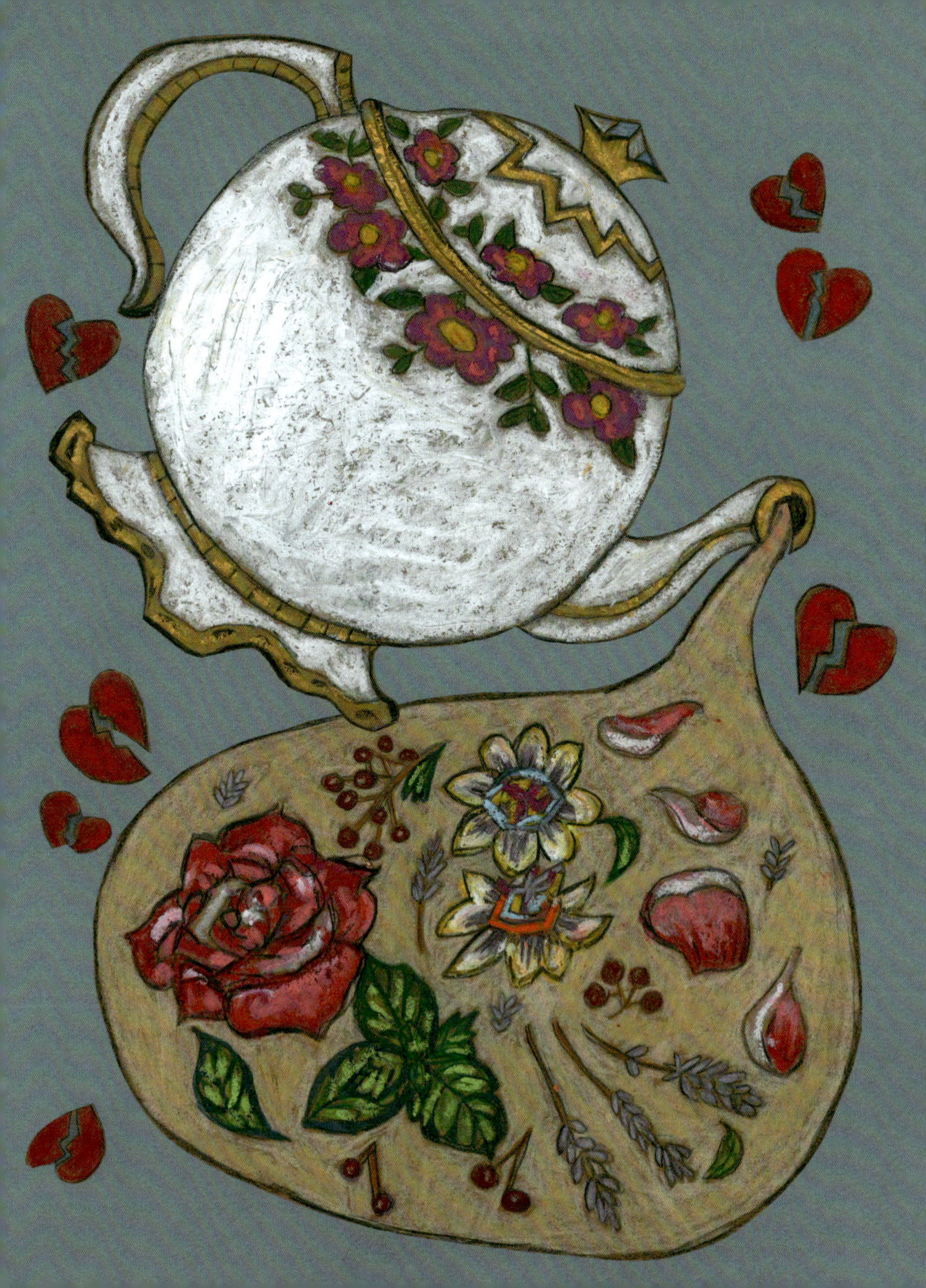

Orpheus's Heartbreak Helper Tea

(Serves 2)

A wonderful tea to help soothe and heal you in a time of heartbreak.
This tea will ease emotional tension, inviting compassion for
yourself back into your heart.

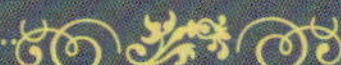

2 teaspoons dried rose petals
1 teaspoon dried hawthorn berries
1 teaspoon dried holy basil leaves
1 teaspoon dried lavender buds
1 teaspoon dried passionflower
2 cups water
Lemon slices (optional)

Combine the rose petals, hawthorn berries, holy basil leaves, lavender buds, and passionflower in a bowl. Notice their soothing colors.

Set the water to boil. Place 1 tablespoon herbal mixture into a teapot or tea infuser.

When the water boils, pour it over the herbs and cover the pot. Let it steep for 7 to 10 minutes. Close your eyes and imagine the warmth of the tea filling your heart with a healing calmness.

Strain the tea into your cups and serve. Toss the spent herbs into the compost bin. Add a slice of lemon for additional flavor, if desired.

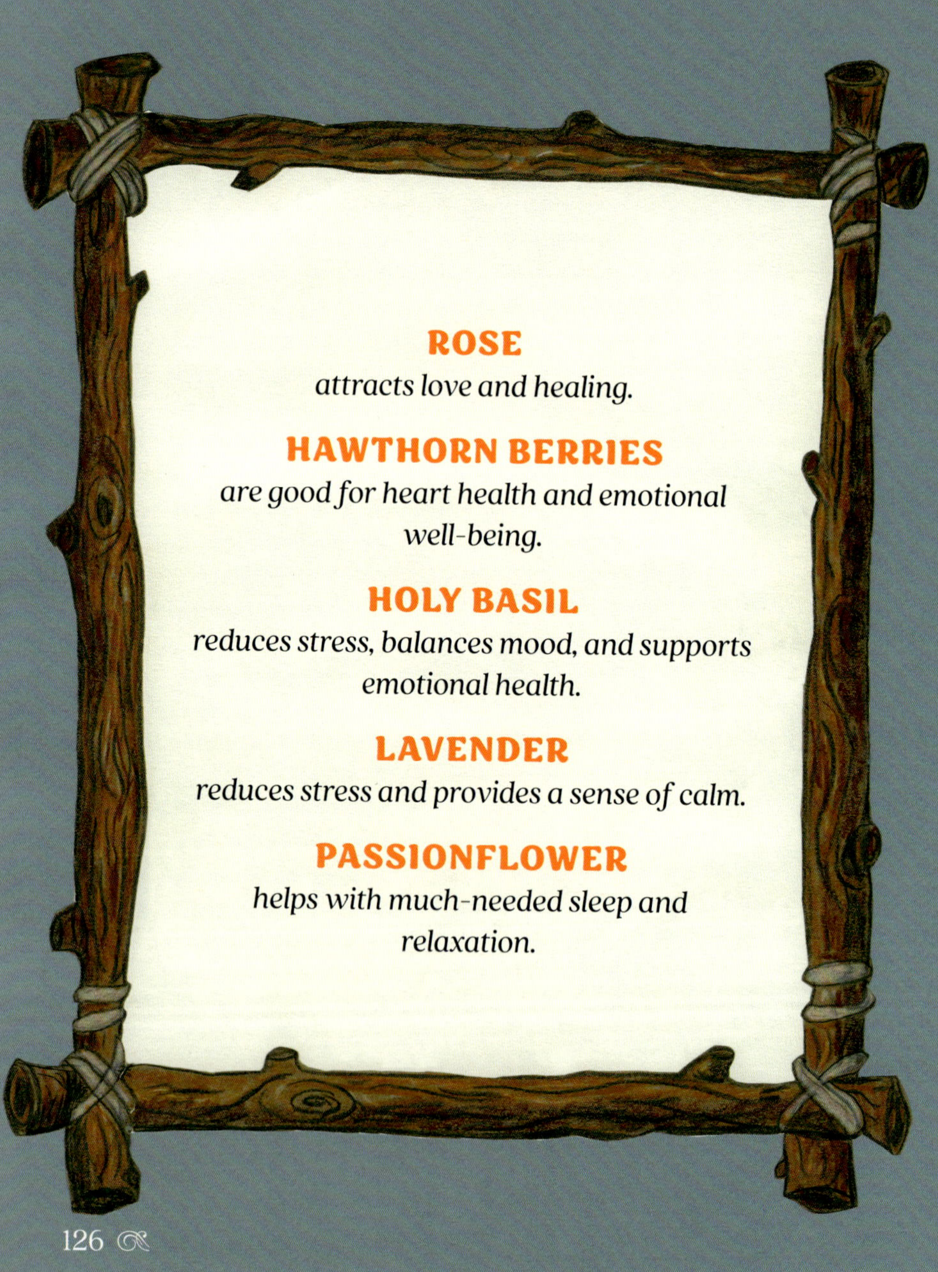

ROSE
attracts love and healing.

HAWTHORN BERRIES
are good for heart health and emotional well-being.

HOLY BASIL
reduces stress, balances mood, and supports emotional health.

LAVENDER
reduces stress and provides a sense of calm.

PASSIONFLOWER
helps with much-needed sleep and relaxation.

Did You Know?

In Greek mythology, one of the most famous tales of heartbreak is the tragic love story of Orpheus and the lovely nymph Eurydice. Their happiness was shattered when Eurydice died from the bite of a venomous snake. The broken-hearted Orpheus journeyed to the underworld and used his music to soften the cold heart of Hades, the god of the dead. Hades agreed to allow Eurydice to return with Orpheus to the living world with one condition: that Orpheus not look back at her until they reached the surface. But just as they were about to step into the light, Orpheus was overcome by both doubt and longing. He glanced back and tragically caused Eurydice to vanish forever.

Tristan and Isolde's Love Potion Tea

(Serves 2)

This wonderful tea invokes the deep, romantic connection
of Tristan and Isolde. Share it with someone dear to you to fully
embrace its heart-opening effects.

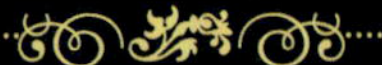

2 teaspoons dried jasmine flowers
1 teaspoon dried rose petals
1 teaspoon dried hibiscus flowers
1 teaspoon dried damiana leaves
1 teaspoon dried lavender buds
1 cinnamon stick
2 cups water

Combine the jasmine flowers, rose petals, hibiscus flowers, damiana leaves, and lavender buds in a bowl.

Bring water to a boil in a pot. Once the water is bubbling, lower the heat to a gentle simmer. Add the herbal mixture and the cinnamon stick to the water to simmer for 10 to 15 minutes. As the petals and leaves dance in the water, close your eyes and breathe deeply.

Strain the tea into your cups. Discard the spent herbs and cinnamon stick into the compost bin. Grasp your warm cup with your hands and imagine it glowing with a soft, warm light, as if you were holding a little sun.

Sip slowly, savoring each drop of this cup of comfort, meant just for you.

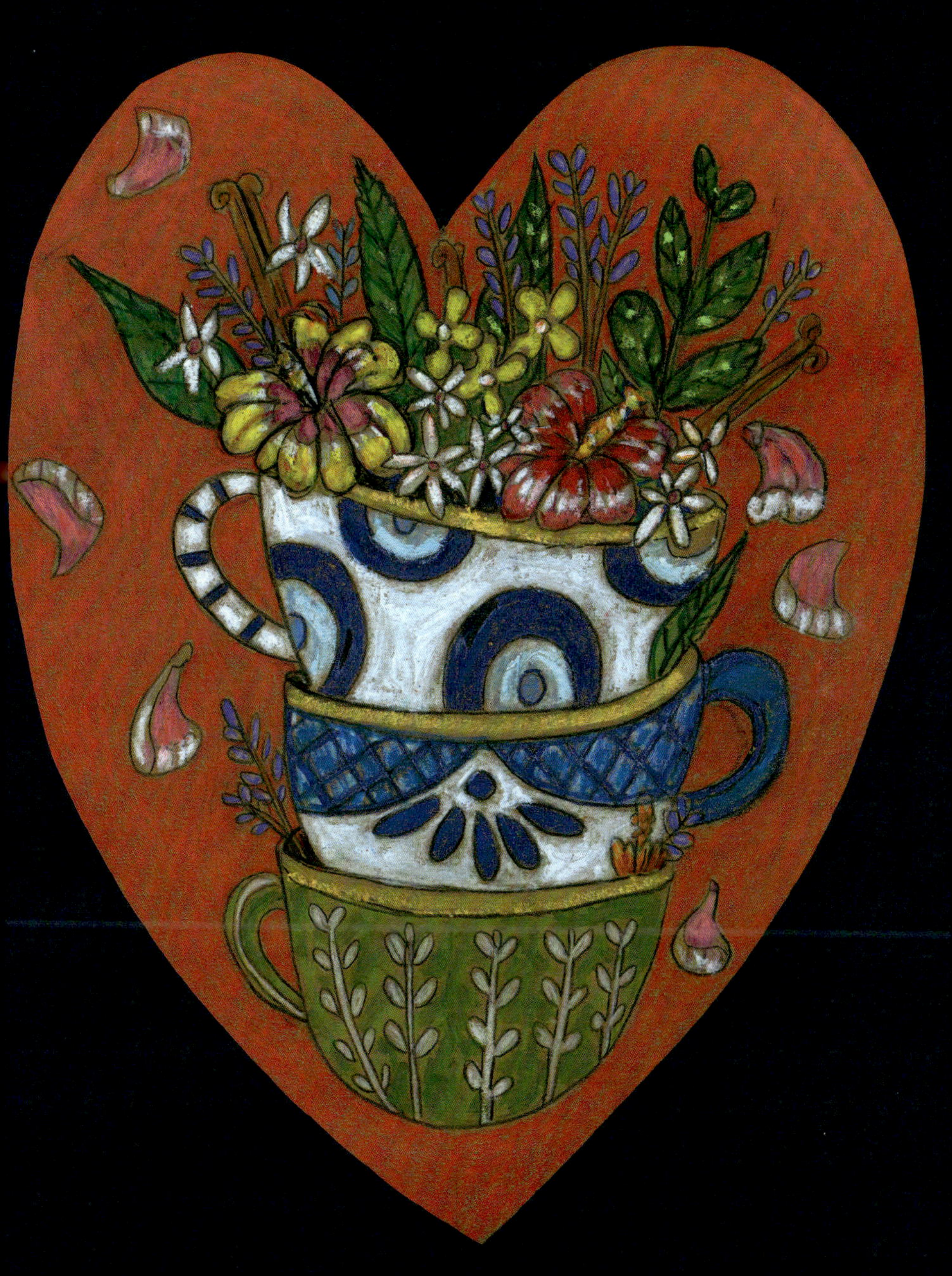

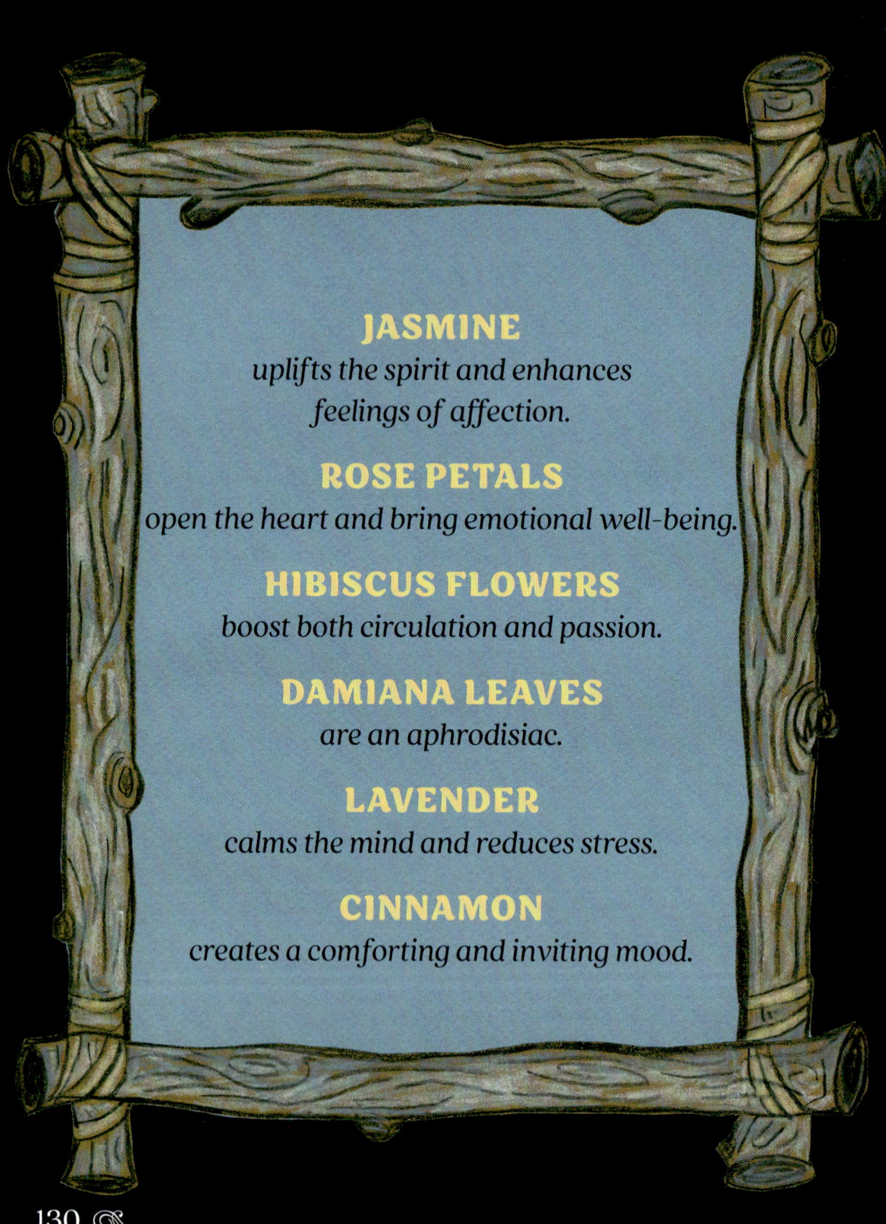

JASMINE
uplifts the spirit and enhances
feelings of affection.

ROSE PETALS
open the heart and bring emotional well-being.

HIBISCUS FLOWERS
boost both circulation and passion.

DAMIANA LEAVES
are an aphrodisiac.

LAVENDER
calms the mind and reduces stress.

CINNAMON
creates a comforting and inviting mood.

Did You Know?

In Arthurian legend, Tristan, a Knight of the Round Table, and Isolde, an Irish princess, accidentally consumed a love potion intended for Isolde and her future husband. This bound them together for eternity, and despite many obstacles, Tristan and Isolde's unwavering love remains one of the most enduring romances in folklore.

Cleopatra's Seducing Body Oil

(Makes ½ cup, enough for one 4-ounce glass bottle)

This is a luxurious oil, crafted to awaken sensuality, nurture self-love, and invite romance.

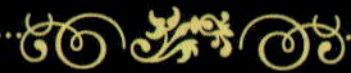

½ cup sweet almond oil (or carrier oil of your choice)
10 drops rose essential oil
5 drops ylang-ylang essential oil
5 drops jasmine essential oil
5 drops myrrh essential oil
1 tablespoon dried rose petals
1 tablespoon dried cinnamon chips

Pour the sweet almond oil into a clean, dry glass bottle or jar. Feel free to use a recycled container.

Carefully add the rose, ylang-ylang, jasmine, and myrrh essential oils to the bottle. Add the dried rose petals and cinnamon chips. Gently swirl the bottle to mix the ingredients.

Hold the bottle in your hands and set your intention for love. Visualize the oil radiating powerful love energy.

Store the bottle in a cool, dark place for at least 1 week, allowing the ingredients to fully infuse the oil with their healing properties.

To use, apply a small amount of the oil to your pulse points. You can even use it as a massage oil. Focus on your intention to attract love as you use it.

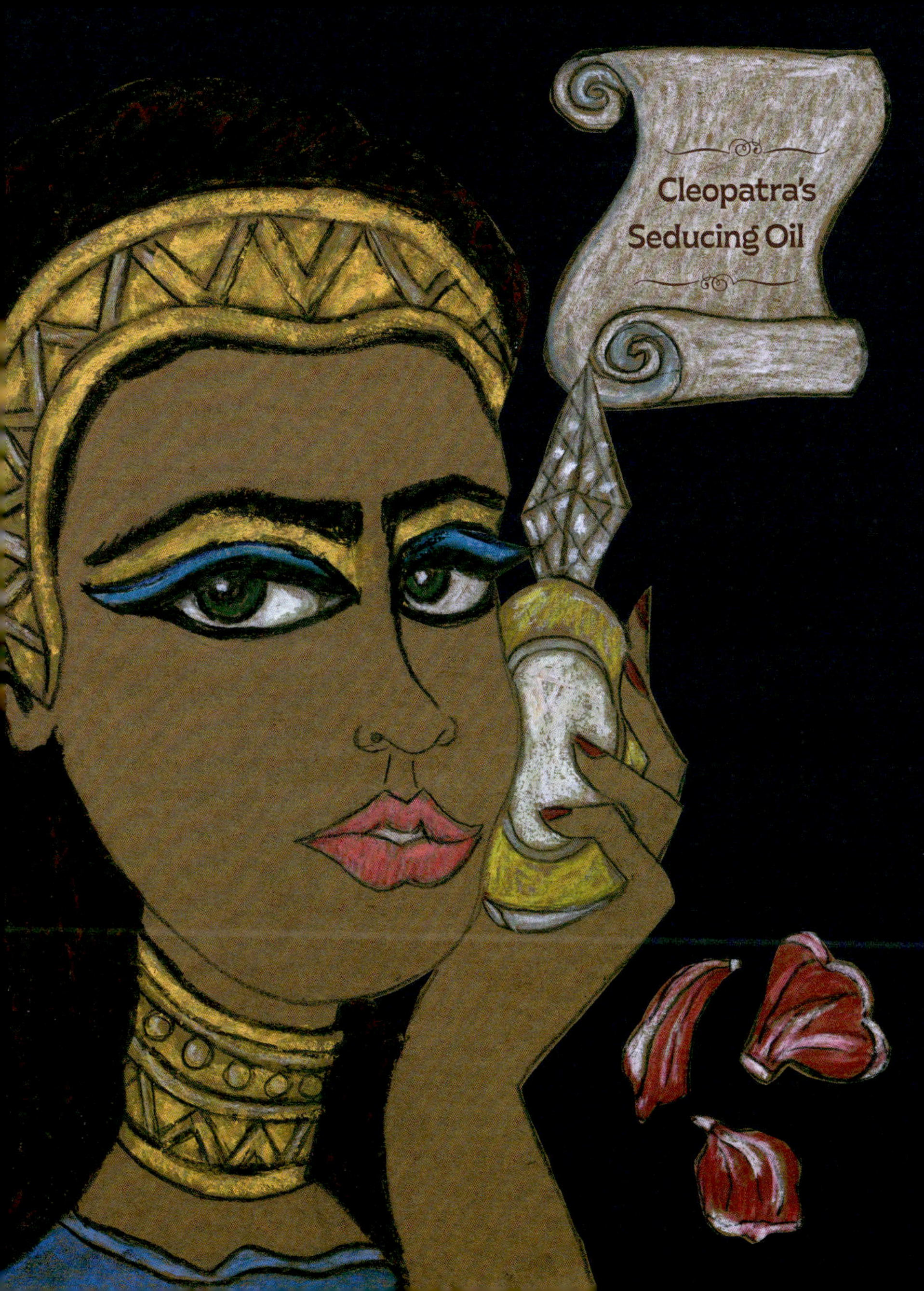

Cleopatra's
Seducing Oil

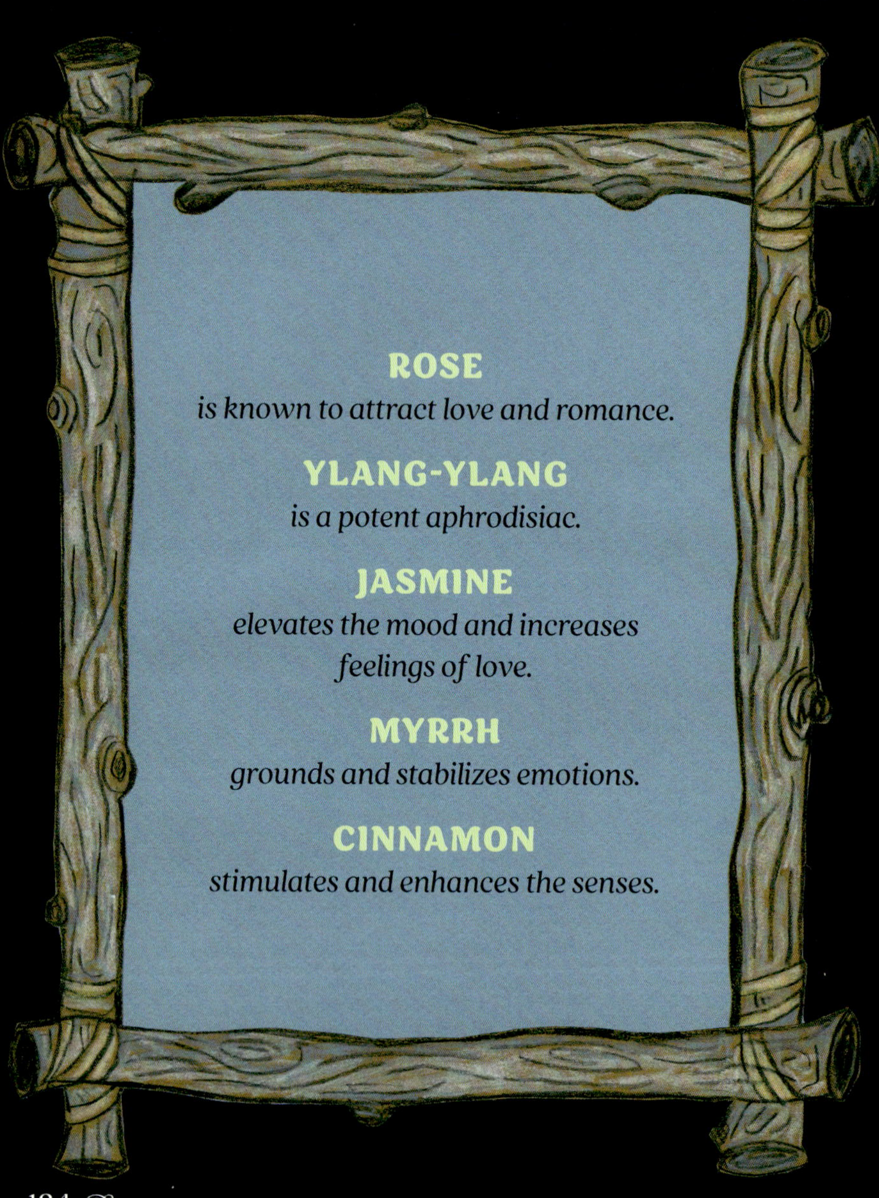

ROSE
is known to attract love and romance.

YLANG-YLANG
is a potent aphrodisiac.

JASMINE
elevates the mood and increases
feelings of love.

MYRRH
grounds and stabilizes emotions.

CINNAMON
stimulates and enhances the senses.

Did You Know?

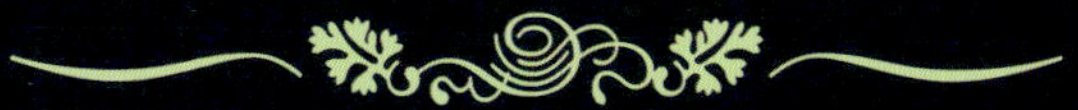

In ancient Egypt, Cleopatra, known for her beauty and charm, crafted perfumed oils such as this one to attract lovers. She famously applied this oil to her skin when meeting Julius Caesar and, later, Mark Antony. The scent of the oil and, of course, her own beauty, seduced these powerful men, leading to legendary romances.

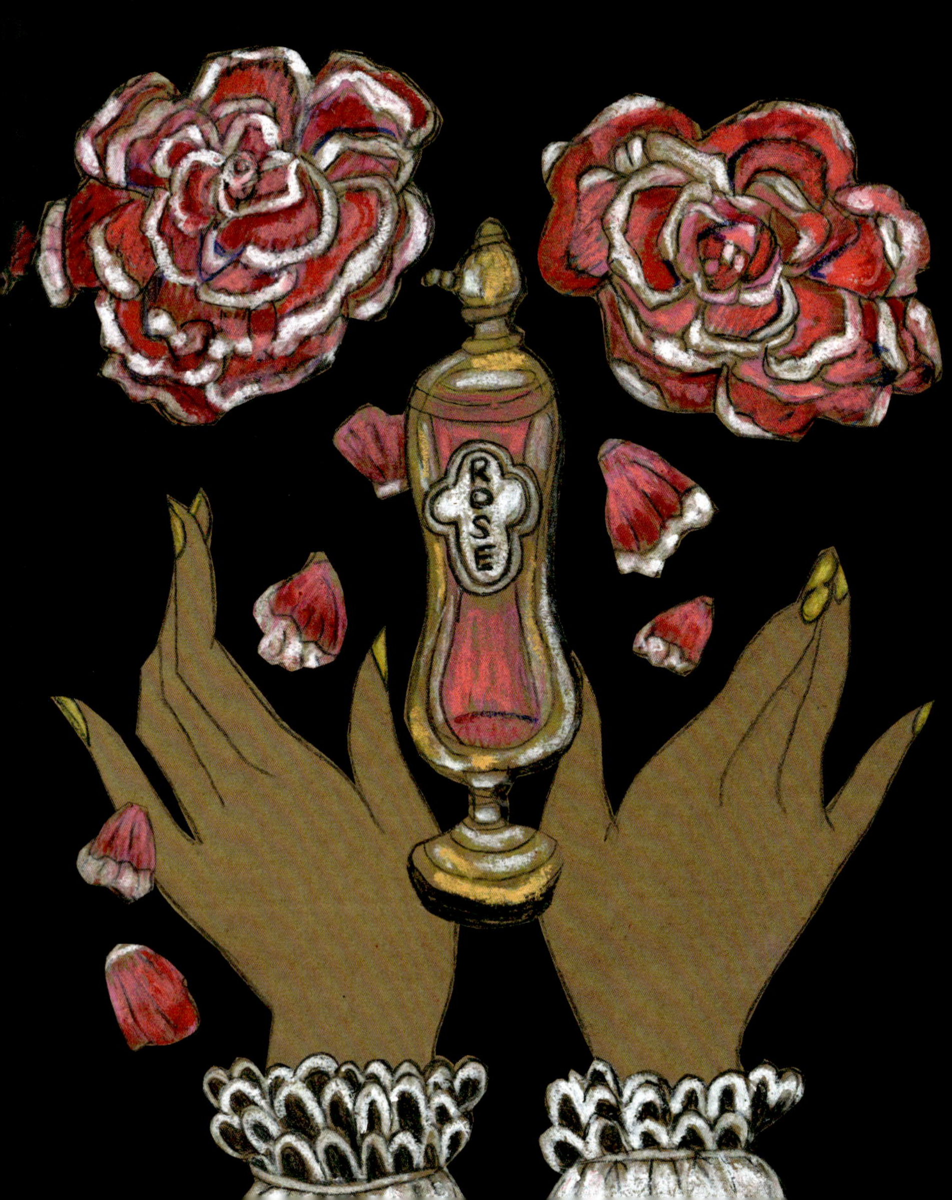

ROSE

Aphrodite's Rose Face Mist

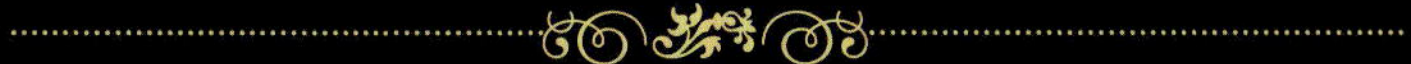

(Makes enough for one 14-ounce spray bottle)

Facial mists are a refreshing way to tone and moisturize your skin. Rose water has anti-inflammatory properties and can help get rid of acne and skin irritations.

Petals from 3 organic roses
1½ cups distilled water
7 drops rose essential oil, or more if desired
Glass spray bottle

Carefully rinse the rose petals in a colander. As you rinse, take a slow breath and imagine any stress washing away with the water.

Place distilled water and rinsed petals into a small saucepan and simmer on low for 10 minutes.

Notice the gentle steam rising. Let it remind you to relax into the moment.

Remove the pot from the heat, stir in the rose essential oil, and let the mixture cool completely.

Strain the liquid through a fine mesh sieve into the spray bottle. Discard the rose petals into the compost bin.

Store in the refrigerator for up to 1 month.

Use your rose water as a facial toner or mild astringent to soothe razor burn after shaving. You can also use it as a face mist whenever you need a refreshing spritz of hydration.

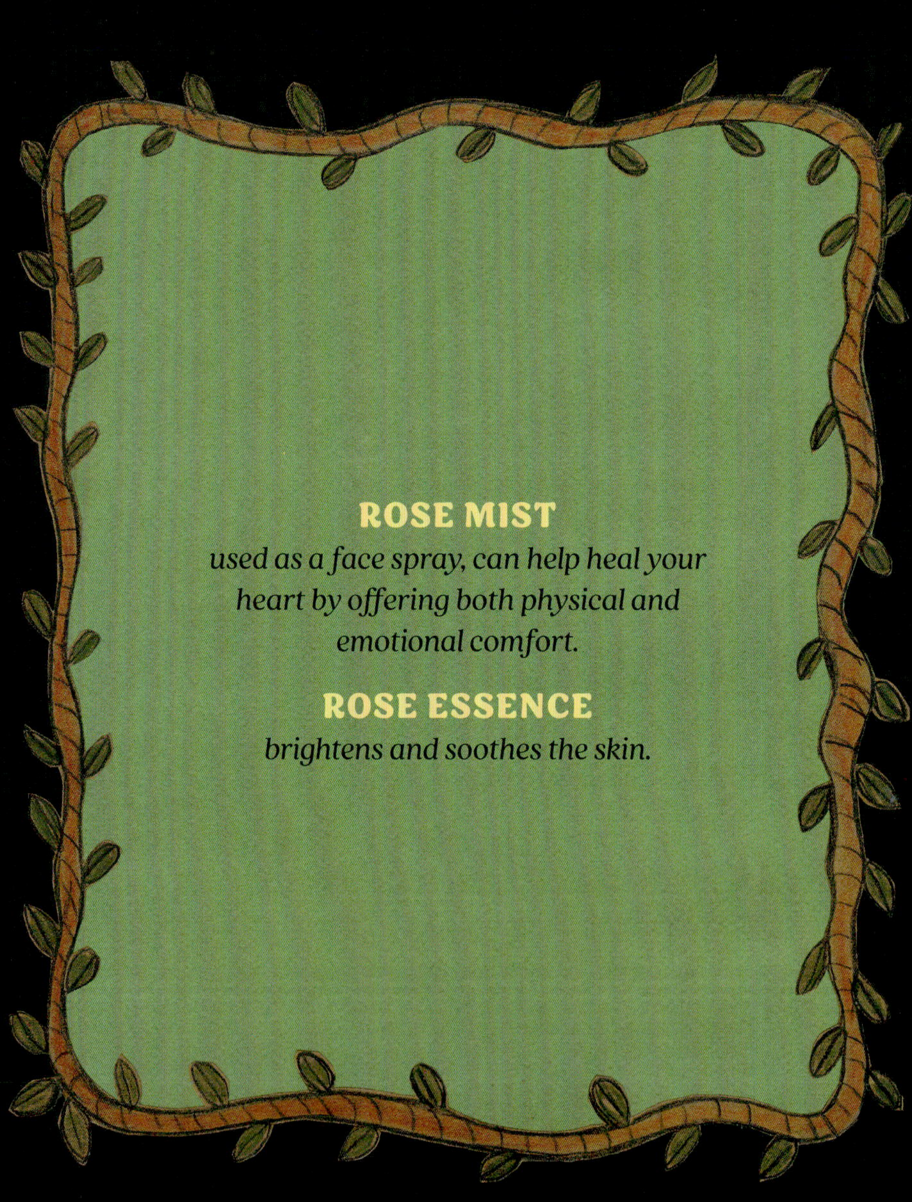

ROSE MIST
used as a face spray, can help heal your
heart by offering both physical and
emotional comfort.

ROSE ESSENCE
brightens and soothes the skin.

Did You Know?

Roses are symbolic of Aphrodite, the ancient Greek goddess of love. When her lover Adonis was mortally wounded, Aphrodite's tears dripped to the ground, and where they landed, roses grew and bloomed.

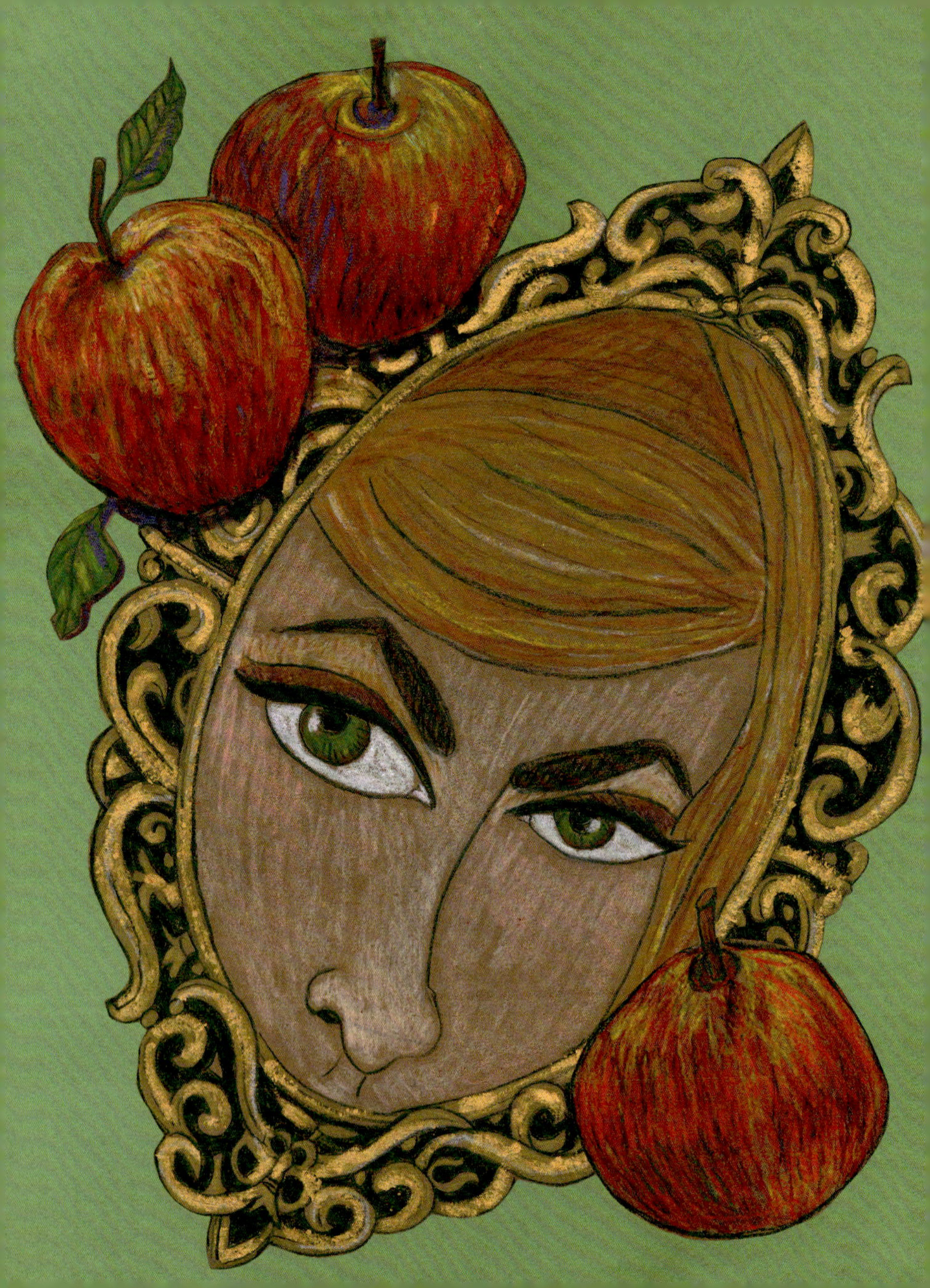

I Am Beautiful Apple Ritual

(Serves 1)

A simple personal ritual inspired by the heart-healing energy of apples.

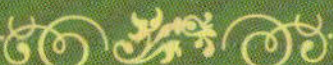

1 fresh apple, any variety, sliced
1 tablespoon maple syrup
Sprinkle of cinnamon
1 cup Tristan and Isolde's Love Potion Tea (page 128)

Place the apple slices neatly on a small plate. Dribble on maple syrup and sprinkle with cinnamon. As you prepare your apple slices, breathe slowly and deeply, reminding yourself that caring for your body is a rewarding and essential act of self-love.

Pour yourself a cup of Tristan and Isolde's Lover's Tea. Sit somewhere quiet and take a moment to appreciate the colors, aromas, and textures of the apple before you begin. As you sip your tea and chew your apple treat, repeat silently or aloud, "I am beautiful inside and out, and I am deserving of love."

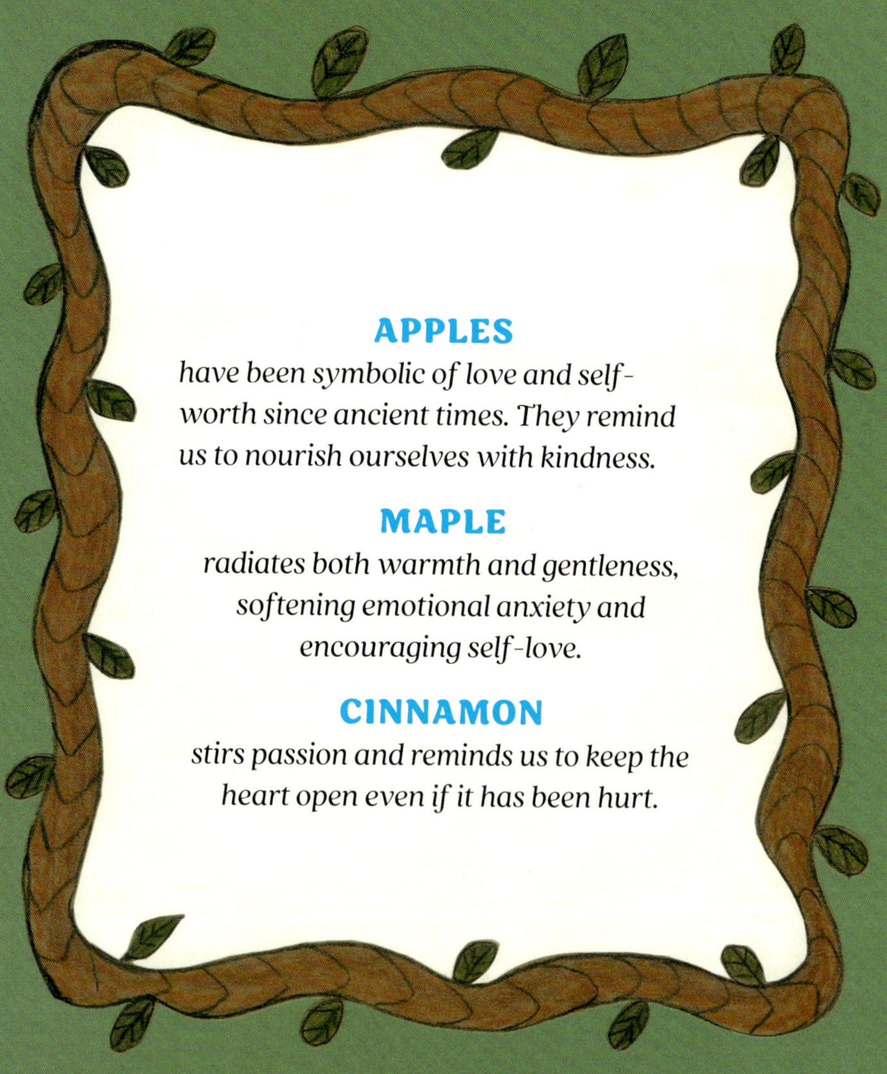

APPLES

have been symbolic of love and self-worth since ancient times. They remind us to nourish ourselves with kindness.

MAPLE

radiates both warmth and gentleness, softening emotional anxiety and encouraging self-love.

CINNAMON

stirs passion and reminds us to keep the heart open even if it has been hurt.

Did You Know?

In Greek mythology, apples were sacred to Aphrodite, the goddess of love. The golden apple that was inscribed "to the fairest" sparked the Trojan War and ultimately made the apple a symbol of the human desire for self-worth. The story reminds us that true beauty is not found in external validation, but in the love and acceptance we must cultivate within, for ourselves.

Rose Heart Soothing Bath Tea

(Makes enough for 1 bath)

A gentle treat for the bath water, to calm the body and open the heart.

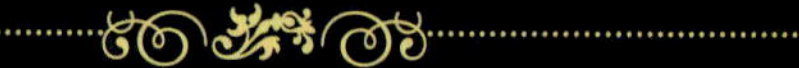

½ cup dried rose petals
½ cup rolled oats
¼ cup Epsom salt or pink Himalayan salt
1 teaspoon almond oil
A few drops rose essential oil
Small muslin or cotton bag with a drawstring

In a small bowl, combine the dried rose petals, oats, and salt. Add almond oil and rose essential oil, stirring gently to blend. Scoop the mixture into the muslin bag and tie it securely.

Hang the bag under the warm running water as you fill your bath, letting the essence of rose and oats swirl through the water.

Before stepping in, take a slow, mindful breath and set an intention for release— imagine the bathwater rinsing away your emotional tension and softening your heart.

As you soak, place a hand over your chest and notice your breath. With each inhale, invite in compassion; with each exhale, let go of heaviness.

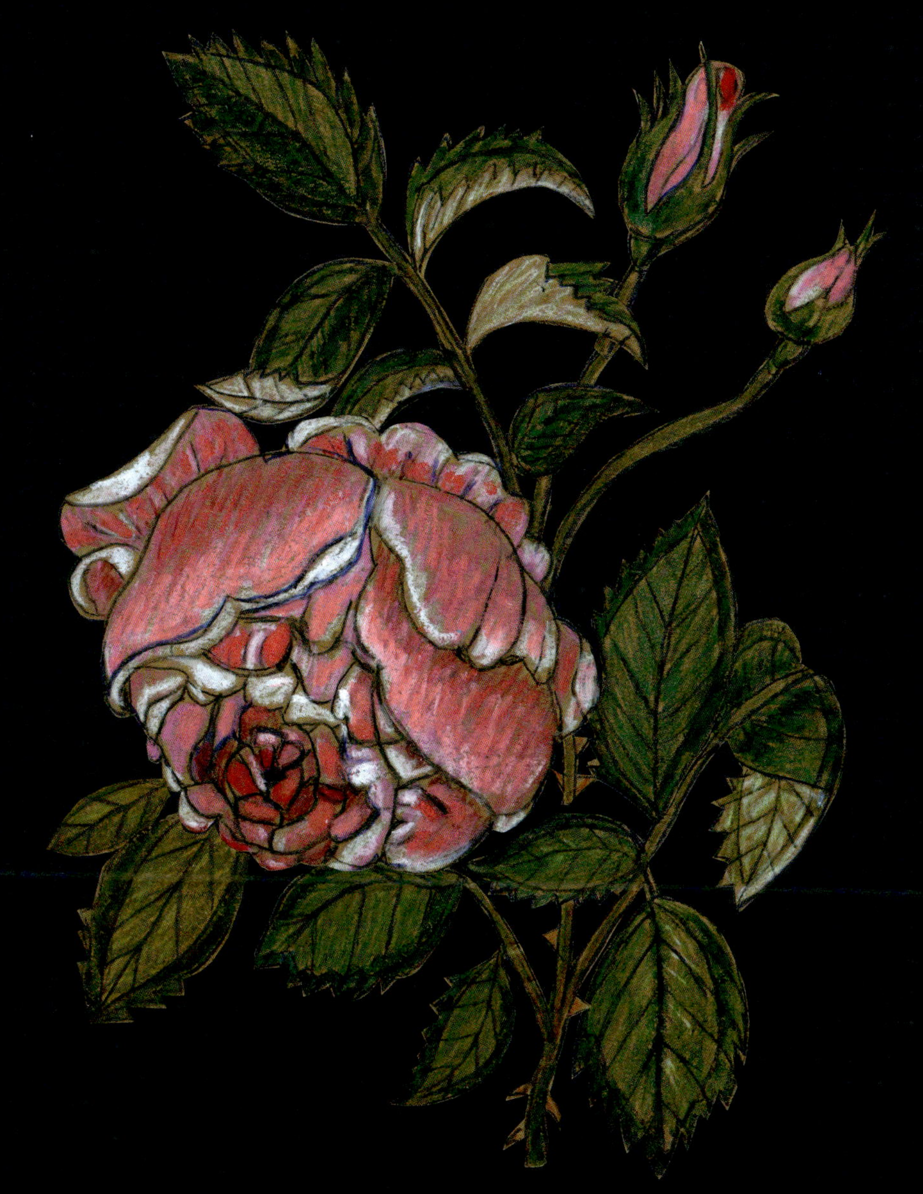

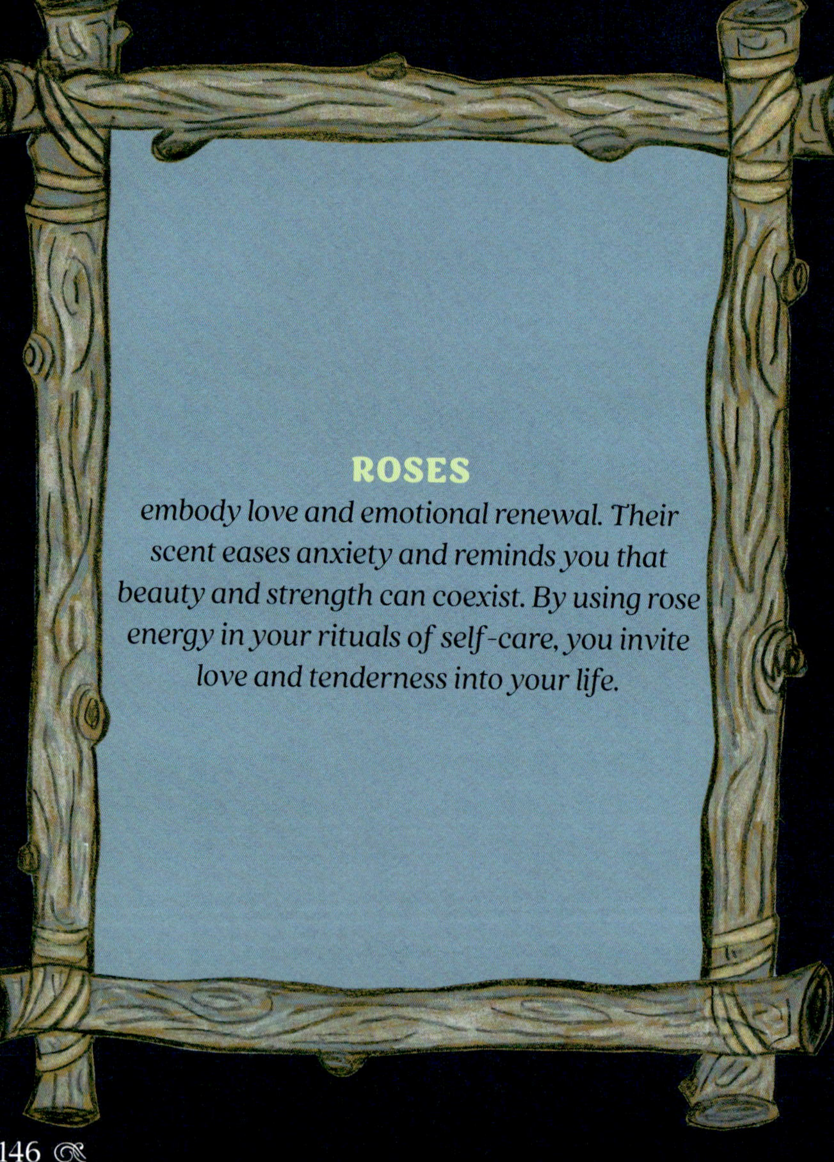

ROSES

embody love and emotional renewal. Their
scent eases anxiety and reminds you that
beauty and strength can coexist. By using rose
energy in your rituals of self-care, you invite
love and tenderness into your life.

Did You Know?

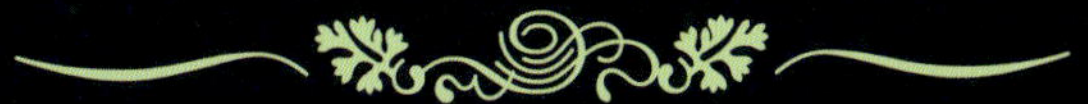

In Victorian times, rose tea was used as a comfort for those mourning the loss of a love, or simply longing for love. The tea's aroma was a reminder that even in heartache, tenderness can persist.

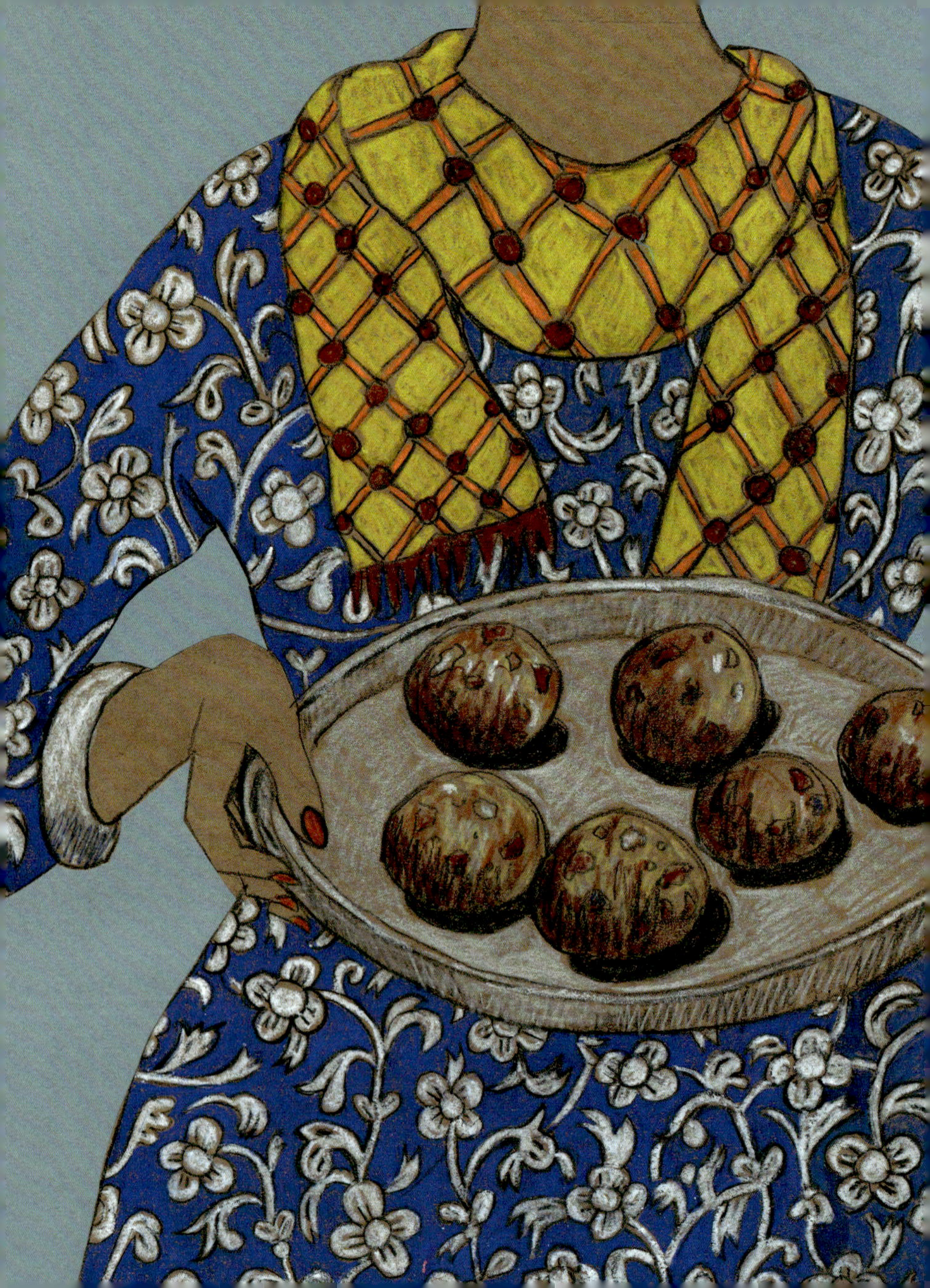

Cherry and Oatmeal Energy Balls

(Makes 8–10 balls)

Enjoy your nutritious energy balls as a quick snack or pre-workout boost!

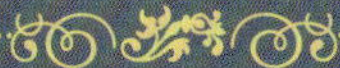

1 cup rolled oats
½ cup chopped dried cherries
¼ cup chia seeds
¼ cup flaxseeds, ground with a mortar and pestle
½ cup nut butter (such as almond or peanut butter)
⅓ cup maple syrup
Pinch of salt

In a large bowl, combine the rolled oats, chopped dried cherries, chia seeds, and ground flaxseeds. In a separate bowl, stir together the nut butter, maple syrup, and salt until smooth. Take a deep breath here, noticing the sweet, nutty aroma and allowing yourself to feel grounded and present in the moment.

Pour the maple mixture into the oat mixture and stir until well combined. Use clean hands to form the mixture into small balls, about 1 inch in diameter. Place the energy balls on a baking sheet lined with parchment paper. As you roll each ball, think of it as a small act of care.

Refrigerate for at least 30 minutes to allow them to firm up. Once set, transfer the energy balls to an airtight container and store in the refrigerator for up to 1 week. You can also freeze them for up to 1 month.

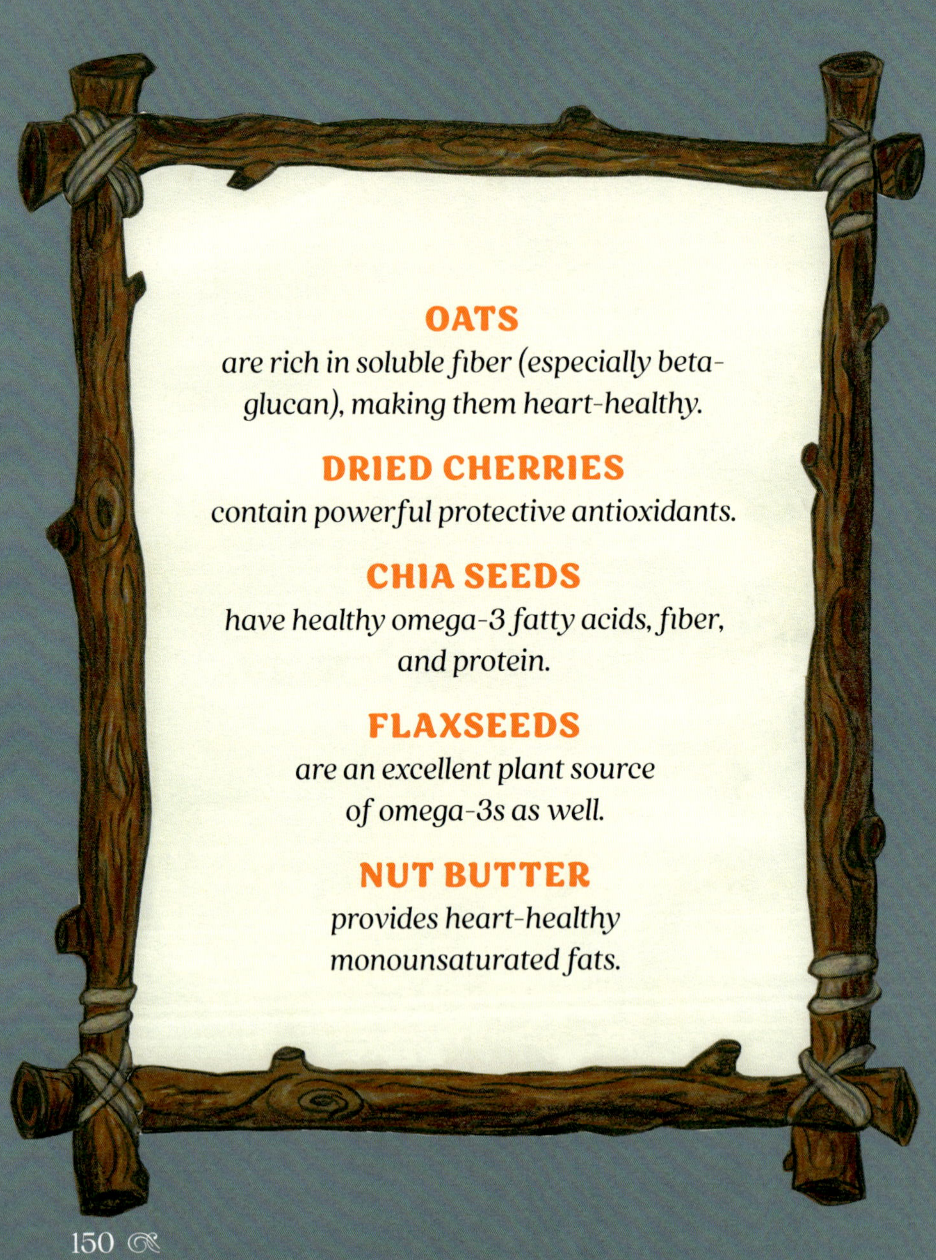

OATS

are rich in soluble fiber (especially beta-glucan), making them heart-healthy.

DRIED CHERRIES

contain powerful protective antioxidants.

CHIA SEEDS

have healthy omega-3 fatty acids, fiber, and protein.

FLAXSEEDS

are an excellent plant source of omega-3s as well.

NUT BUTTER

provides heart-healthy monounsaturated fats.

Did You Know?

In ancient Greece, cherries were used by the soldiers of Lucullus, a Roman general who brought the fruit back from Asia. The soldiers believed the fruit carried the strength of Mars, the god of vitality. Oats were a staple of Celtic warriors and Scottish highlanders, who were fed oat porridge for strength and courage before heading into battle.

Strawberrycello

(Makes approximately twelve 2-ounce servings)

This is one of our favorites. Strawberrycello is a toast to romance with its ruby glow and warmth. It is best savored with loved ones.

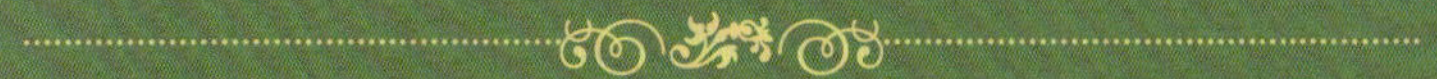

    3 cups vodka
    1 pound fresh strawberries, stems removed,
        trimmed, and sliced
    1 cup sugar
    1 cup water
    1 large glass jar with lid

In a large glass jar with a lid, combine vodka and strawberries. Cover and store in the refrigerator for 2 weeks. Each time you open the fridge, take a moment to gently shake the jar and notice the deepening color.

Strain the vodka mixture through a fine mesh sieve and transfer the liquid to a separate container. Discard the berries into your compost bin.

Combine the sugar and water in a small saucepan. Bring it to a gentle simmer, stirring until the sugar dissolves. As the syrup warms, breathe in the sweet scent rising with the steam, letting it lift your spirits.

Cool the syrup to room temperature, then stir it into the strained vodka mixture. Chill the mixture for several hours before serving.

Enjoy your Strawberrycello in 2-ounce shot glasses.

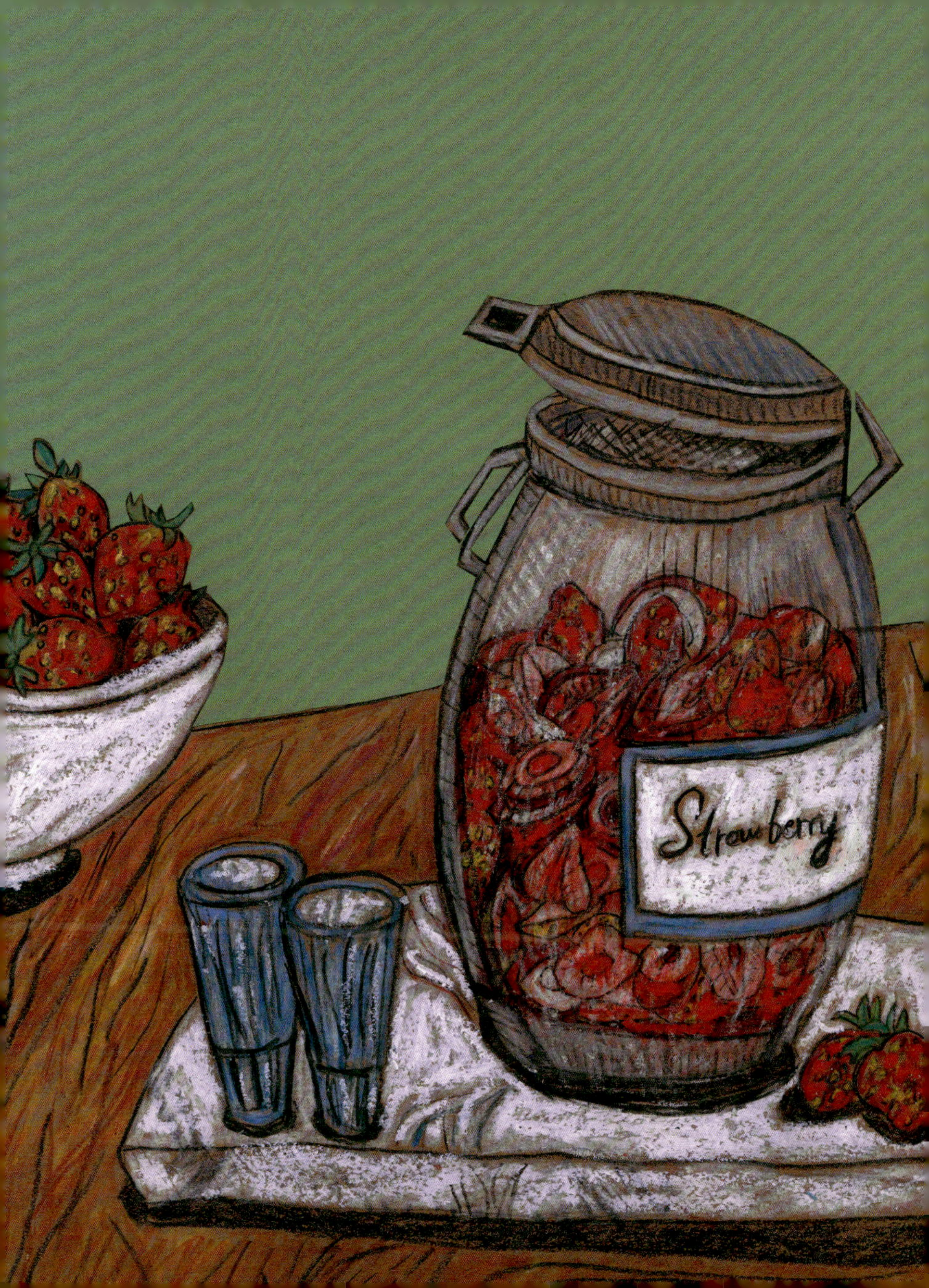
Strawberry

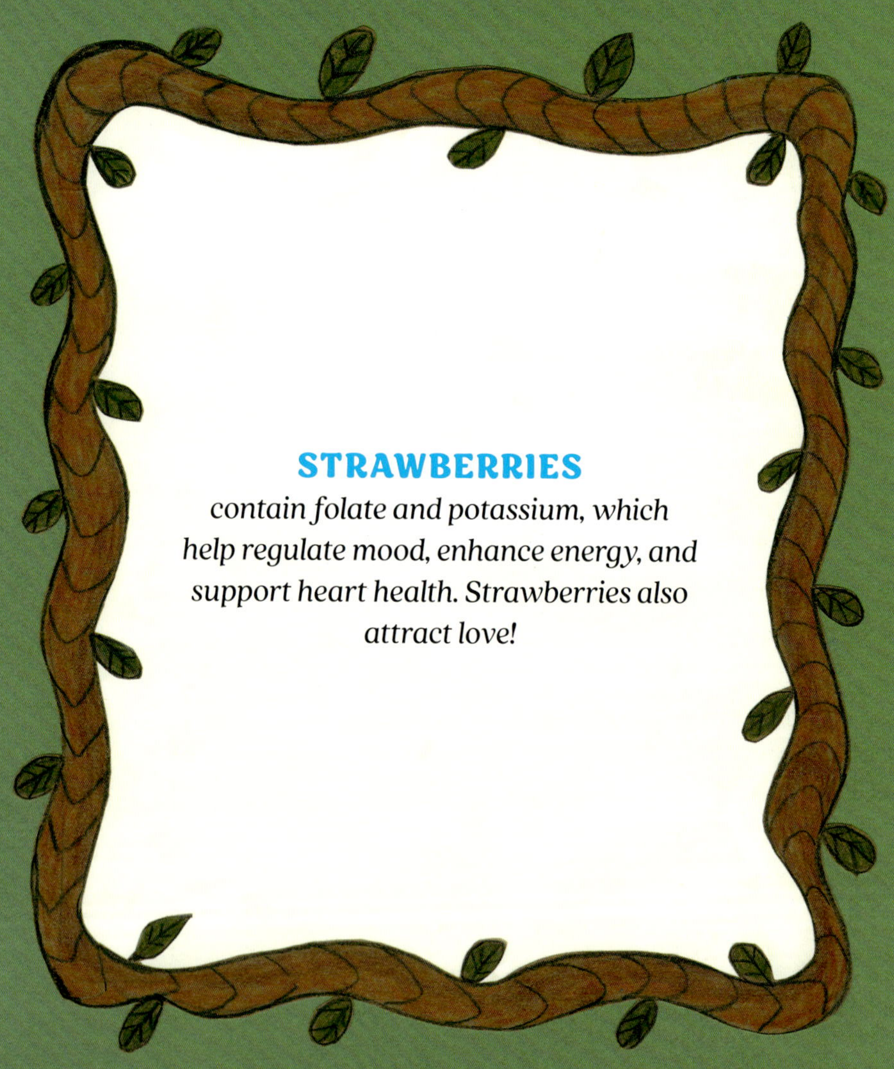

STRAWBERRIES

contain folate and potassium, which help regulate mood, enhance energy, and support heart health. Strawberries also attract love!

Did You Know?

In Roman mythology, strawberries represent Venus, the goddess of love, and thus embody all the qualities of romance.

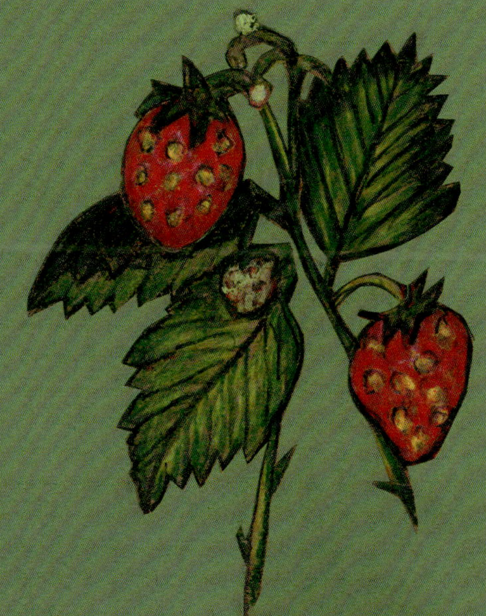

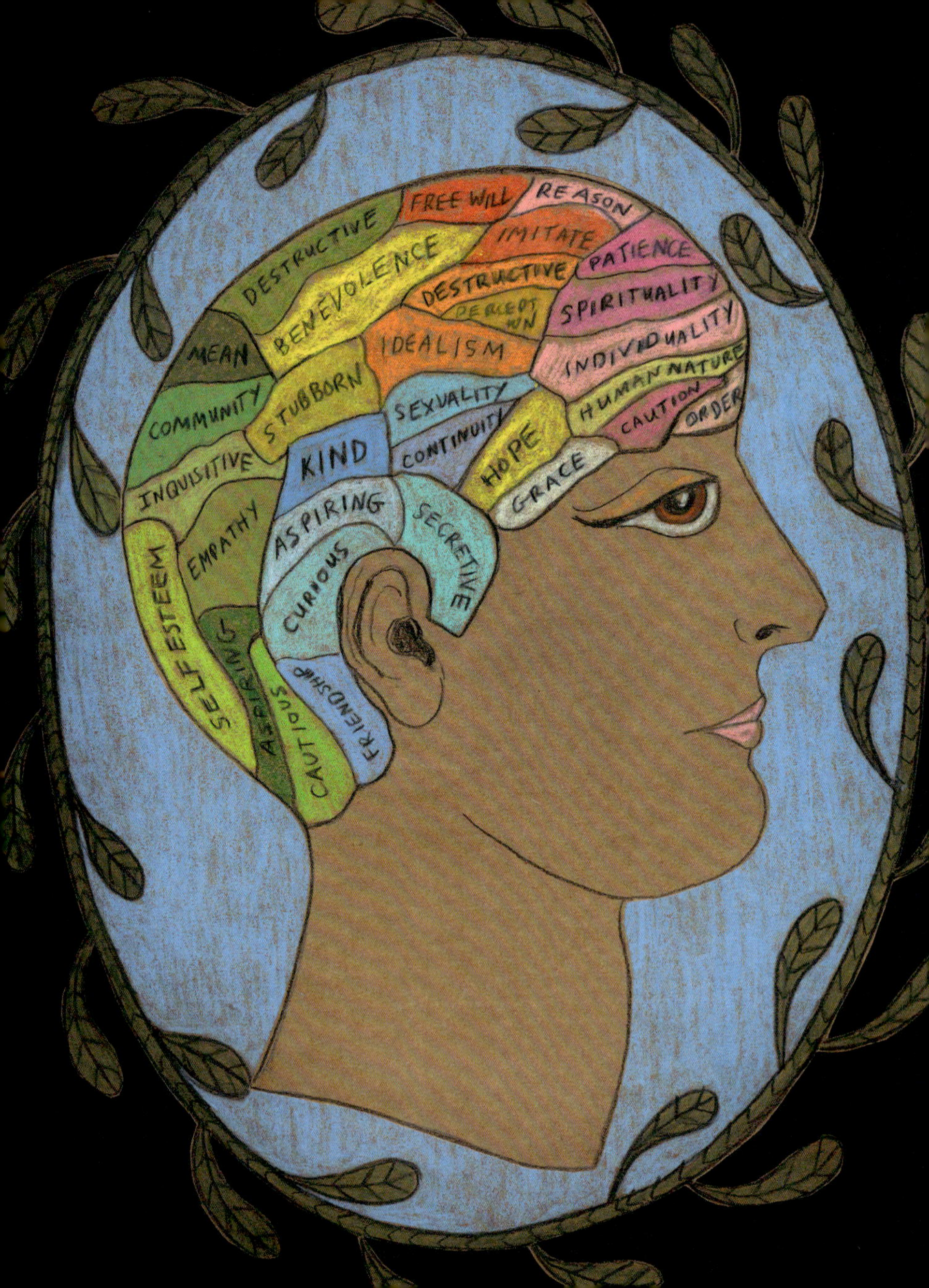

DESTRUCTIVE
FREE WILL
REASON
IMITATE
BENEVOLENCE
PATIENCE
DESTRUCTIVE
PERCEPTION
SPIRITUALITY
MEAN
IDEALISM
INDIVIDUALITY
COMMUNITY
STUBBORN
HUMAN NATURE
SEXUALITY
CAUTION
ORDER
INQUISITIVE
KIND
CONTINUITY
HOPE
GRACE
SELF ESTEEM
EMPATHY
ASPIRING
SECRETIVE
ASPIRING
CURIOUS
CAUTIOUS
FRIENDSHIP

CHAPTER 5

HEAL YOUR MIND

Our minds are like a garden—sometimes blooming with inspiration, other times tangled with anxiety. The key is to gently tend to your inner landscape, clearing the weeds of stress and planting seeds of wellness. In this chapter, we help you create space for peace to take root.

Throughout history, herbs have been trusted allies of the mind. Here you will find teas, baths, oils, and tonics designed to nourish your mind and refresh your spirit by taking moments to pause and ground yourself. We seek stillness amid the noise, to let small rituals become moments of peace in a hectic world.

Our chapter starts with *Pitys's White Pine Longevity Tea*, a brew of resilience from the wisdom of the forest.

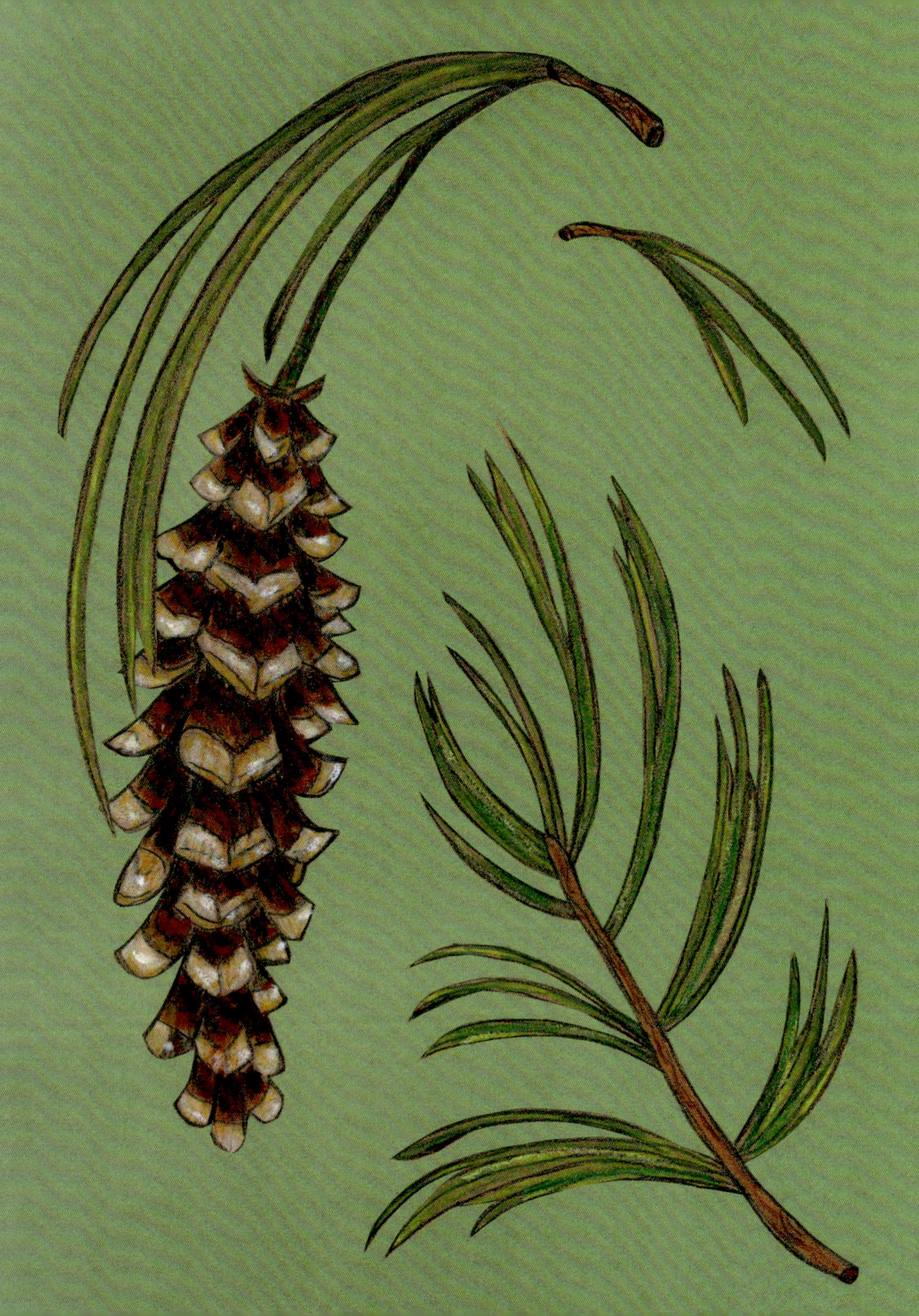

Pitys's White Pine Longevity Tea

(Serves 2)

This tea is a soothing, forest-inspired brew that calms your mind and supports the body's resilience. It protects and renews you with each sip.

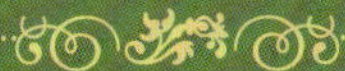

Handful fresh white pine needles,
  or 1-2 tablespoons dried
2 cups water

Be sure to collect fresh white pine needles from a healthy tree. Remember to be mindful of the environment, taking only what you need.

Rinse the pine needles under cool running water to remove any dirt or impurities. As you do this, think to yourself, "These healing needles will cleanse me."

Bring water to a boil in a pot or kettle. Once it bubbles, remove it from the heat.

Add white pine needles to the water. Cover the pot and let the needles steep for 10 to 15 minutes.

Strain the tea into cups with a fine mesh strainer. Remember to add the needles to your compost bin. Stir gently and enjoy this unique tea.

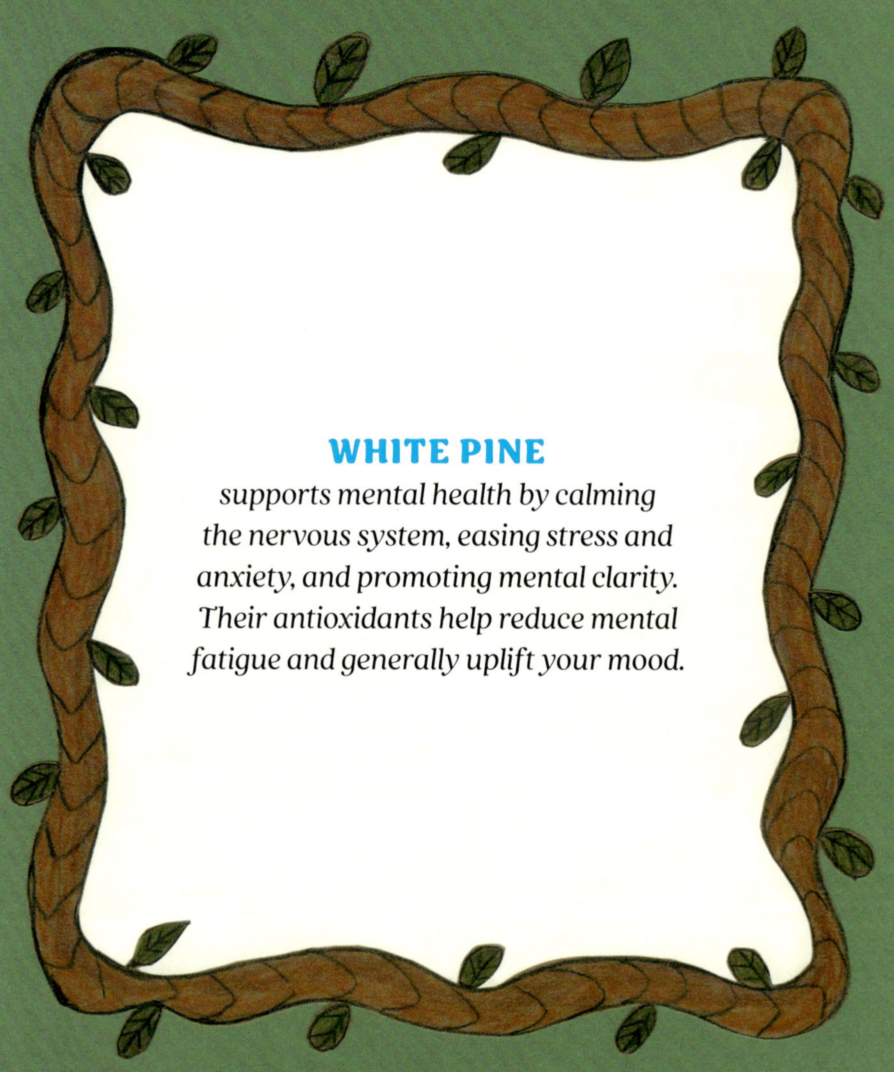

WHITE PINE

supports mental health by calming the nervous system, easing stress and anxiety, and promoting mental clarity. Their antioxidants help reduce mental fatigue and generally uplift your mood.

Did You Know?

White pine (*Pinus strobus*) needles have anti-inflammatory and antiseptic qualities, and they support the upper respiratory system, stomach, liver, and kidneys. In Greek mythology, Pitys is the nymph linked with pine trees. Pursued relentlessly by the god Pan, she prayed for escape, and the gods transformed her into a pine tree to protect her. Can you imagine how incredibly annoying Pan must have been for her to take such drastic measures to avoid him?!

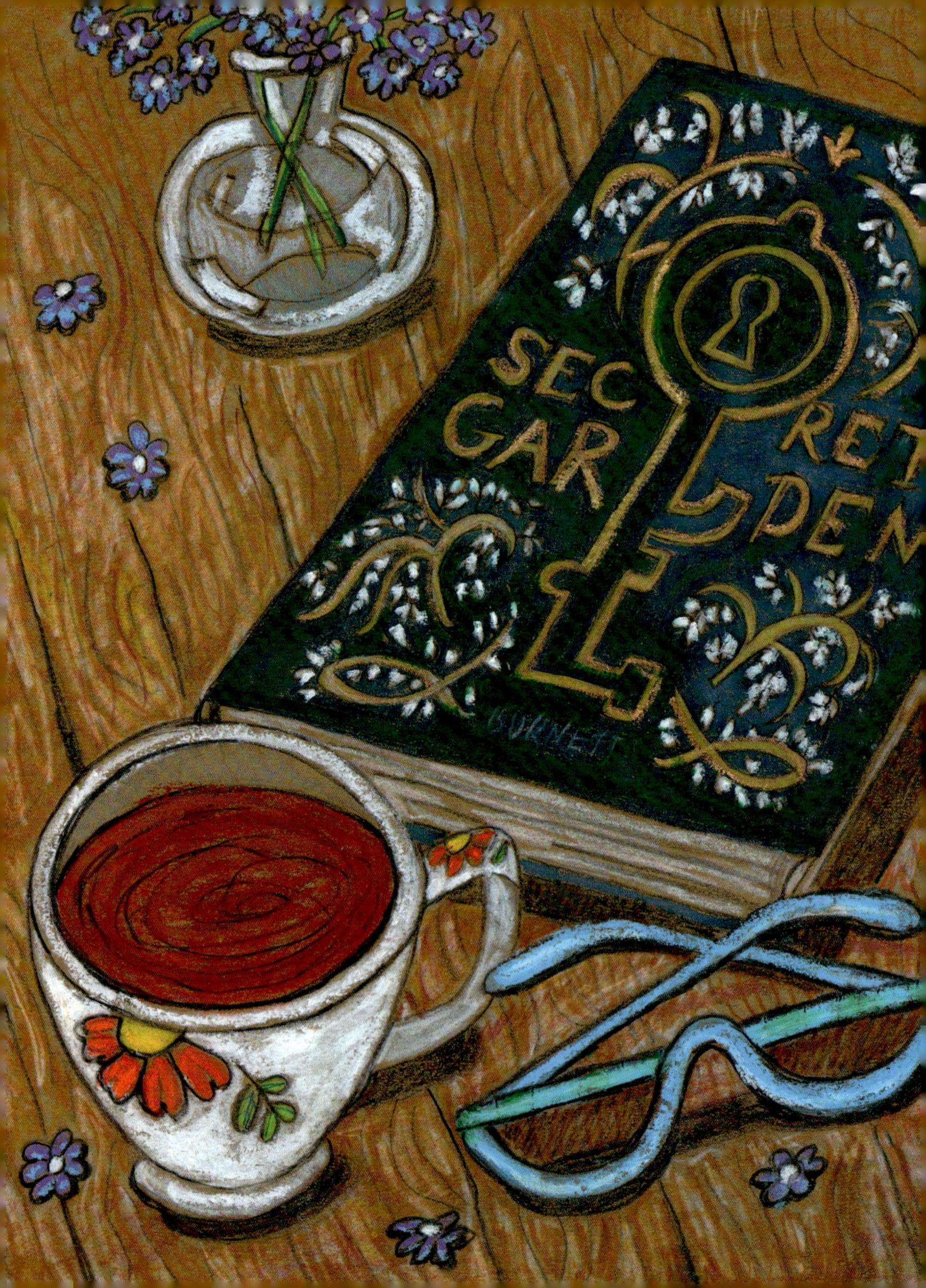

SEC
GAR
RET
DEN
BURNETT

Secret Garden Tea

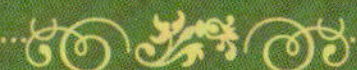

(Makes 2 cups)

This gentle floral blend invites a deep sense of calm and mental clarity.

1 teaspoon dried catmint leaves
1 teaspoon dried chamomile flowers
1 teaspoon dried lavender buds
1 teaspoon dried skullcap leaves
1 teaspoon dried passionflower
2 cups water
Lemon or lime slice (optional)

Combine the catmint leaves, chamomile flowers, lavender buds, skullcap leaves, and passionflower in a bowl.

Bring water to a boil.

Place 1 tablespoon of the herbal mixture into a tea infuser or teapot. Pour the water over the herbs and cover.

Let the tea steep for 7 to 10 minutes. As it steeps, take a deep breath and let the aroma relax you and clear your thoughts.

Strain the tea through a fine mesh sieve and serve. Discard the herbs into your compost bin.

Add a slice of lemon or lime for additional flavor, if you desire.

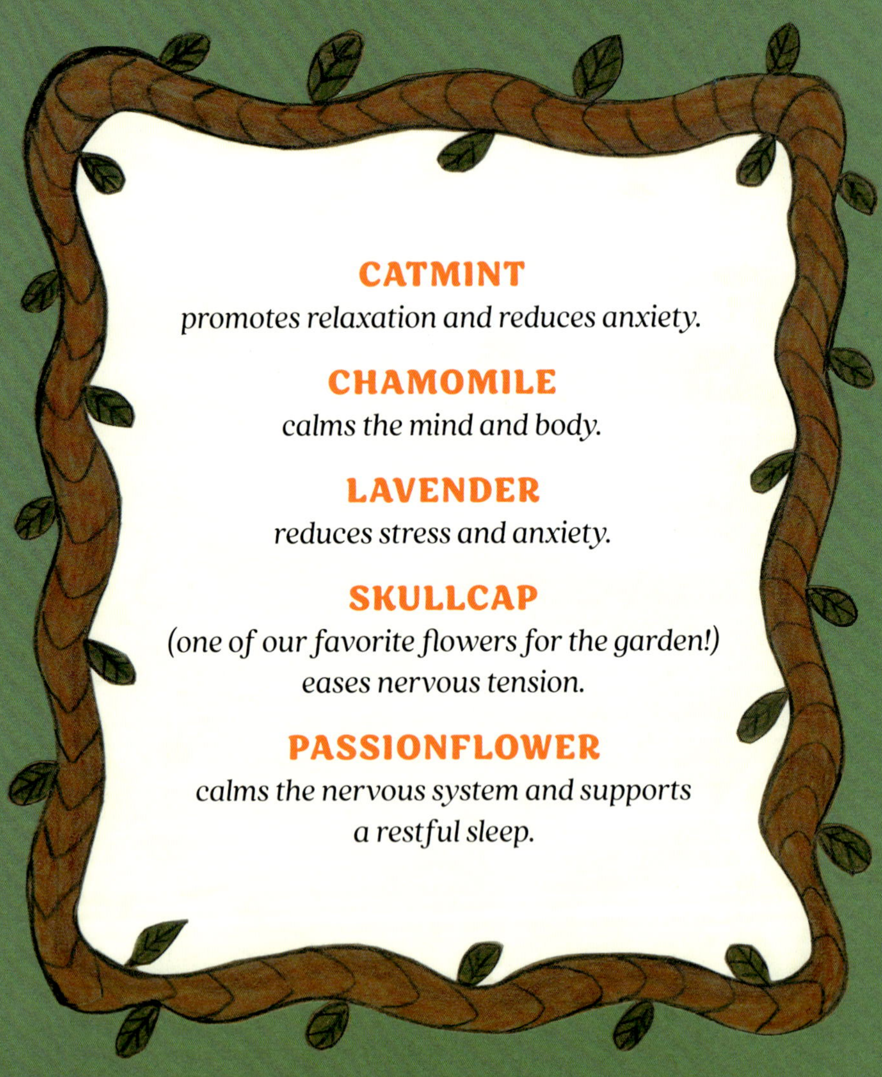

CATMINT

promotes relaxation and reduces anxiety.

CHAMOMILE

calms the mind and body.

LAVENDER

reduces stress and anxiety.

SKULLCAP

*(one of our favorite flowers for the garden!)
eases nervous tension.*

PASSIONFLOWER

*calms the nervous system and supports
a restful sleep.*

Did You Know?

Traditionally, a secret garden offers a private, peaceful refuge from the stresses of daily life. Surrounded by greenery, lovely scents, and the songs of birds who visit it, this retreat invites stillness, reflection, and calm. In this tranquil space, the mind quiets, worries fade, and a feeling of serenity blossoms. Such gardens are inspired by Frances Hodgson Burnett's classic novel *The Secret Garden.*

Joséphine's Violet Serenity Bath Salts

(Makes enough for 3—4 baths)

This blend calms the mind by combining violet's gentle tranquility with lemon balm's uplifting clarity, while the sea salts ease physical tension.

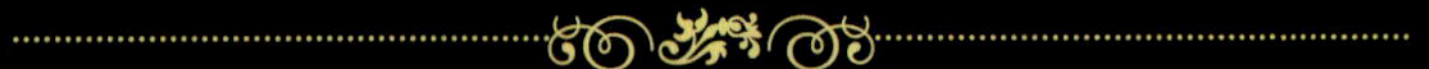

1 cup Epsom salt
1 cup Himalayan pink salt
½ cup baking soda
10-15 drops violet essential oil
10-15 drops lemon balm essential oil

In a large bowl, combine the Epsom salt, pink salt, and baking soda. Stir well to combine. Add the violet essential oil and lemon balm essential oil to the salt mixture. Mix thoroughly to ensure the oils are evenly distributed.

As you stir, take a few slow breaths and set an intention for a relaxing and restorative bath. Transfer the bath salts into a clean, airtight jar or container.

Add ½ to 1 cup of bath salts to the warm water in your tub. As you soak, allow your body to release tension, as if the water is washing away all your stress.

For optimal serenity, soak for at least 15 to 20 minutes.

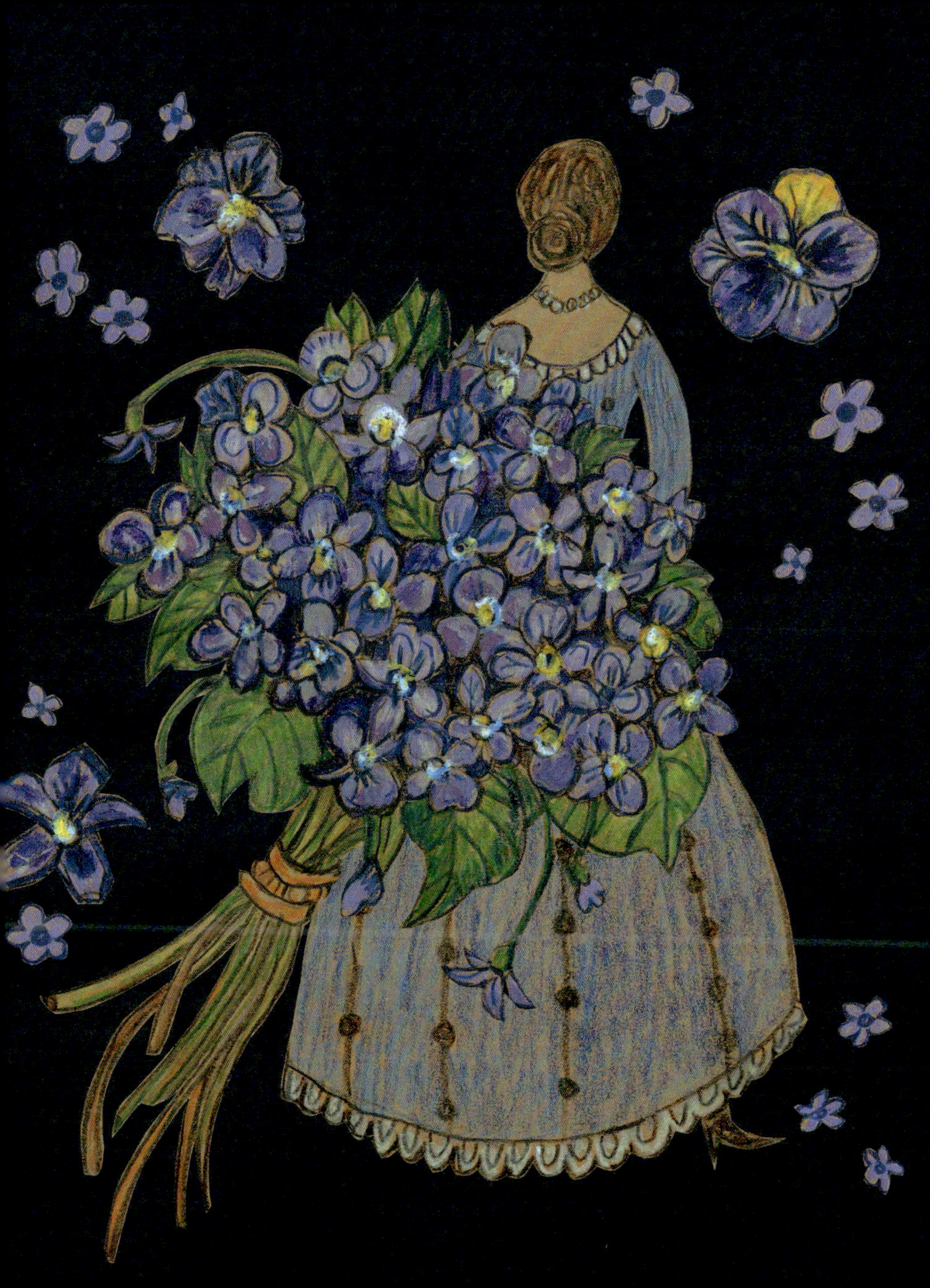

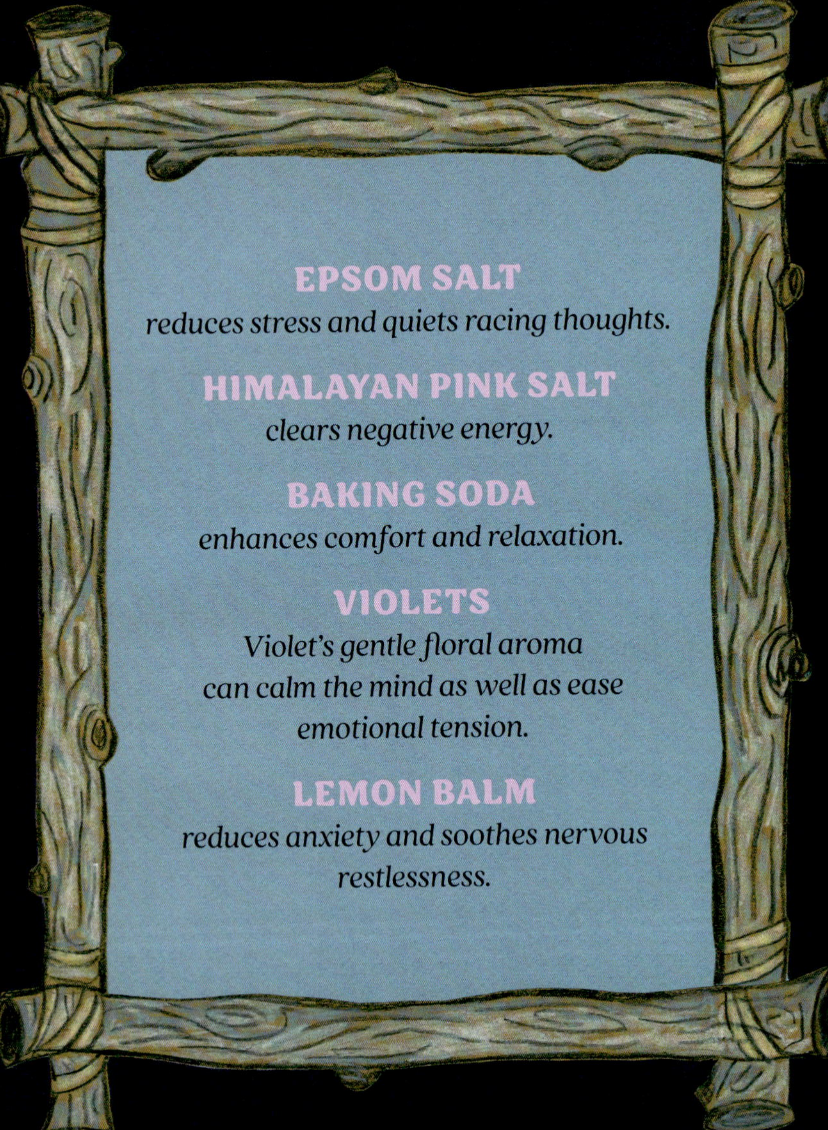
EPSOM SALT
reduces stress and quiets racing thoughts.

HIMALAYAN PINK SALT
clears negative energy.

BAKING SODA
enhances comfort and relaxation.

VIOLETS
Violet's gentle floral aroma
can calm the mind as well as ease
emotional tension.

LEMON BALM
reduces anxiety and soothes nervous
restlessness.

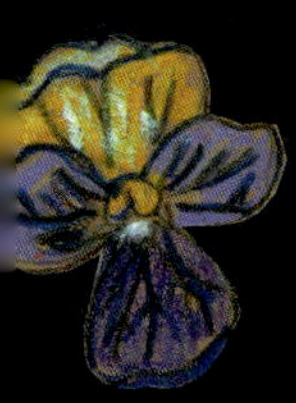
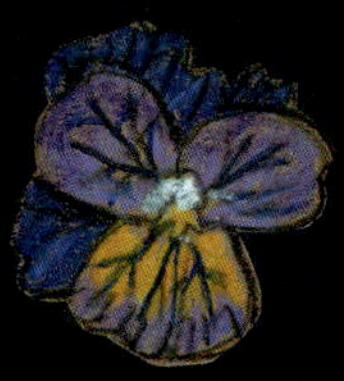

Did You Know?

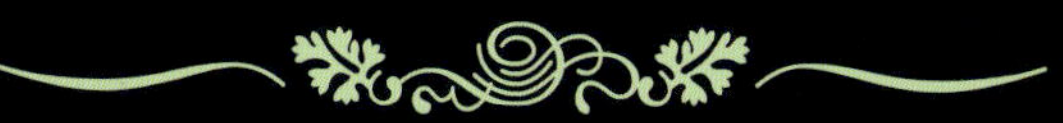

Empress Joséphine, the beloved wife of
Napoleon Bonaparte, adored violets for their
delicate fragrance and beauty. She filled
her gardens at Malmaison with them, and
she wore violets so often that she became
famously associated with them.

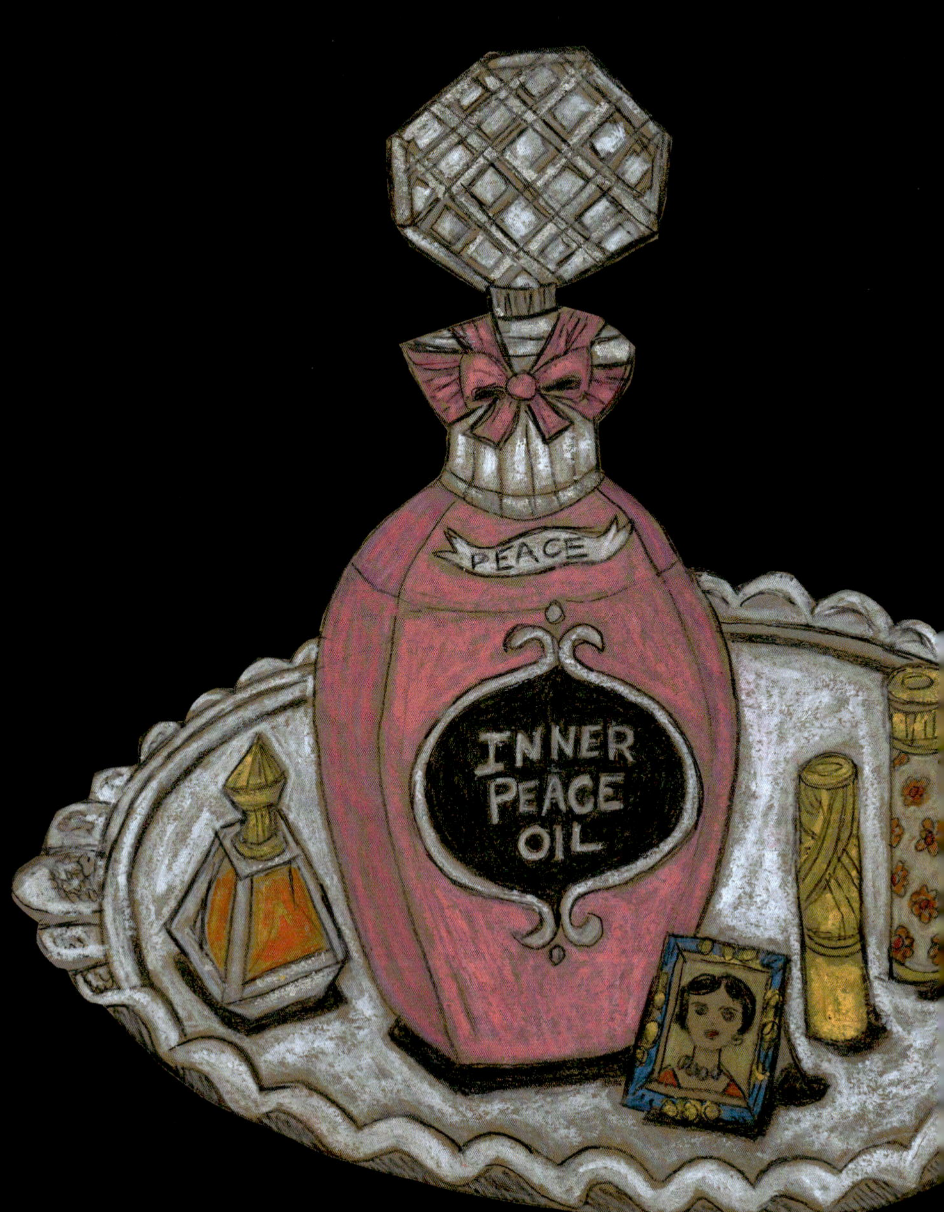
PEACE
INNER
PEACE
OIL

Thetis's Inner Peace Anointing Oil

(Makes one 6-ounce bottle)

This concoction soothes the mind by blending uplifting citrus and grounding floral essences that promote relaxation, clarity, and inner peace.

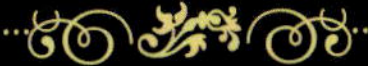

> 6 ounces jojoba oil
> 9 drops grapefruit essential oil
> 9 drops lemongrass essential oil
> 9 drops lavender essential oil
> 9 drops rose geranium essential oil
> 9 drops frankincense essential oil
> 1 glass bottle or dropper bottle, at least 6 ounces

Fill a glass bottle or dropper bottle with jojoba oil. Add 9 drops of each essential oil.

Secure the cap tightly on the bottle and shake the bottle to blend the oils.

Apply a small dab on your wrists and neck. Take a deep breath in, allowing a sense of peace to surround you. Exhale slowly, releasing any tension.

Store your anointing oil in a cool, dark place to maintain its potency. Shake gently before each use to re-blend the oils. Use the oil during meditation or yoga practices, or add a few drops to your bath water for a calming soak.

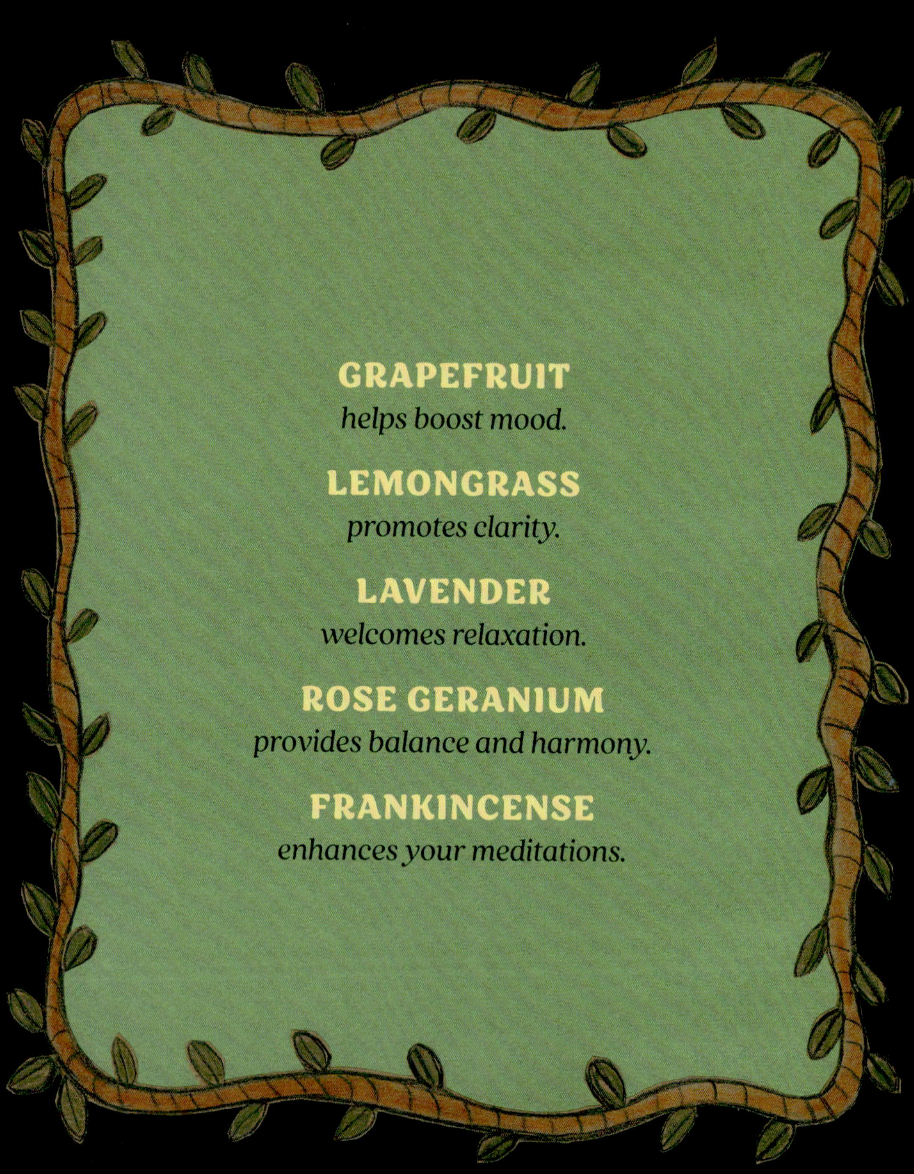

GRAPEFRUIT

helps boost mood.

LEMONGRASS

promotes clarity.

LAVENDER

welcomes relaxation.

ROSE GERANIUM

provides balance and harmony.

FRANKINCENSE

enhances your meditations.

Did You Know?

In Greek mythology, the hero Achilles was anointed with a sacred oil by his mother, the sea-nymph Thetis, in order to shield him from the mortal wounds of war. However, because his heel wasn't anointed by the oil, it remained vulnerable, eventually leading to his downfall.

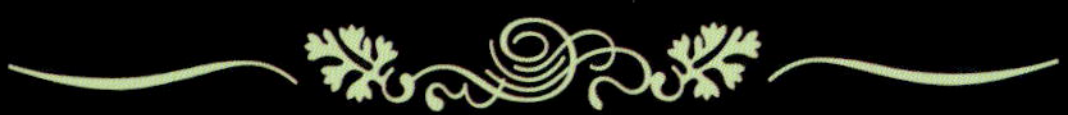

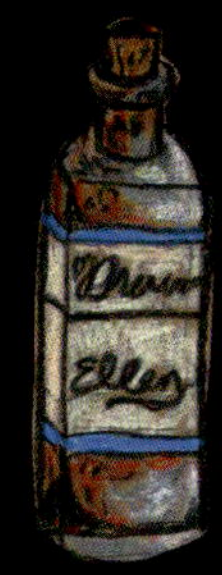

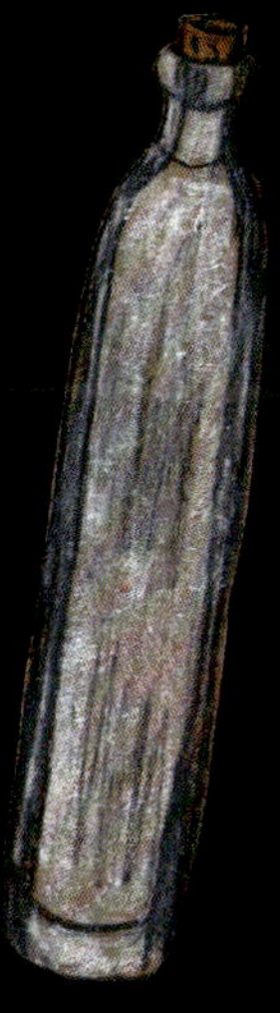

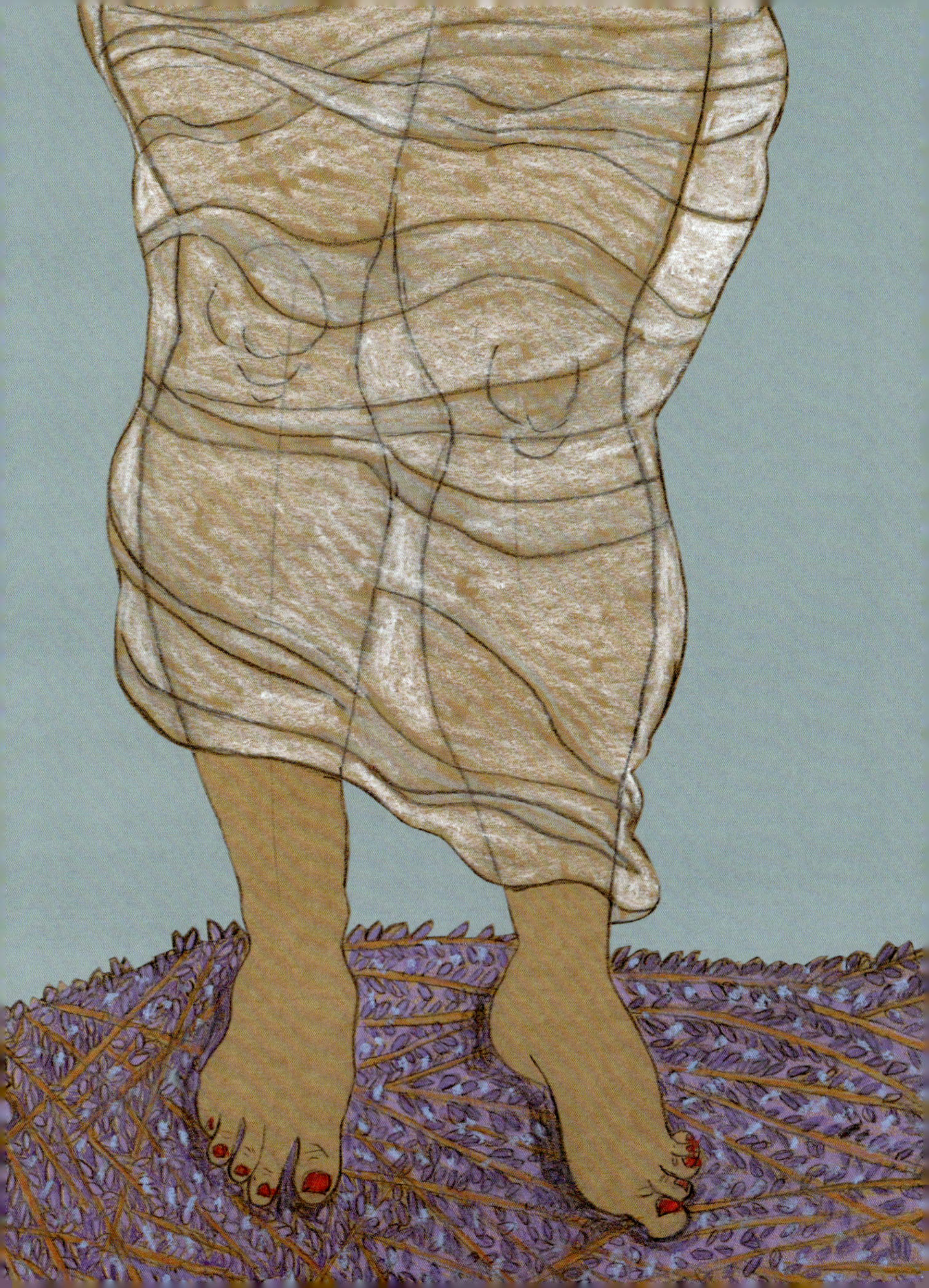

Lavender and Rosemary Foot Soak

(Makes enough for 1 foot bath)

Rosemary awakens and clarifies the mind, while lavender soothes and settles it—making them a perfect pairing for balance and calm relaxation without grogginess.

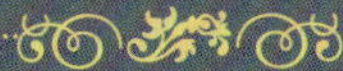

½ cup Epsom salt
½ cup sea salt or Himalayan pink salt
1 cup dried lavender flowers
7 drops lavender essential oil
7 drops rosemary essential oil
Warm water

In a small bowl, combine the Epsom salt and sea salt (or Himalayan salt). Add dried lavender flowers, then the essential oils. Mix well.

Fill a foot basin or tub with warm water, enough to soak your feet comfortably.

Pour the salt and lavender mixture into the warm water, stirring gently to dissolve.

Before soaking your feet, take a slow, deep breath and imagine releasing the stresses of the day. Immerse your feet in the warm water and relax for 15 to 20 minutes. Enjoy the soothing aroma and the benefits of the salts. Allow the warm water to carry away your tension.

After soaking, rinse your feet with clean water and pat them dry. You can moisturize with your favorite lotion for added softness.

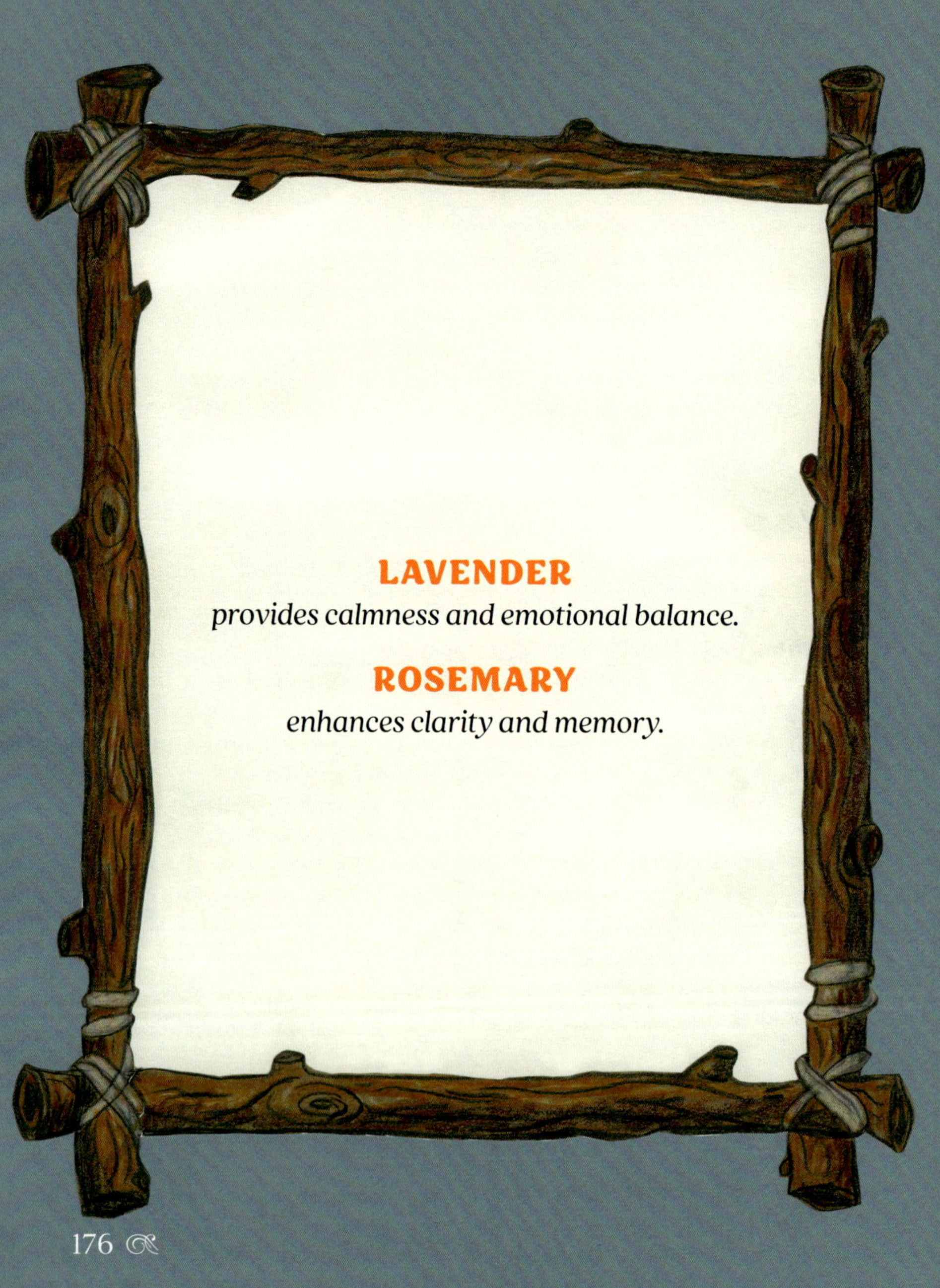

LAVENDER
provides calmness and emotional balance.

ROSEMARY
enhances clarity and memory.

Did You Know?

In ancient Greece, students wore rosemary garlands while studying to strengthen their memory. In *Hamlet*, Shakespeare referenced rosemary as the herb of remembrance. Romans were known to use lavender in baths for refreshing the scent of their bodies and relaxation. It was also kept in pillows by the Romans to protect their dreams and bring restful sleep.

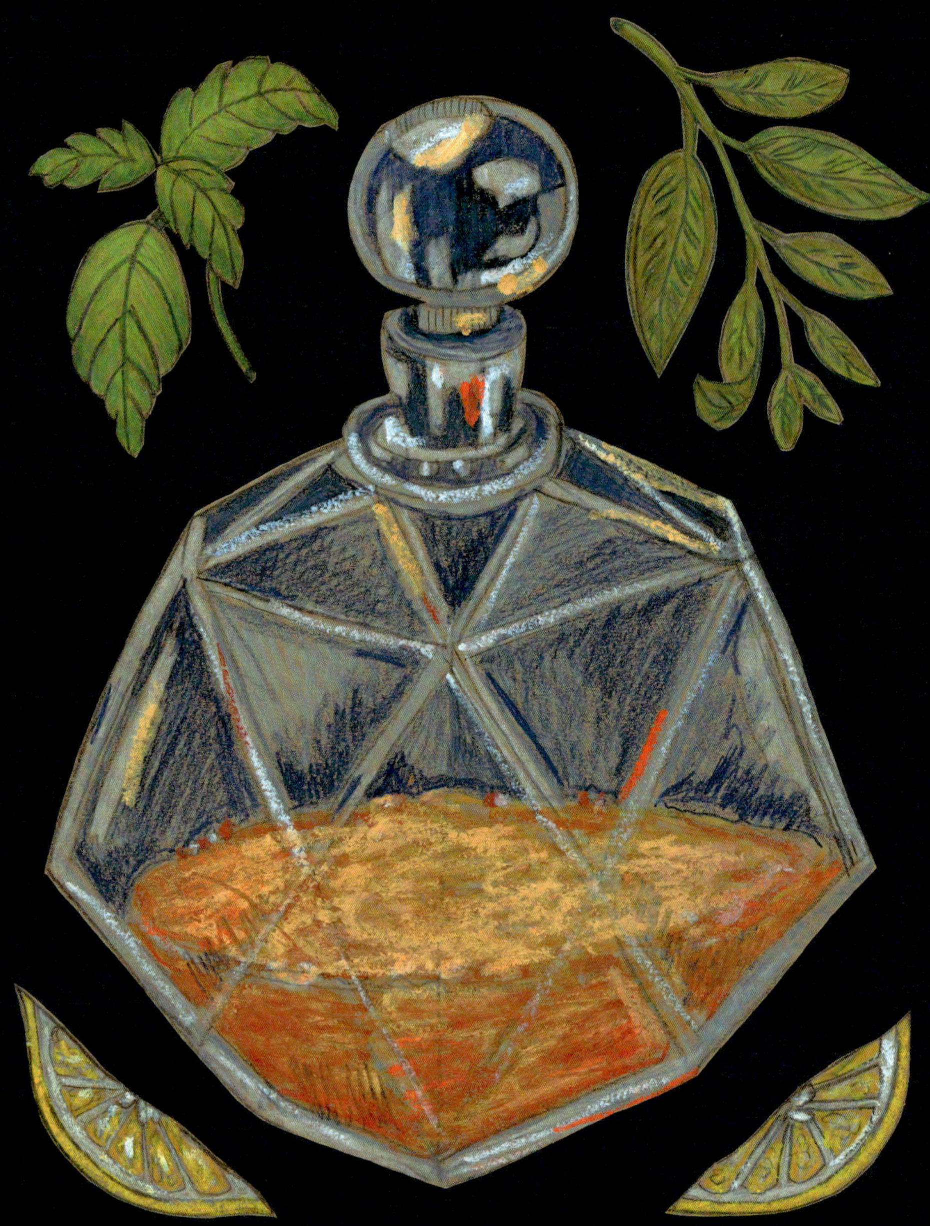

Sage and Holy Basil Whiskey Elixir

(Serves 1 adult)

Take a breath before sipping this hearty concoction, noticing the warmth in your hands and offering gratitude for this moment of stillness.

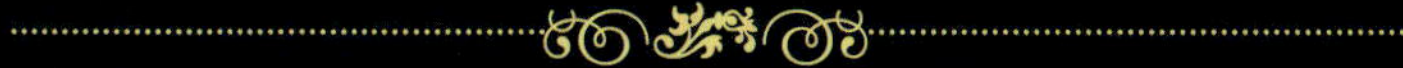

1 cup water
2-3 fresh sage leaves
2-3 fresh holy basil leaves, or 1 teaspoon dried
1-2 teaspoons agave sweetener, to taste
2 ounces whiskey
Juice of ½ lemon
Cinnamon stick and lemon slice for garnish

Bring water to a boil.

Place the sage and holy basil leaves in a teapot or tea infuser. Pour the hot water over the herbs and let them steep for about 5 minutes. As the leaves infuse, breathe slowly and imagine the steam carrying away tension from your body.

After steeping, strain the tea. Deposit the spent herbs into the compost bin.

Pour the tea into a clean mug. Then, stir in the agave. Add the whiskey and lemon juice and stir.

Garnish with a cinnamon stick and a slice of lemon.

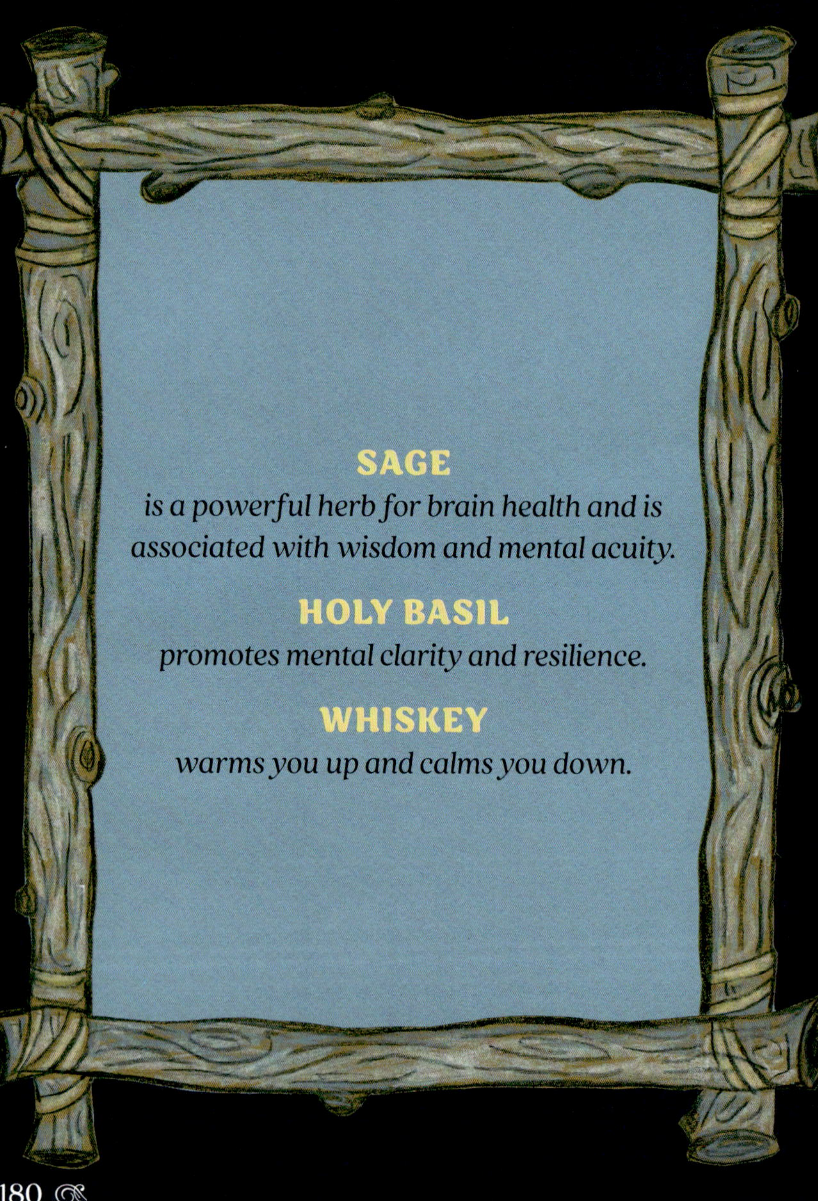

SAGE

is a powerful herb for brain health and is
associated with wisdom and mental acuity.

HOLY BASIL

promotes mental clarity and resilience.

WHISKEY

warms you up and calms you down.

Did You Know?

Gaelic poets would drink *uisge beatha* ("water of life"—the early name for whiskey) before reciting their poetry, which must have made for a colorful performance! Whiskey was used to clear the mind and spark the bard's memories, helping them recall long oral histories and write their poetry.

Blueberry and Cinnamon Boba Tea

(Serves 2)

Before sipping, pause. Hold the glass in both hands and offer a moment of gratitude for the ingredients and the calm they bring.

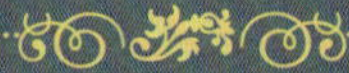

1 cup tapioca pearls (boba)
1 cup fresh blueberries, and a few additional berries for garnish
¼ cup water
4 tablespoons maple syrup, divided (or to taste)
1 tablespoon lemon juice
2 cups brewed black tea (cooled)
1 cup almond milk (or any plant-based milk)
1 teaspoon ground cinnamon

Boil a large pot of water. Add the tapioca pearls. Cook according to package instructions, usually for about 5 to 7 minutes or until they float to the surface.

Drain pearls and rinse under cold water. Set aside. As you rinse, imagine the water sweeping away any tension you hold.

In a small saucepan, combine blueberries, ¼ cup water, 2 tablespoons maple syrup, and lemon juice. Cook over medium heat, stirring occasionally, until the blueberries break down, about 5 to 7 minutes.

Strain liquid through a fine mesh sieve into a small bowl. Let cool. Discard the berries into the compost bin.

In a large pitcher, stir together the cooled black tea, almond milk, 2 remaining tablespoons of maple syrup (more or less, to your taste), and ground cinnamon.

Add a few tablespoons of cooked boba pearls to the bottoms of 2 serving glasses. Pour in the tea mixture. Drizzle blueberry syrup mixture on top and stir to combine. Add ice, if desired, and garnish with additional blueberries or a sprinkle of cinnamon.

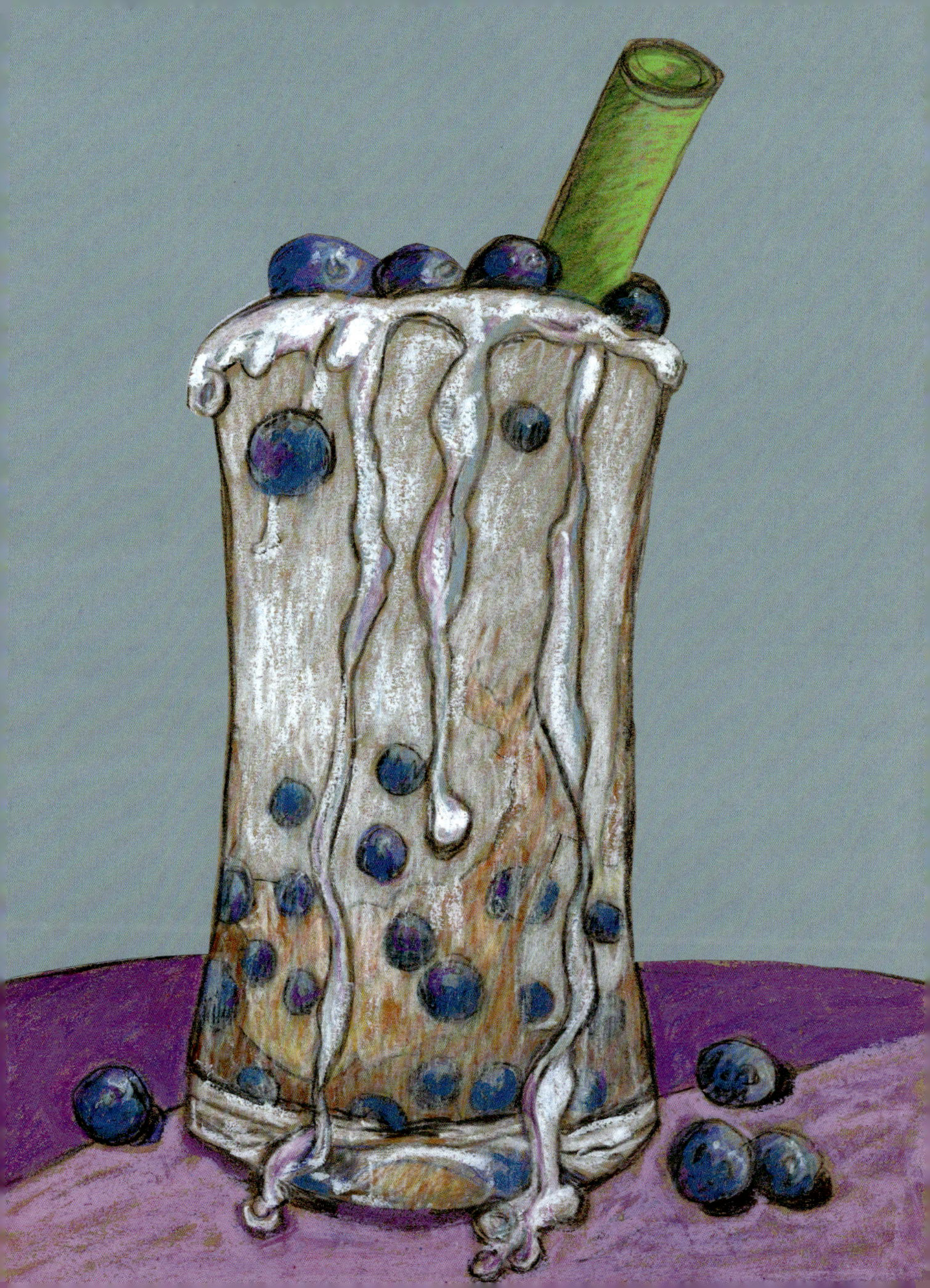

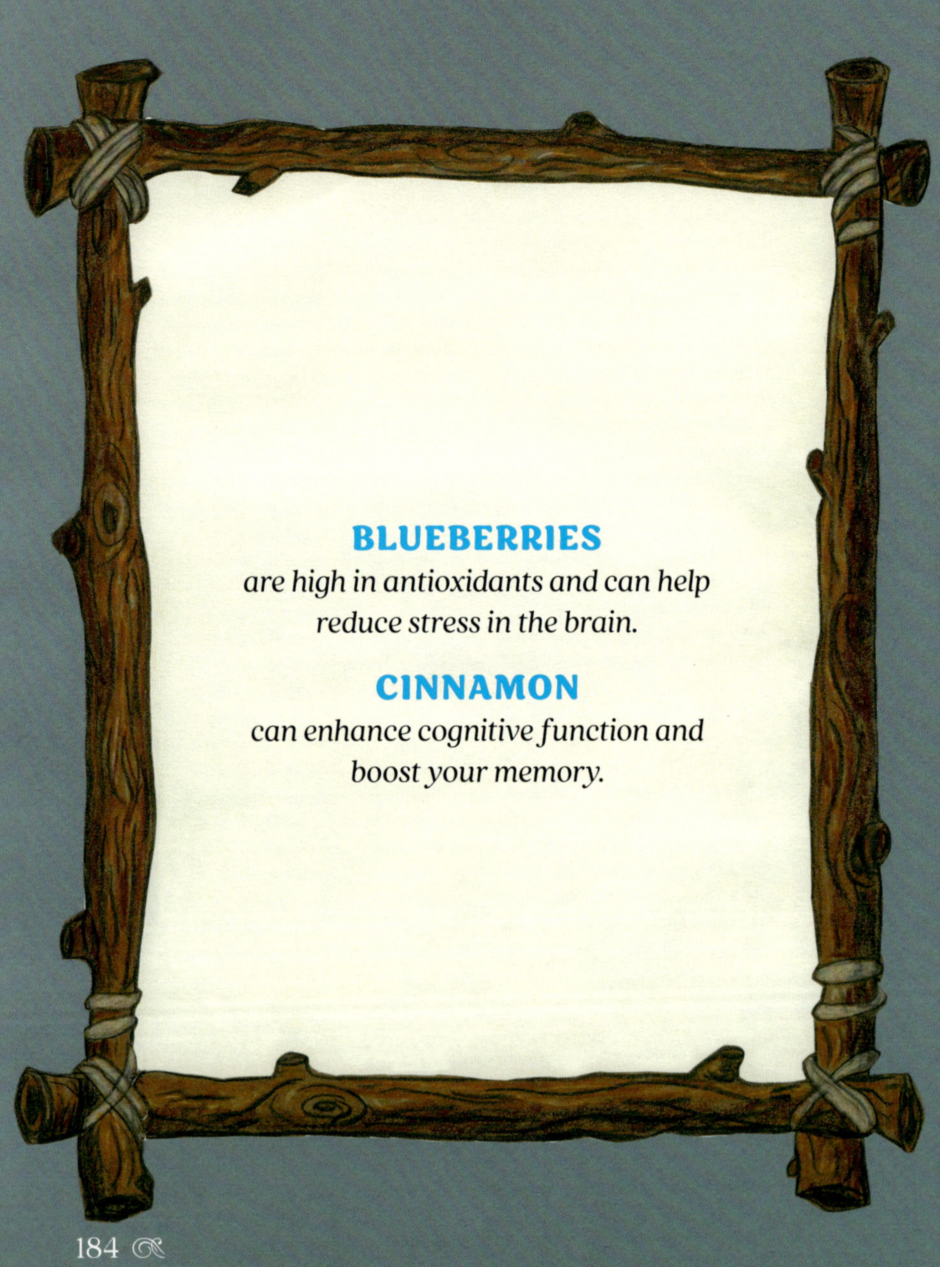

BLUEBERRIES

are high in antioxidants and can help reduce stress in the brain.

CINNAMON

can enhance cognitive function and boost your memory.

Did You Know?

Many Indigenous tribes of North America believed blueberries to be gifts from the Great Spirit. The Cherokee tribe used blueberry root and leaves in teas for calming.

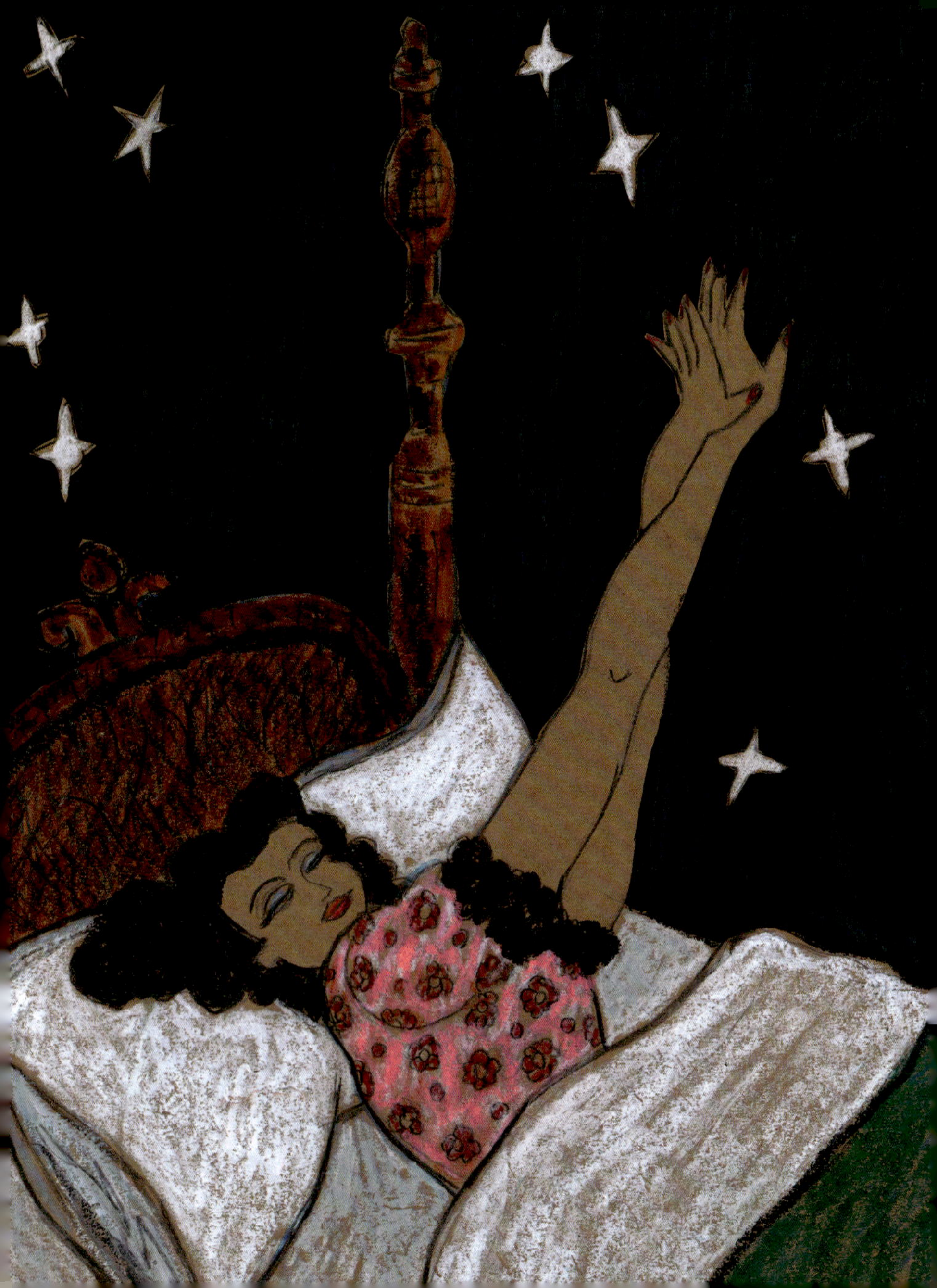

CHAPTER 6

HEAL YOUR SLEEP

Sleep is the great restorer—the time when the body mends and the mind escapes through dreams. This chapter invites you to treat bedtime as a sacred ritual, a gentle return to balance after the stress of the day. Wellness begins when you dim the lights, steep some calming tea, breathe deeply, and give yourself permission to rest.

Across time and cultures, sleep has had many rituals: lavender tucked into pillows, chamomile brewed for relaxation, mugwort brewed by dreamers seeking visions. These traditions remind us that rest is transformation and renewal.

Here you'll find teas, treats, and bedtime creations to quiet the body and calm the mind—each one an invitation to slow down and let bedtime become a gift you give to yourself. (Confession: Sleeping is our favorite thing!)

We start our guide to restful nights with *Little Briar Rose Sleepy Time Tea*, a gentle blend to lull you into a fairytale-inspired dreamland.

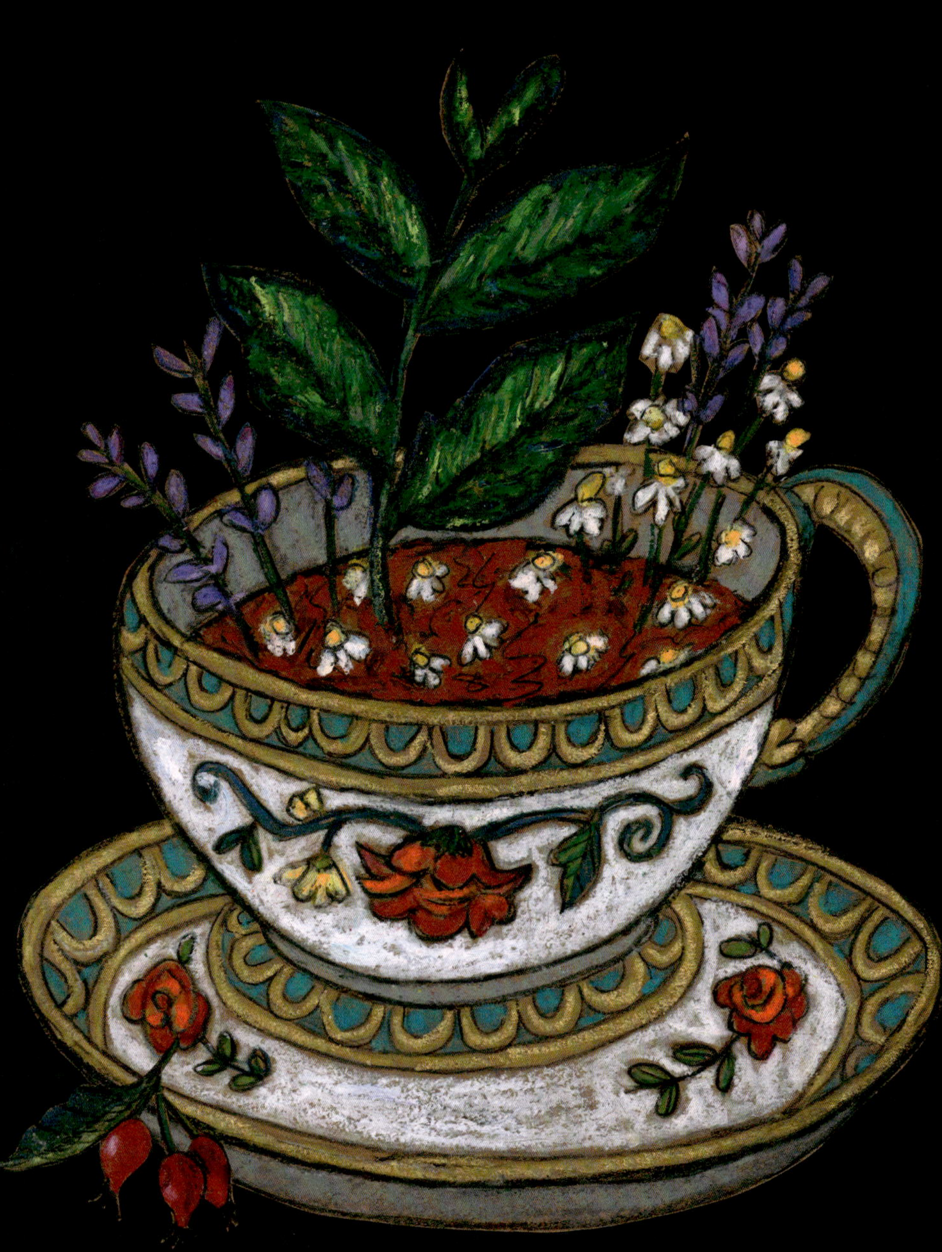

Little Briar Rose Sleepy Time Tea

(Serves 2)

This gentle blend of calming herbs soothes the mind, relaxes the body, and guides you into a peaceful, restorative sleep.

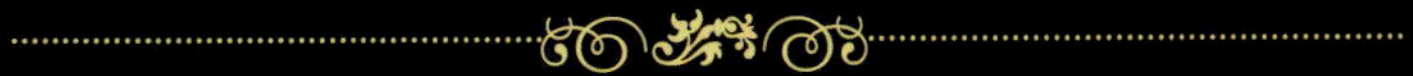

1 teaspoon dried chamomile flowers
1 teaspoon dried peppermint leaves
1 teaspoon dried lavender buds
1 teaspoon dried rose hips
1 teaspoon dried valerian root
1 teaspoon dried passionflower
2 cups water

Combine the dried herbs into a bowl. As you mix, take a deep breath and notice the scent of each herb.

Bring the water to a boil in a pot. While the water heats, use this time to slow down and take a few deep breaths.

Once the water is boiling, reduce the heat to a gentle simmer. Add the herbal mixture to the water. Let the mixture simmer for 10 to 15 minutes. As the herbs steep, imagine their calming energies soothing your nervous system.

Let the rising steam invite you to release any tension you're holding.

Strain the tea with a fine mesh sieve. Toss the herbs into your compost bin. As you serve your tea, set an intention for rest and restoration.

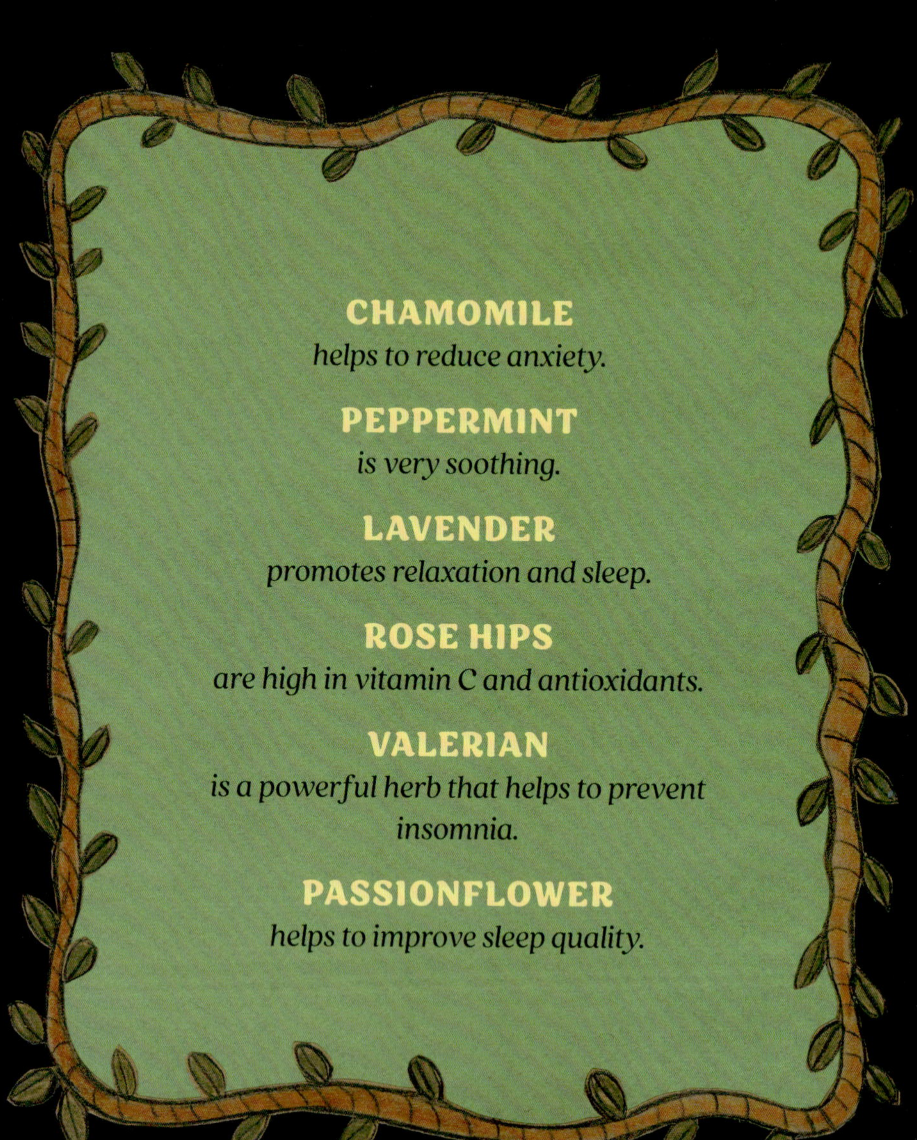

CHAMOMILE
helps to reduce anxiety.

PEPPERMINT
is very soothing.

LAVENDER
promotes relaxation and sleep.

ROSE HIPS
are high in vitamin C and antioxidants.

VALERIAN
is a powerful herb that helps to prevent
insomnia.

PASSIONFLOWER
helps to improve sleep quality.

Did You Know?

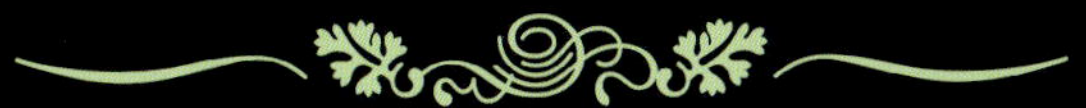

"Little Briar Rose," a fairy tale by the Brothers Grimm, tells the story of a beautiful princess named Briar Rose who's been cursed by a vengeful fairy. The fairy's spell dictates that on Briar Rose's fifteenth birthday, she will prick her finger on a spindle and fall into a deep sleep lasting one hundred years. In order to prevent this fate, her father, the king, orders all spindles in the kingdom to be destroyed. On her fifteenth birthday, Briar Rose finds a spindle that has been overlooked and does indeed prick her finger. The entire kingdom falls asleep with her and is surrounded by a thick briar hedge. After a century, a handsome prince bravely ventures through the hedge, and upon finding her, he breaks the fairy's curse by awakening Briar Rose with a kiss.

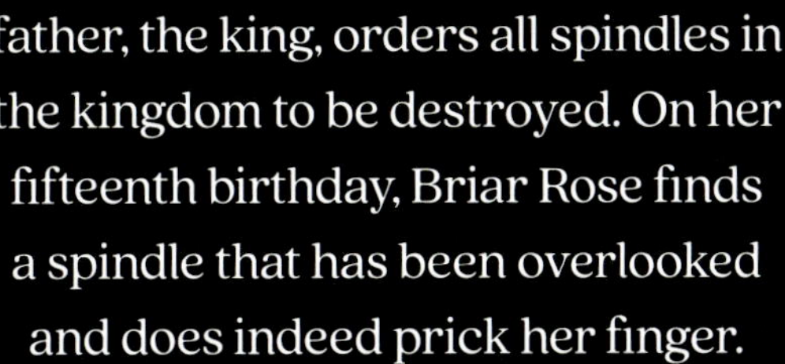

191

Lucid Dream Tea

(Serves 2)

**A calming herbal tea to support vivid dreams and a peaceful rest.
Best enjoyed 30 to 60 minutes before bed.**

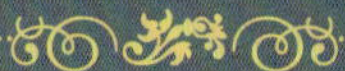

1 teaspoon dried mugwort (avoid during pregnancy)
1 teaspoon dried chamomile
1 teaspoon dried passionflower
½ teaspoon dried peppermint
A few dried rose petals
2 cups water

Place the herbs into a bowl and combine. Take your time as you mix. Your day is over; there is no reason to rush!

Bring water to a gentle boil.

Place the herbal blend into a teapot or tea infuser. Pour boiling water over the herbs and cover for 7 to 10 minutes. While the tea steeps, close your eyes and focus on the rhythm of your breath.

Strain the tea through a fine mesh sieve into your favorite mug, discarding the herbs into the compost bin.

Serve and slip slowly, noticing the flavors unfolding with each sip before bed. Keep a journal by your bedside to jot down any dreams you remember.

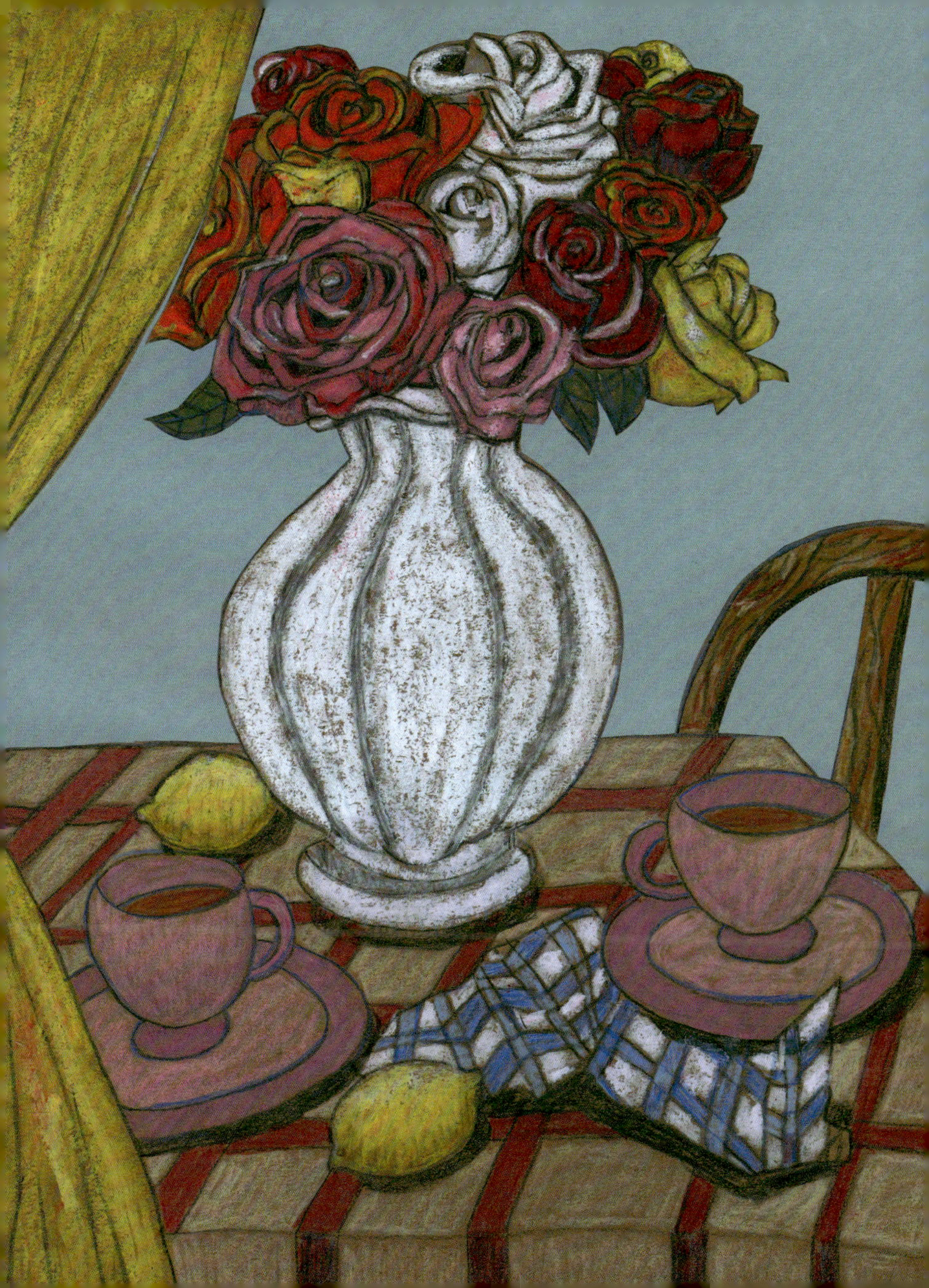

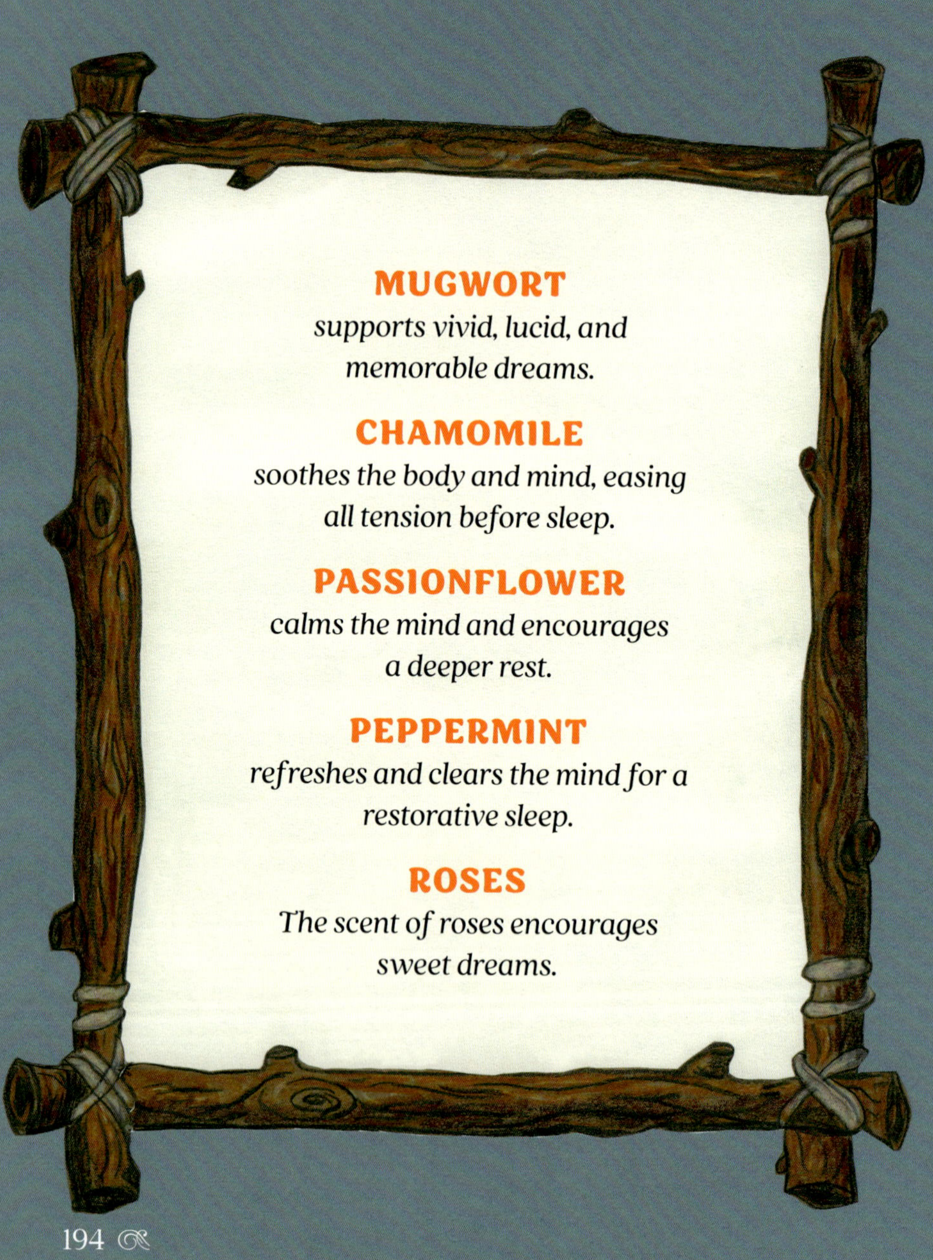

MUGWORT

supports vivid, lucid, and
memorable dreams.

CHAMOMILE

soothes the body and mind, easing
all tension before sleep.

PASSIONFLOWER

calms the mind and encourages
a deeper rest.

PEPPERMINT

refreshes and clears the mind for a
restorative sleep.

ROSES

The scent of roses encourages
sweet dreams.

Did You Know?

In European folklore, mugwort has long been known as the "dreaming herb." It was often brewed as a tea before sleep.

Midsummer Night's Dream Ritual

(Makes enough for 1 ritual)

A mindful evening practice for vision, rest, and inner magic. This ritual is especially potent at the summer equinox, but it may be practiced anytime. Place the herbs and the amethyst crystal in a cotton sachet bag and tuck under your pillow.

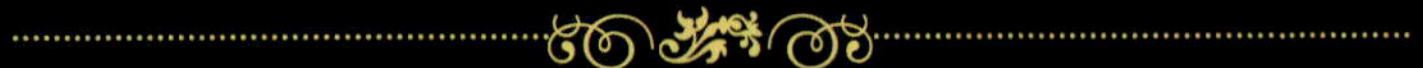

1 cup calming herbal tea, such as Little Briar Rose Sleepy Time Tea (page 189)

1 candle (choose white for tranquility)

1 small bowl water

1 handful fresh or dried herbs, such as lavender, mugwort, chamomile, rose petals, or a mix

1 amethyst crystal

1 cotton sachet bag

1 piece of paper and a pen

As your herbal tea steeps, tidy your bed and allow the quiet to settle around you. Inhale the aroma of your tea, drawing in a sense of calmness.

Light your candle. Bring your awareness to the present moment.

Dip your fingers into the bowl of water and lightly touch your forehead, heart, and wrists—pausing with each touch to say quietly: "I will sleep peacefully."

Place the herbs and the amethyst crystal in a sachet bag and tuck under your pillow.

What dream or message would you like to receive tonight? Write your dream request on the paper. Fold it gently and put it under your pillow with the herbs.

Blow out the candle and say: "I welcome my dreams."

Crawl into bed without checking your smartphone, the news, or any media. (Yes, you can do it!)

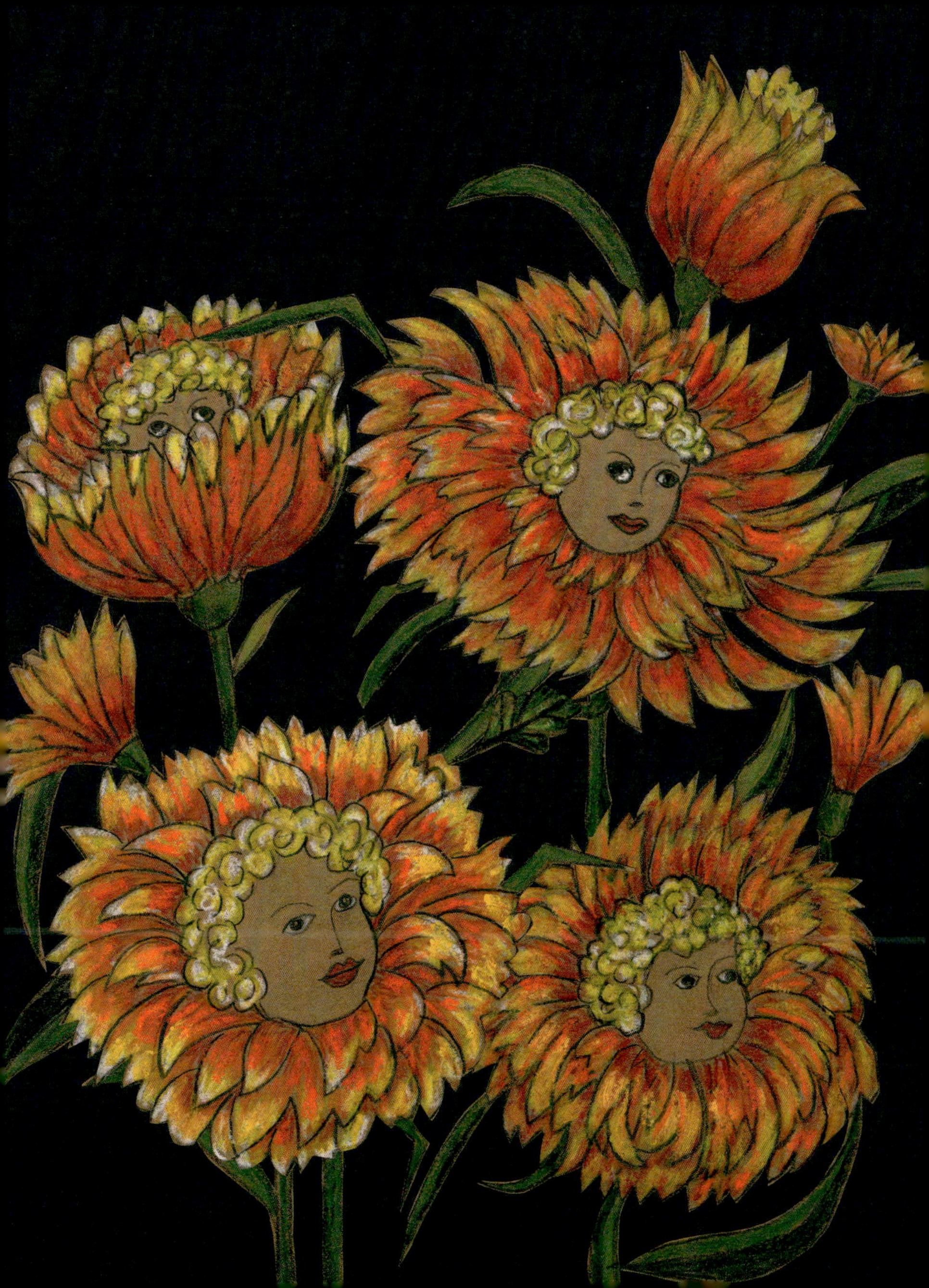

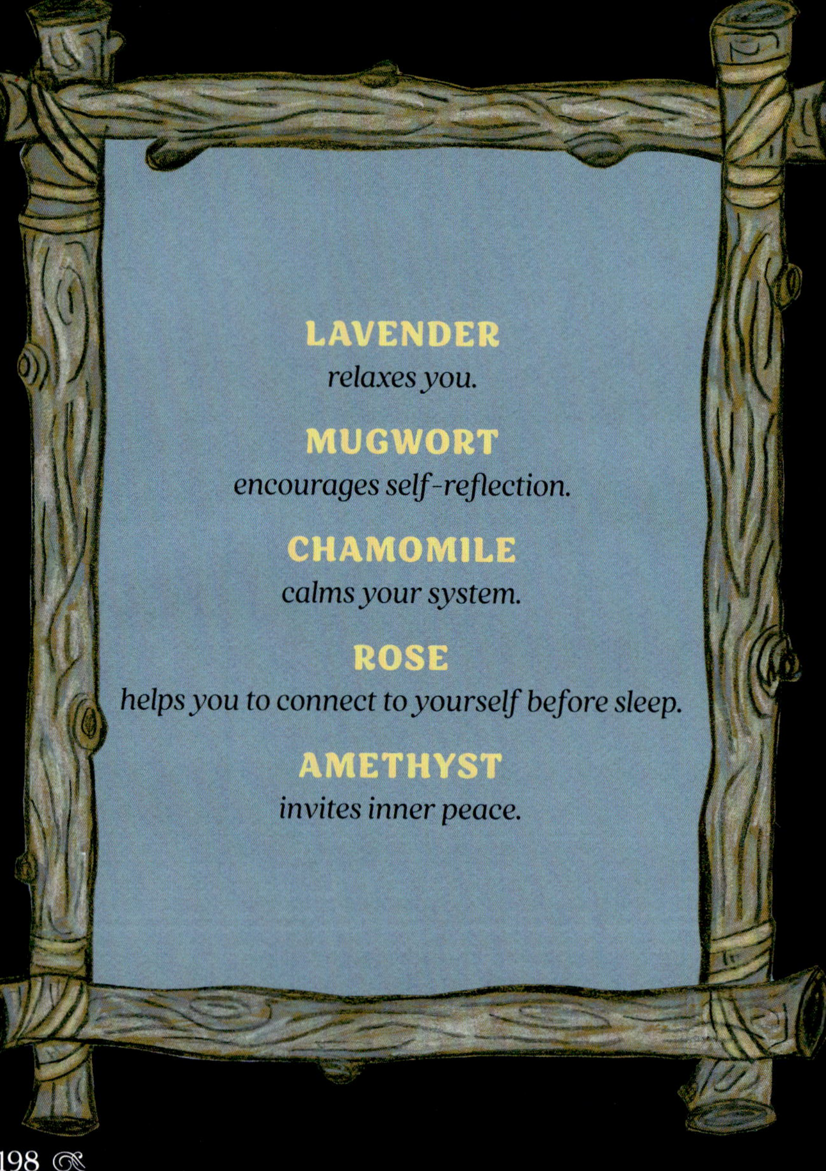

LAVENDER
relaxes you.

MUGWORT
encourages self-reflection.

CHAMOMILE
calms your system.

ROSE
helps you to connect to yourself before sleep.

AMETHYST
invites inner peace.

Did You Know?

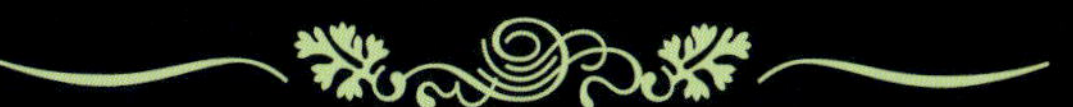

Shakespeare drops some great herbal references in "A Midsummer Night's Dream." The most famous one is the "love-in-idleness" flower (a wild pansy or viola), which Oberon uses to make the magical love potion. In this play, Cupid's arrow struck this flower, turning its petals purple and giving it the power to make anyone fall in love with the first person they see upon awakening.

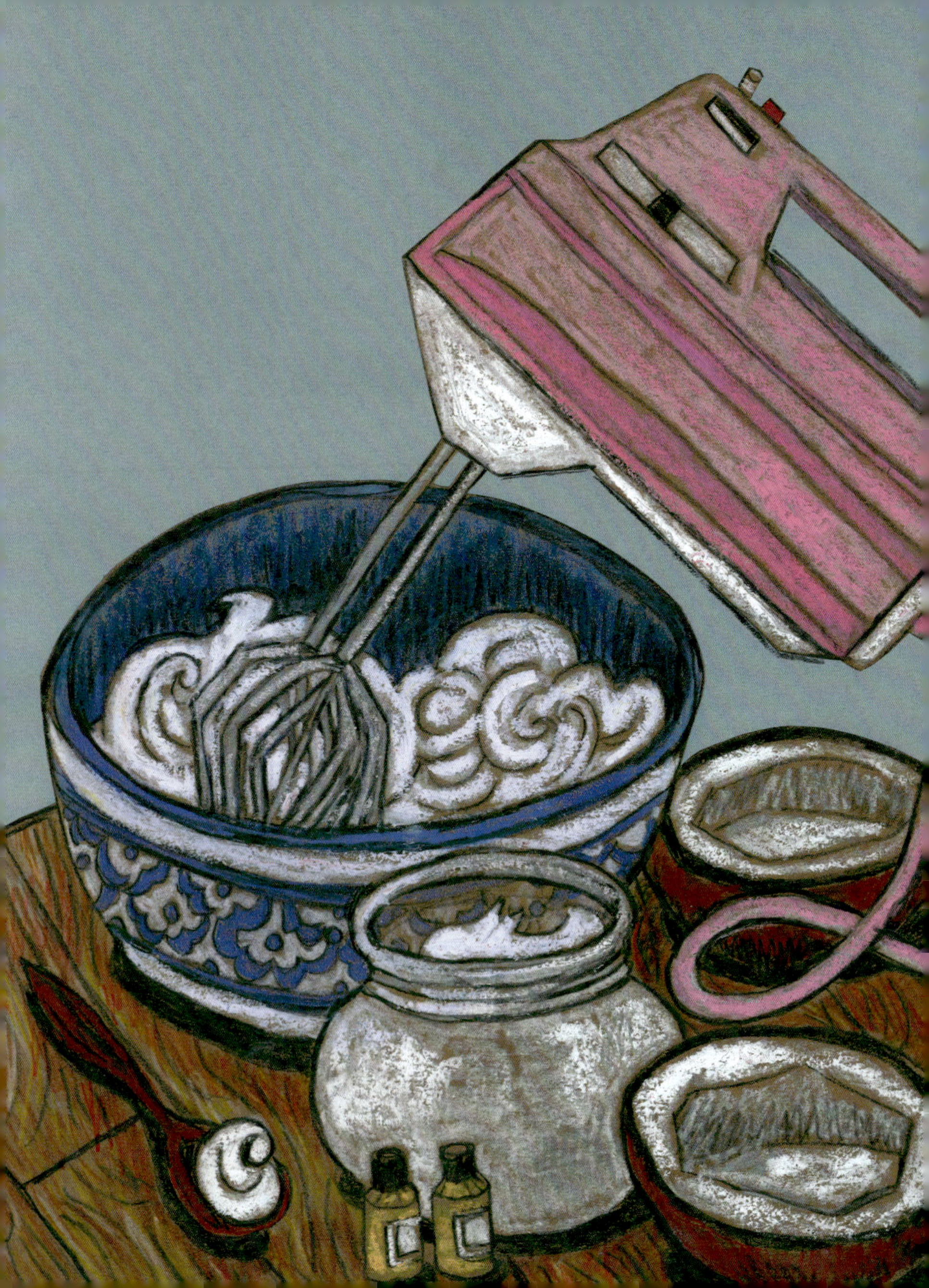

Whipped Coconut Oil Moisturizer

(Makes approximately ¾ cup moisturizer)

**Indulge in this luxurious whipped coconut moisturizer.
It's wonderful for skin nourishment and a peaceful night's sleep.**

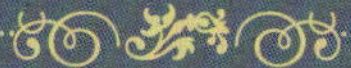

½ cup coconut oil at room temperature (solid state)
7 drops rose essential oil
7 drops lavender essential oil
Electric hand mixer
Small glass jar with lid

Scoop the coconut oil into a bowl. Using your hand mixer, whip the coconut oil on medium speed. Let your thoughts settle into the rhythm of the beaters, watching as the texture transforms into something light and airy. This will take about 3 to 5 minutes.

As you continue to whip the coconut oil, add the drops of rose essential oil one by one. Follow with the lavender essential oil.

Scrape the whipped moisturizer into a small glass jar, taking a moment to admire its texture. Seal it tightly and place it somewhere cool and dry.

Apply moisturizer to the body, especially your hands and the soles of your feet, just before bed.

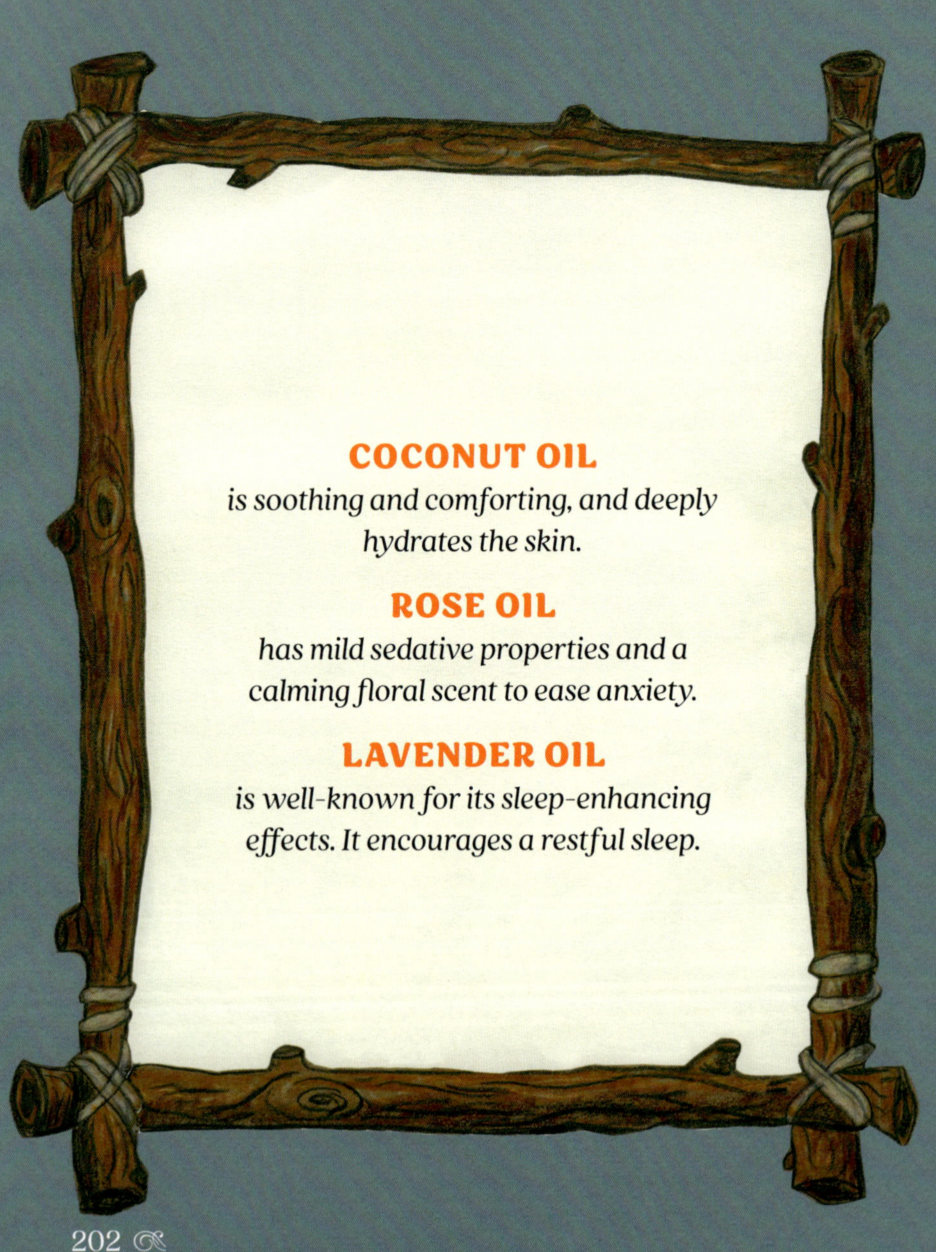

COCONUT OIL
is soothing and comforting, and deeply hydrates the skin.

ROSE OIL
has mild sedative properties and a calming floral scent to ease anxiety.

LAVENDER OIL
is well-known for its sleep-enhancing effects. It encourages a restful sleep.

Did You Know?

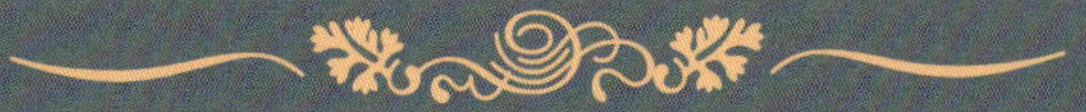

Coconut oil is used in Ayurvedic medicine and Polynesian healing traditions for evening massages to calm the body and soften the skin. In Ancient Rome, women scented their baths and beds with rose oil to attract love and rest. And in medieval Europe, rose petals were tucked into pillows to ward off nightmares.

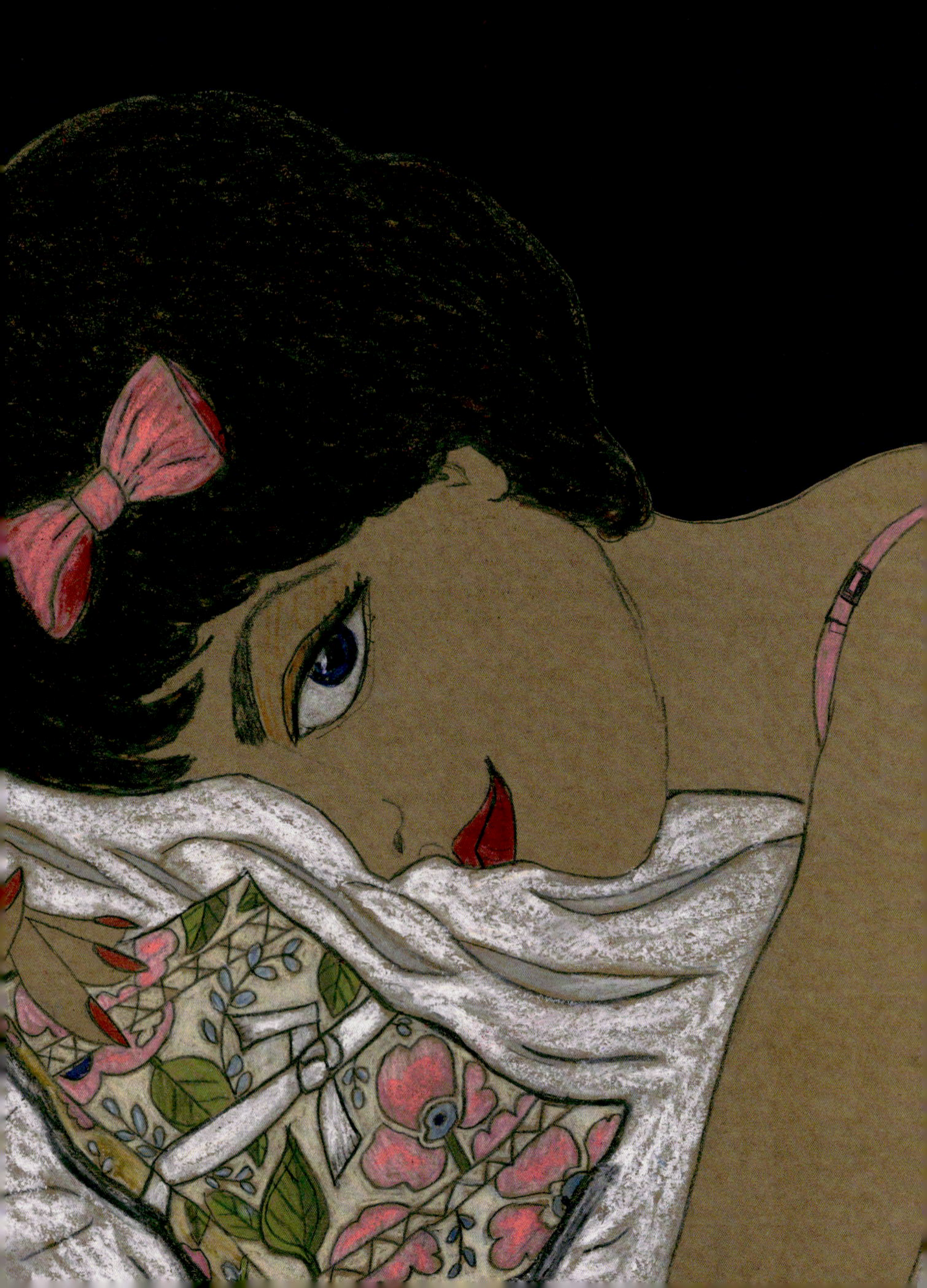

Dream Pillow

(Makes 1 pillow)

Enhance your sleep by tucking this fragrant sachet beneath your pillow, allowing its calming aroma to guide you toward restful slumber.

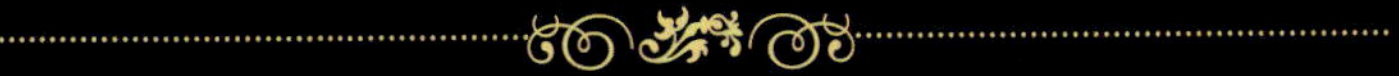

2 teaspoons dried rose petals
2 teaspoons dried chamomile flowers
1 teaspoon cloves
1 teaspoon dried meadowsweet
3-4 sprigs lavender
2-3 drops bergamot essential oil, applied to a
    small piece of cotton cloth
1 muslin bag, 3 × 4 inches, with drawstring, or 2 fabric squares,
    3 × 4 inches, with needle and thread

As you gather your ingredients, notice their colors, textures, and scents. Let this small act set the tone for rest and peace.

Place the rose petals, chamomile flowers, cloves, meadowsweet, lavender, and bergamot-dabbed cloth into your muslin bag. Close securely. Or create a small pillow by using your needle and thread to stitch two pieces of fabric together along three edges, leaving one side open to fill with the flower mixture. Fill pillow, then stitch final edge closed. Use any scrap fabric, preferably from natural materials like cotton or muslin.

Slip your creation under your pillow. As you lay your head down, take a moment to breathe in the soothing aroma as it leads you into dreamland. This calming ritual will prepare your body for a night of inspiring dreams.

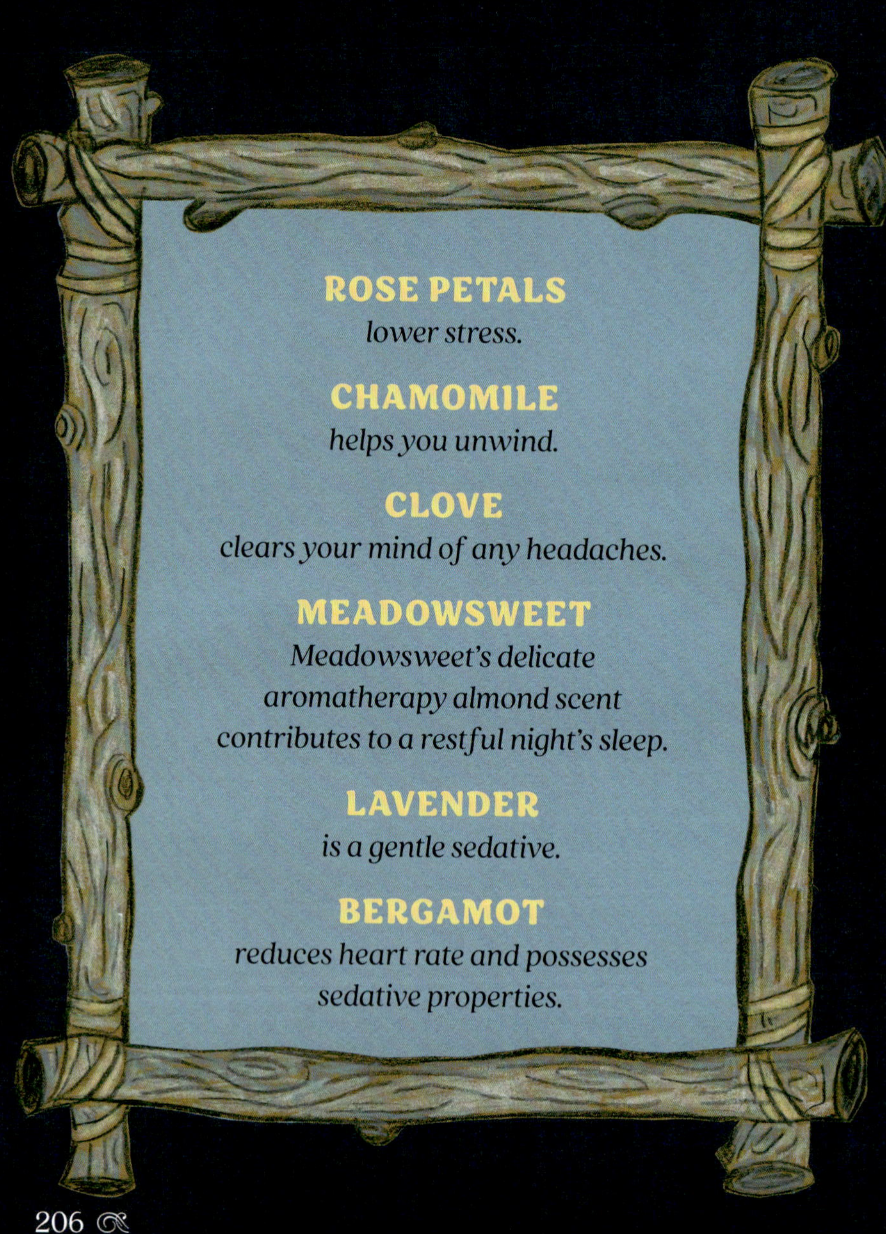

ROSE PETALS
lower stress.

CHAMOMILE
helps you unwind.

CLOVE
clears your mind of any headaches.

MEADOWSWEET
Meadowsweet's delicate
aromatherapy almond scent
contributes to a restful night's sleep.

LAVENDER
is a gentle sedative.

BERGAMOT
reduces heart rate and possesses
sedative properties.

Did You Know?

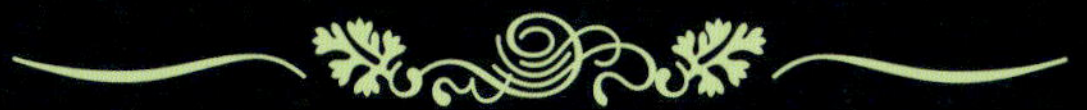

In both Celtic and Appalachian folklore, placing protective herbs under the pillow was said to guard the sleeper from bad spirits, fairy mischief, and nightmares. Often, these herbs were sewn into little cloth pillows, just like the one you created!

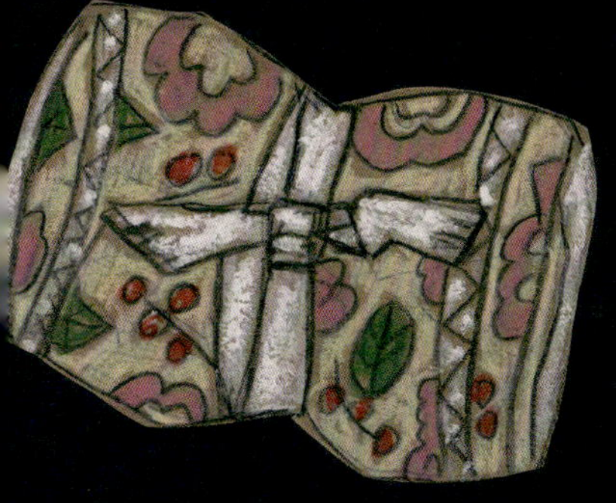

Lavender and Pistachio Chocolate Bark

(Makes 2–4 servings)

A yummy, soothing, and sensory treat. This chocolate bark blends the floral calmness of lavender, the grounding crunch of pistachios, and the soothing comfort of dark chocolate.

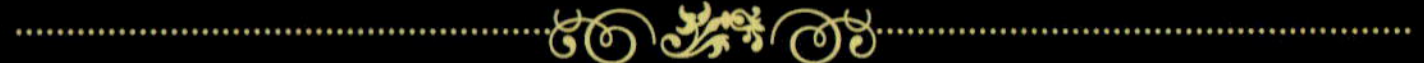

7 ounces dark chocolate, at least 70% cocoa
2 tablespoons culinary dried lavender
3½ ounces chopped pistachios
Pinch of sea salt

Line a baking sheet with parchment paper. Let this moment be a quiet ritual of creating with care.

Break the dark chocolate into small pieces and place them in a microwave-safe bowl.

Microwave in 30-second intervals, stirring gently between each interval until the chocolate is melted and smooth.

Stir the dried lavender into the melted chocolate.

Pour chocolate onto the prepared baking sheet. Gently spread it into an even layer about ¼ inch thick. Sprinkle the chopped pistachios across the surface. Follow with a pinch of sea salt.

Place the baking sheet in the refrigerator for about 30 minutes, or until the chocolate has fully hardened. Once set, break the bark into small, uneven pieces for nibbling. Store in an airtight container at room temperature, or in the fridge, for up to 2 weeks.

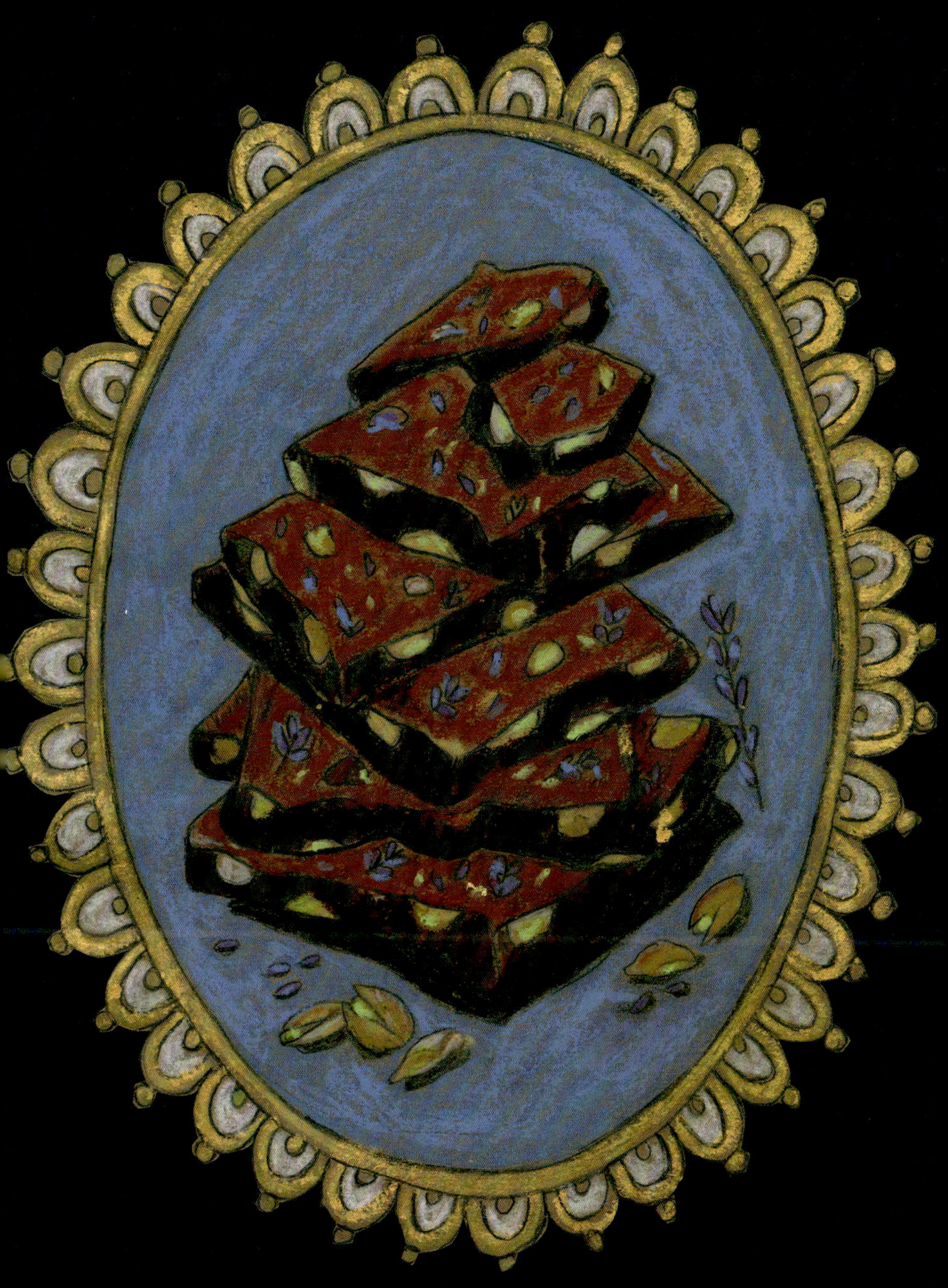

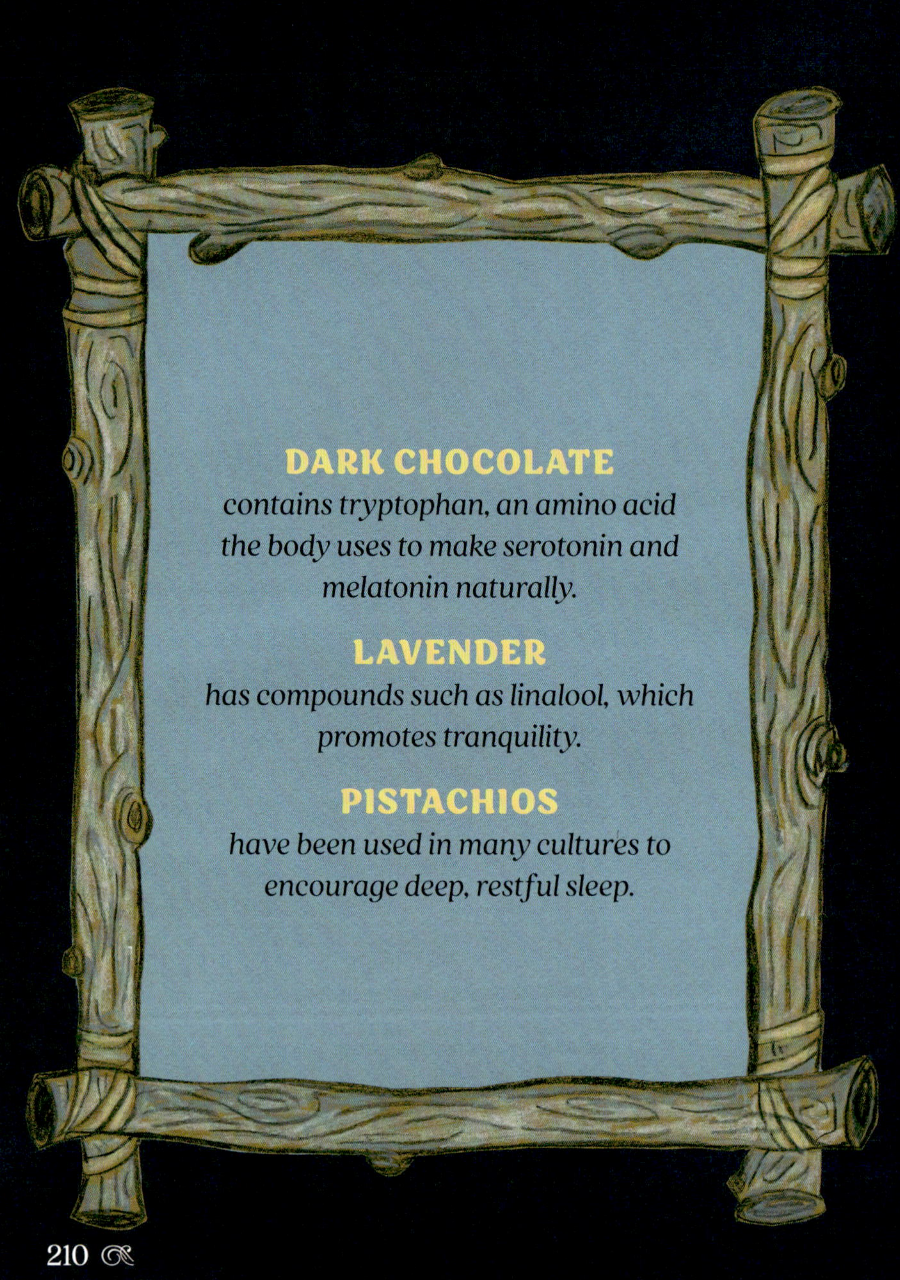

DARK CHOCOLATE

contains tryptophan, an amino acid
the body uses to make serotonin and
melatonin naturally.

LAVENDER

has compounds such as linalool, which
promotes tranquility.

PISTACHIOS

have been used in many cultures to
encourage deep, restful sleep.

Did You Know?

Victorian England prized lavender for its sedative qualities.

Ancient Ayurvedic texts regard pistachios as an ideal snack for evening consumption to prevent restlessness.

In some monastic traditions, monks would eat dark chocolate—based tonics to help calm their minds for nighttime prayers.

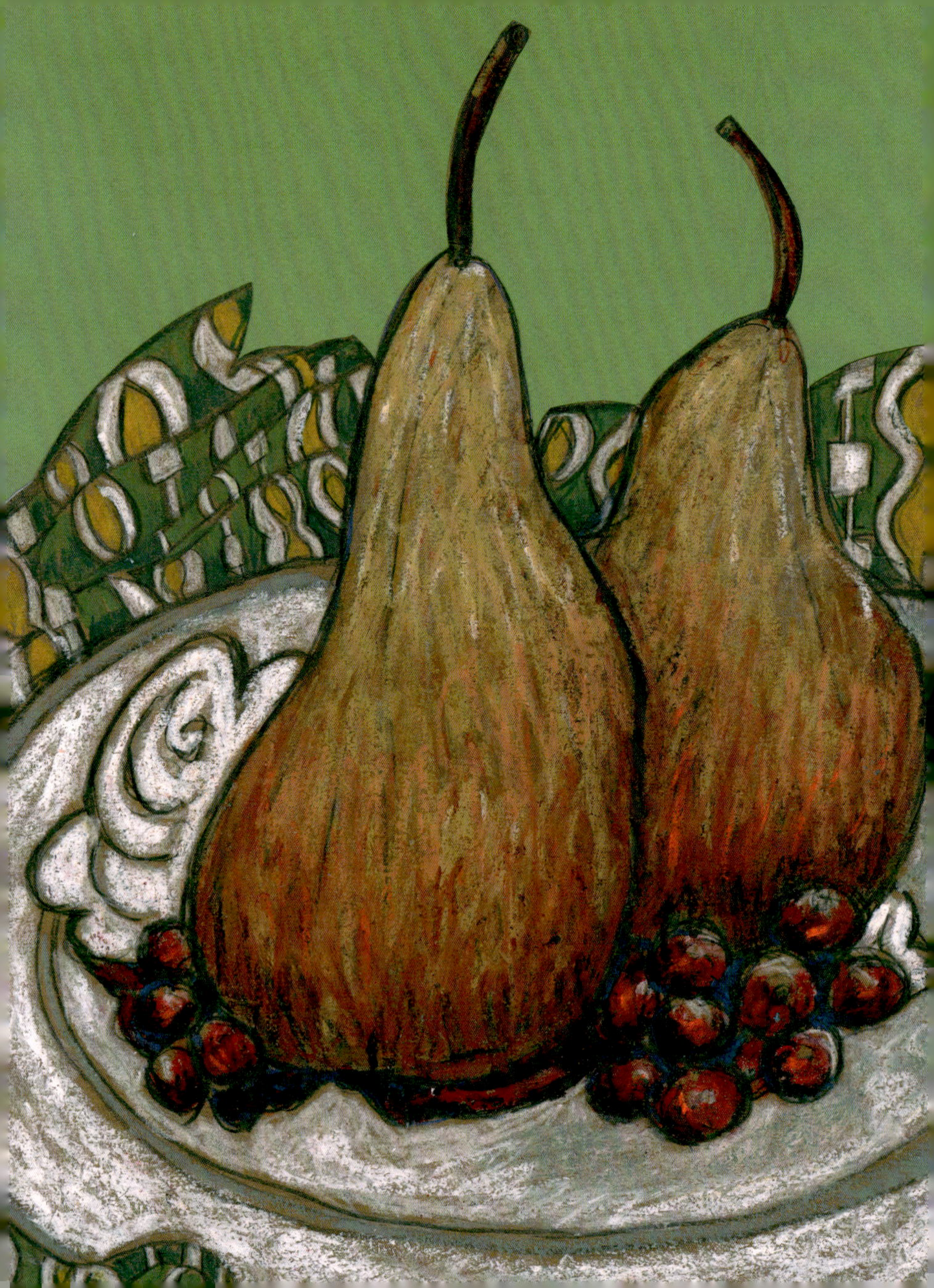

Hibiscus Poached Pears

(Serves 4)

A fragrant and elegant dessert.

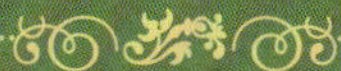

4 firm Bosc pears
Juice of 2 lemons (about 5 tablespoons)
1½ cups dried hibiscus flowers
1½ cups packed brown sugar
1 tablespoon allspice berries
1 tablespoon chopped fresh ginger
2 cinnamon sticks
2 whole cloves
1 dried bay leaf
1 piece orange peel, about 2-3 inches
10 cups water

Gently peel the pears using a vegetable peeler, keeping the stems intact for elegance.

In a large saucepan, combine the lemon juice, dried hibiscus, brown sugar, allspice berries, ginger, cinnamon sticks, cloves, bay leaf, orange peel, and 10 cups water. Bring the mixture to a rolling boil over high heat, stirring occasionally to ensure the sugar dissolves. Reduce the heat to a gentle simmer.

Carefully submerge the peeled pears in the simmering liquid. Cover and cook gently for about 30 minutes. Allow the gorgeous fragrance to fill your kitchen.

Once the pears are tender, remove the saucepan from heat and let the pears cool slowly in the poaching liquid for 10 to 15 minutes.

About a half hour before you are ready to serve, remove the pears from the liquid. Bring the poaching liquid back to a rolling boil and reduce until syrupy, about 25 minutes, stirring occasionally.

Place one pear on each plate and spoon over the hibiscus syrup. Enjoy and take pride in the delicious dessert you've just created.

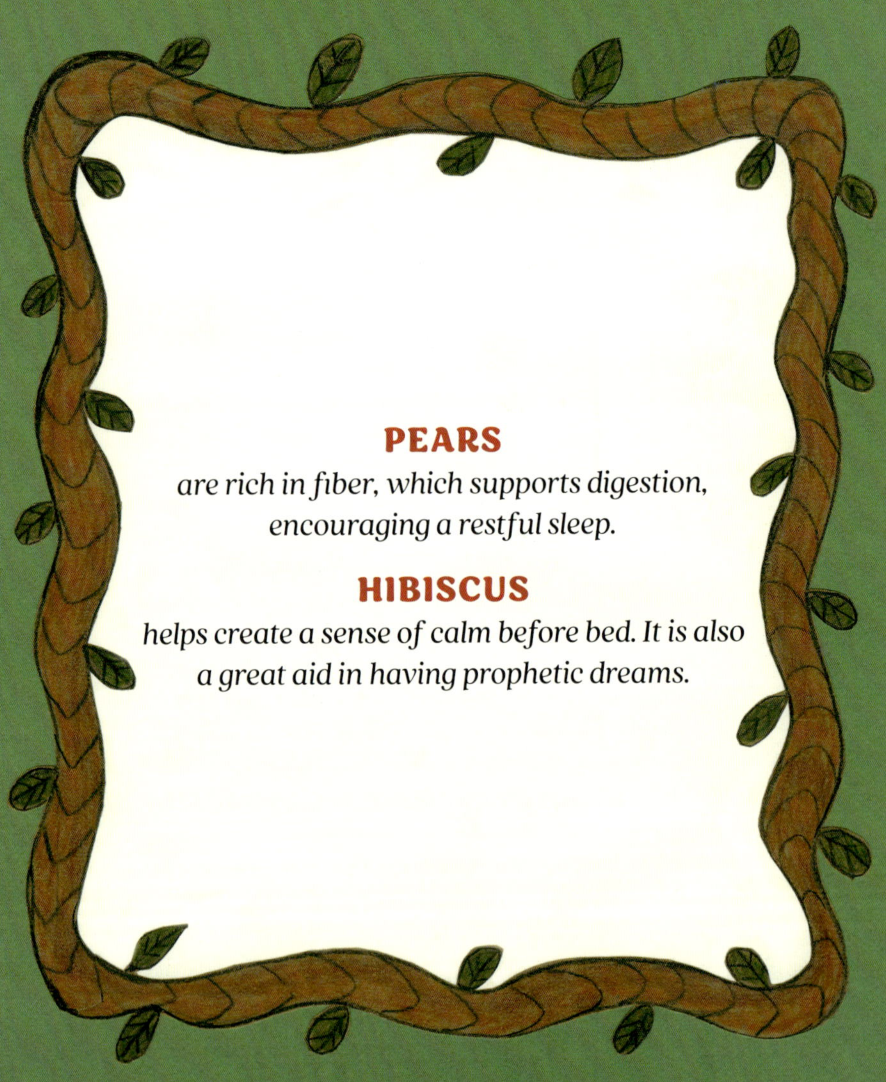

PEARS

are rich in fiber, which supports digestion, encouraging a restful sleep.

HIBISCUS

helps create a sense of calm before bed. It is also a great aid in having prophetic dreams.

Did You Know?

In West Africa, hibiscus tea has long been used in nighttime preparations to promote sleep. In ancient Europe, pears were stewed with warming spices and wine, helping to soothe the body and soul.

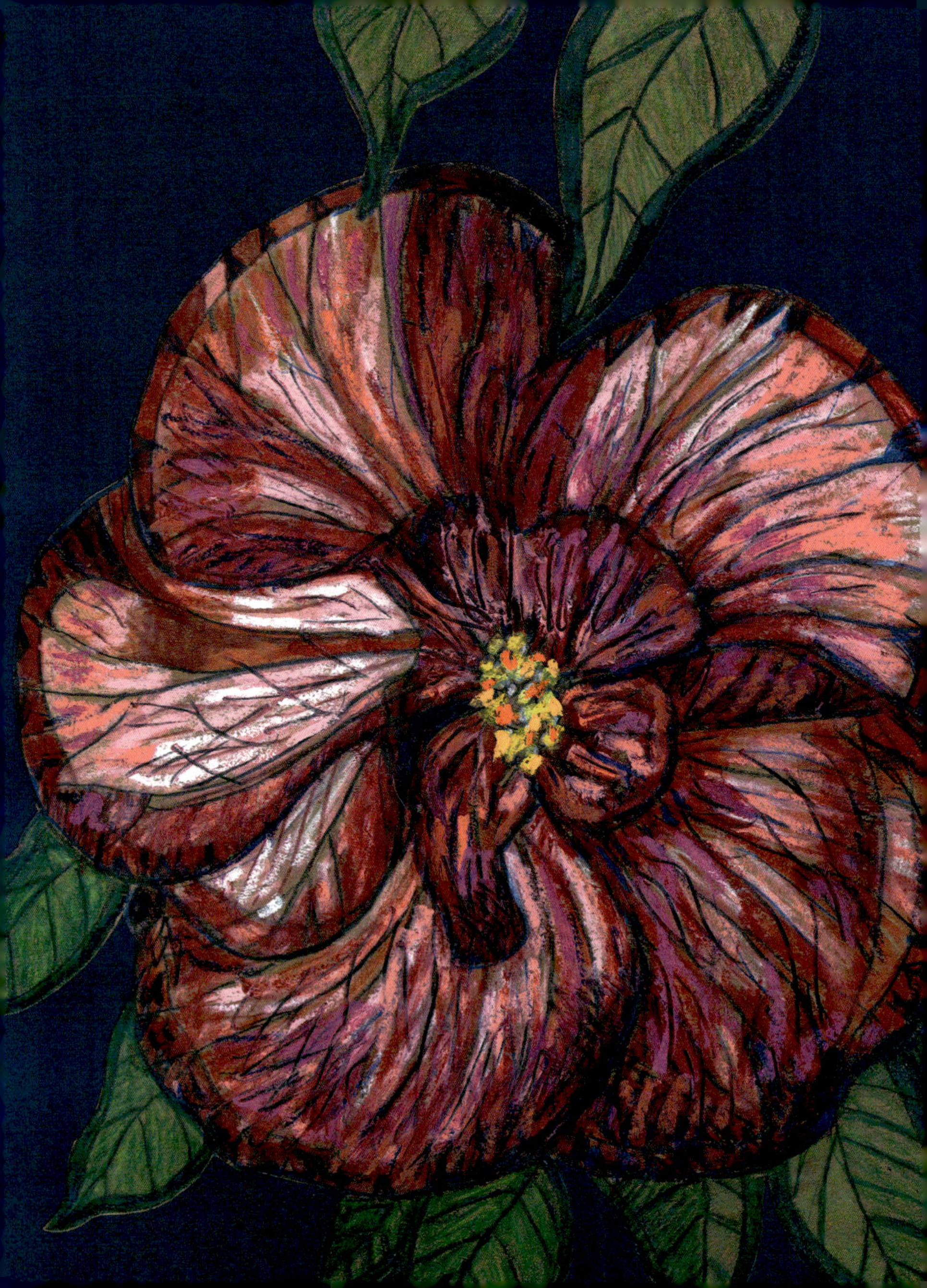

CHAPTER 7

HEAL YOUR SKIN AND HAIR

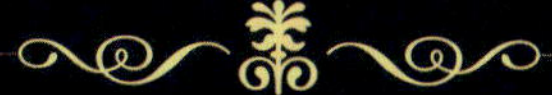

These rituals for taking care of your hair and skin are not vanity but devotion. They are gentle acts that restore balance, soften time's damages, and invite the return of your natural radiance.

For centuries, people have turned to plants for beauty and renewal. Egyptian queens bathed in rose water; Roman women brewed chamomile for beautiful skin; herbalists crushed nettle and aloe into healing tonics. Each act, though simple, reminds us that beauty is born from care and—most importantly—self-love. In this chapter, you'll find teas to pamper the complexion, bath blends to soothe the body, and balms and masks to heal your skin and hair. Each ingredient offers its own unique contribution to your most beautiful self.

Slow down a bit. Create with gratitude and remember now and then to take a deep breath. Let's start with our yummy *Glowing Beauty Tea* for youthful skin and hair that dazzles. You deserve it!

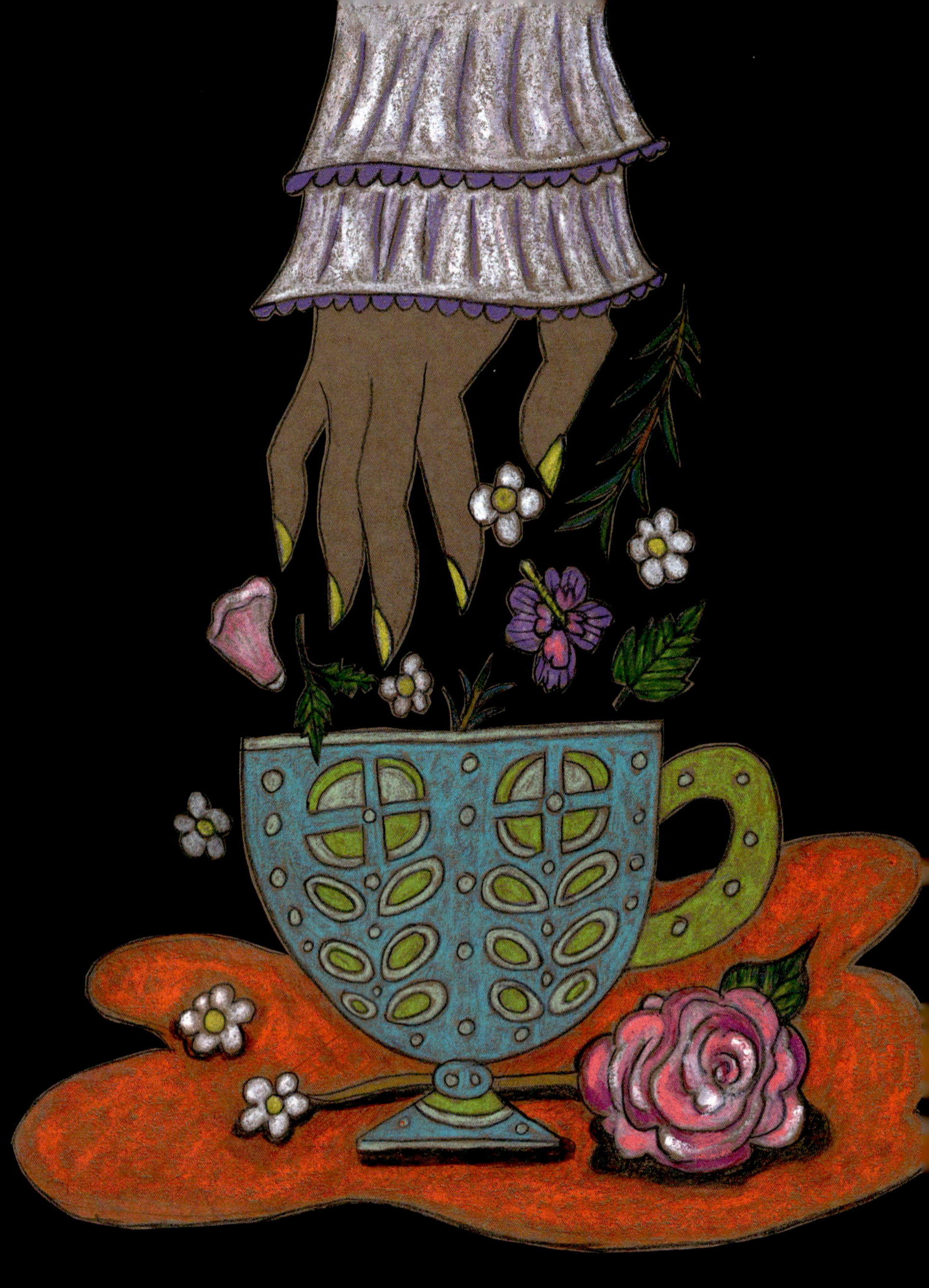

Glowing Beauty Tea

(Serves 2)

A gentle, nourishing blend designed to promote glowing
skin and healthy hair from the inside out.

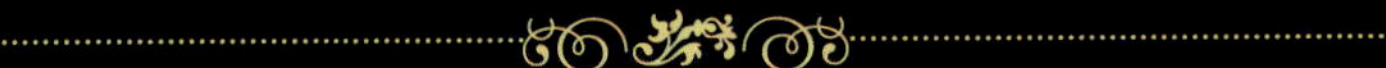

1 teaspoon dried nettle leaves
1 teaspoon dried rose petals
1 teaspoon dried hibiscus flowers
1 teaspoon chamomile flowers
½ teaspoon rosemary leaves
2 cups water

Combine the nettle leaves, rose petals, hibiscus flowers, chamomile flowers, and rosemary leaves in a bowl.

Bring water to a boil.

Place herb mixture into a teapot or tea infuser. Pour the hot water over the herbs and cover to steep for 7 to 10 minutes. Strain through a fine mesh sieve into cups, discarding spent herbs into your compost bin.

As you sip your tea, take a moment to appreciate how each plant supports your natural radiance.

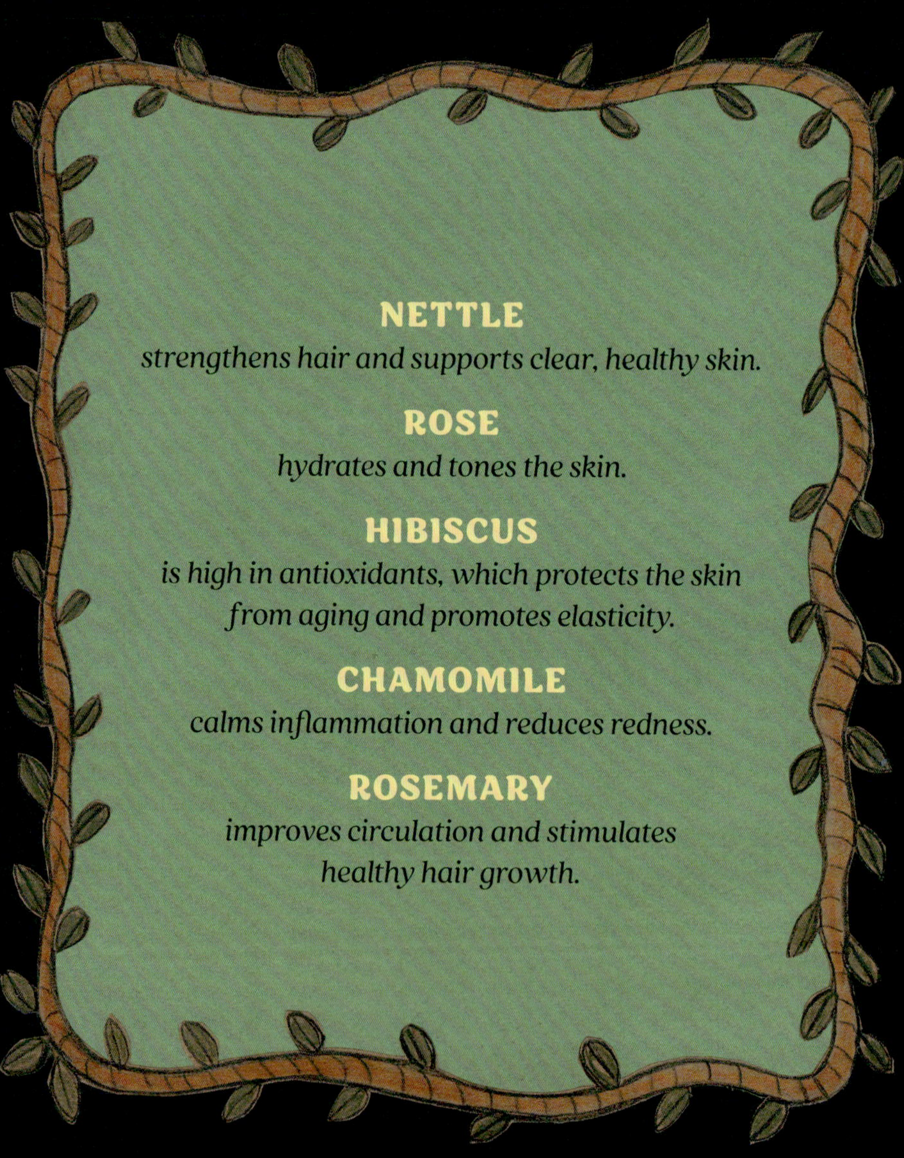

NETTLE
strengthens hair and supports clear, healthy skin.

ROSE
hydrates and tones the skin.

HIBISCUS
is high in antioxidants, which protects the skin
from aging and promotes elasticity.

CHAMOMILE
calms inflammation and reduces redness.

ROSEMARY
improves circulation and stimulates
healthy hair growth.

Did You Know?

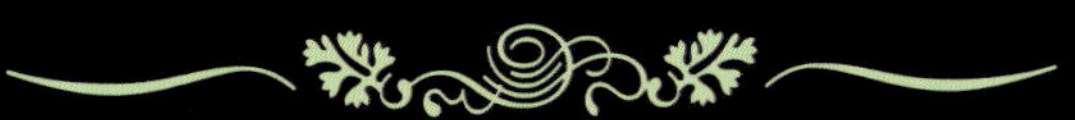

In ancient Egypt, hibiscus was used in teas for radiant skin and shiny hair, and rose water was Cleopatra's secret for soft skin. Nettle was used in recipes in medieval Europe for strengthening the hair. Chamomile was added to herbal baths by Roman women for soft, glowing skin. Rosemary was known as the "herb of remembrance" in literature and linked to youth and clear skin.

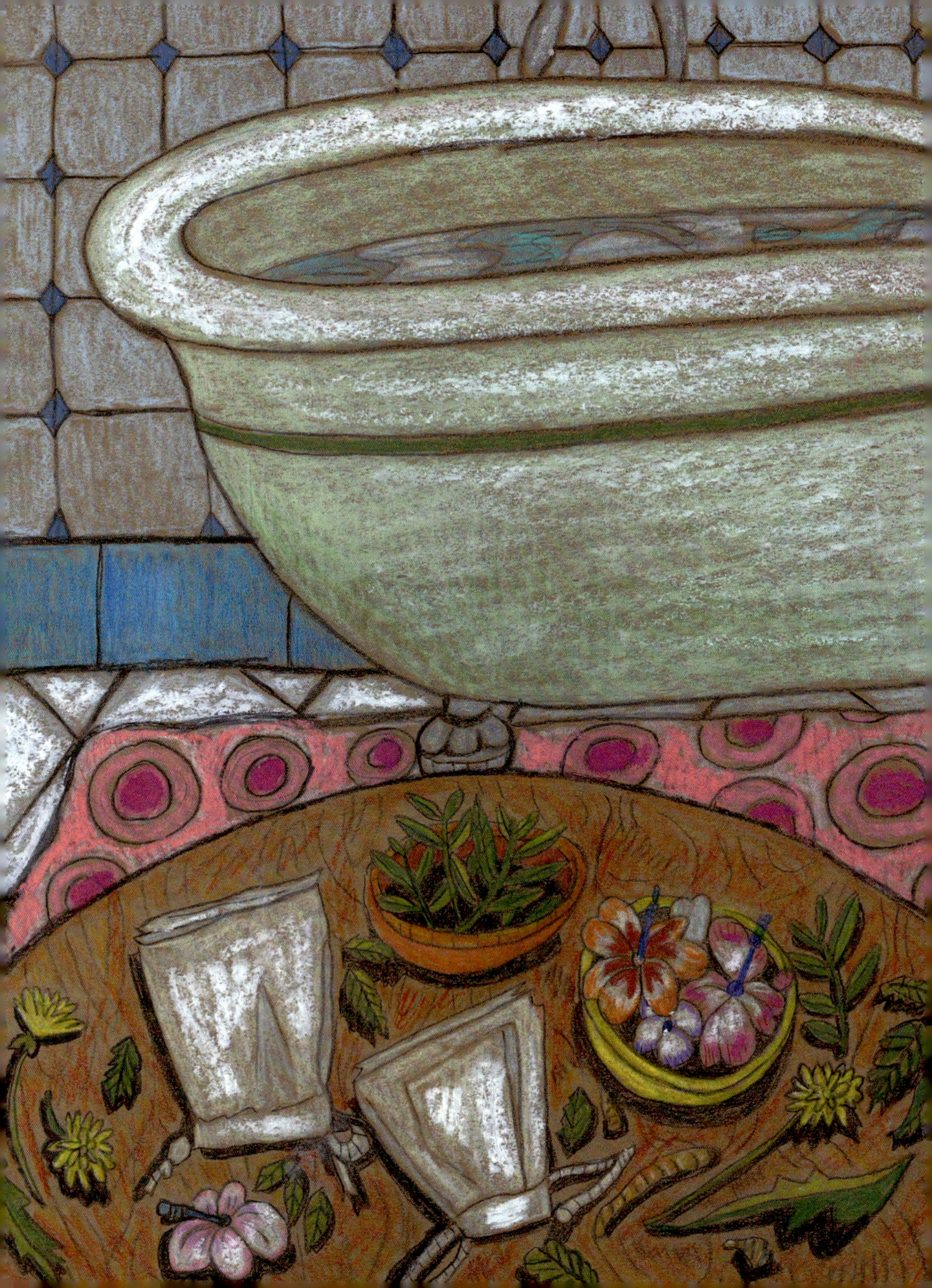

Phoenix Renewal Bath Tea

(Makes 1 bath)

For glowing skin and revitalized hair.

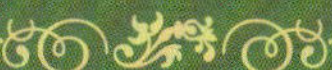

1 teaspoon dried nettle leaves
1 teaspoon dried dandelion root
1 teaspoon dried lemon verbena
1 teaspoon dried peppermint leaves
1 teaspoon dried hibiscus flowers
4 cups water
1 sachet bag with drawstring

In a bowl, combine the nettle leaves, dandelion root, lemon verbena, peppermint leaves, and hibiscus flowers. Spoon the mixture into your bath sachet bag and tie closed.

Bring water to a boil in a pot, then remove from the heat. Place the bag into the hot water and let it steep for 10 to 15 minutes, creating a richly colored infusion. Pour the entire brew—bag and all—into your warm bath.

As you soak, close your eyes and imagine the bath cleansing away stress while restoring your skin's softness and your hair's natural shine.

Soak for 20 minutes. After your bath, empty the contents of the sachet into your compost bin.

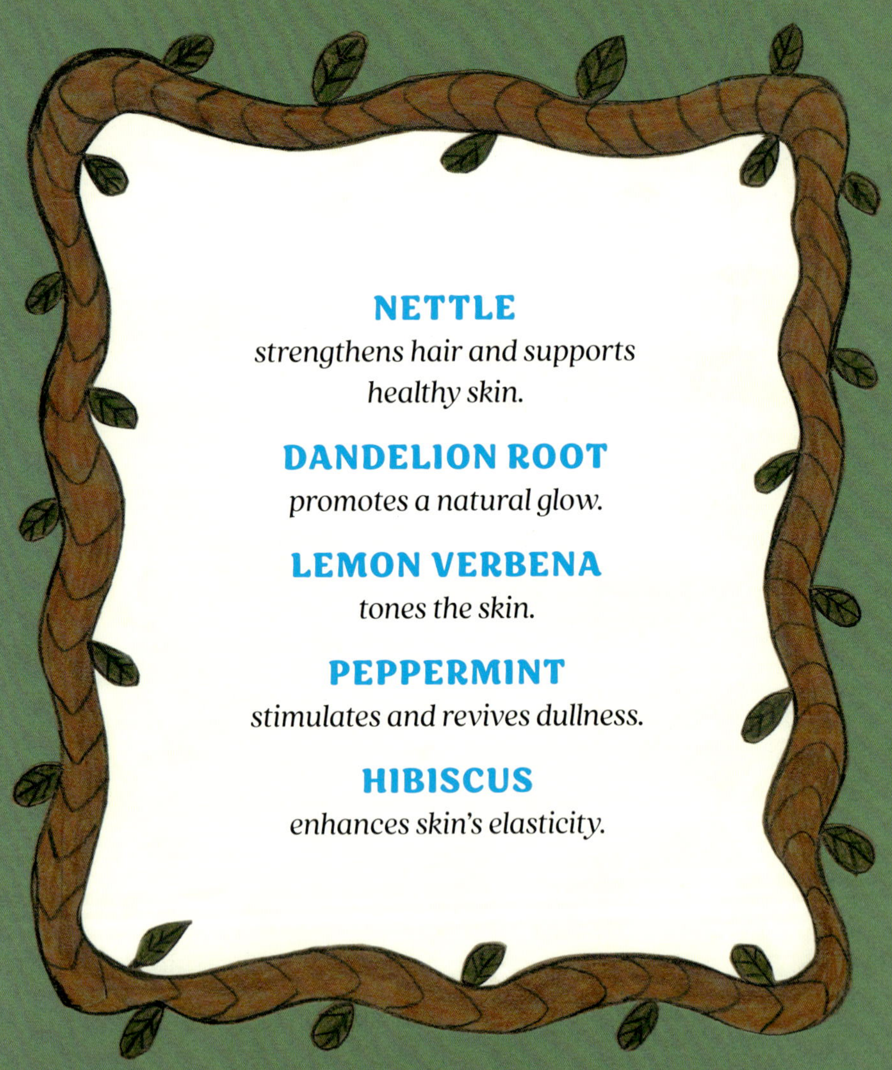

NETTLE
strengthens hair and supports healthy skin.

DANDELION ROOT
promotes a natural glow.

LEMON VERBENA
tones the skin.

PEPPERMINT
stimulates and revives dullness.

HIBISCUS
enhances skin's elasticity.

Did You Know?

In Japanese folklore, hot springs infused with herbs and minerals were used to heal not only physical but emotional wounds.

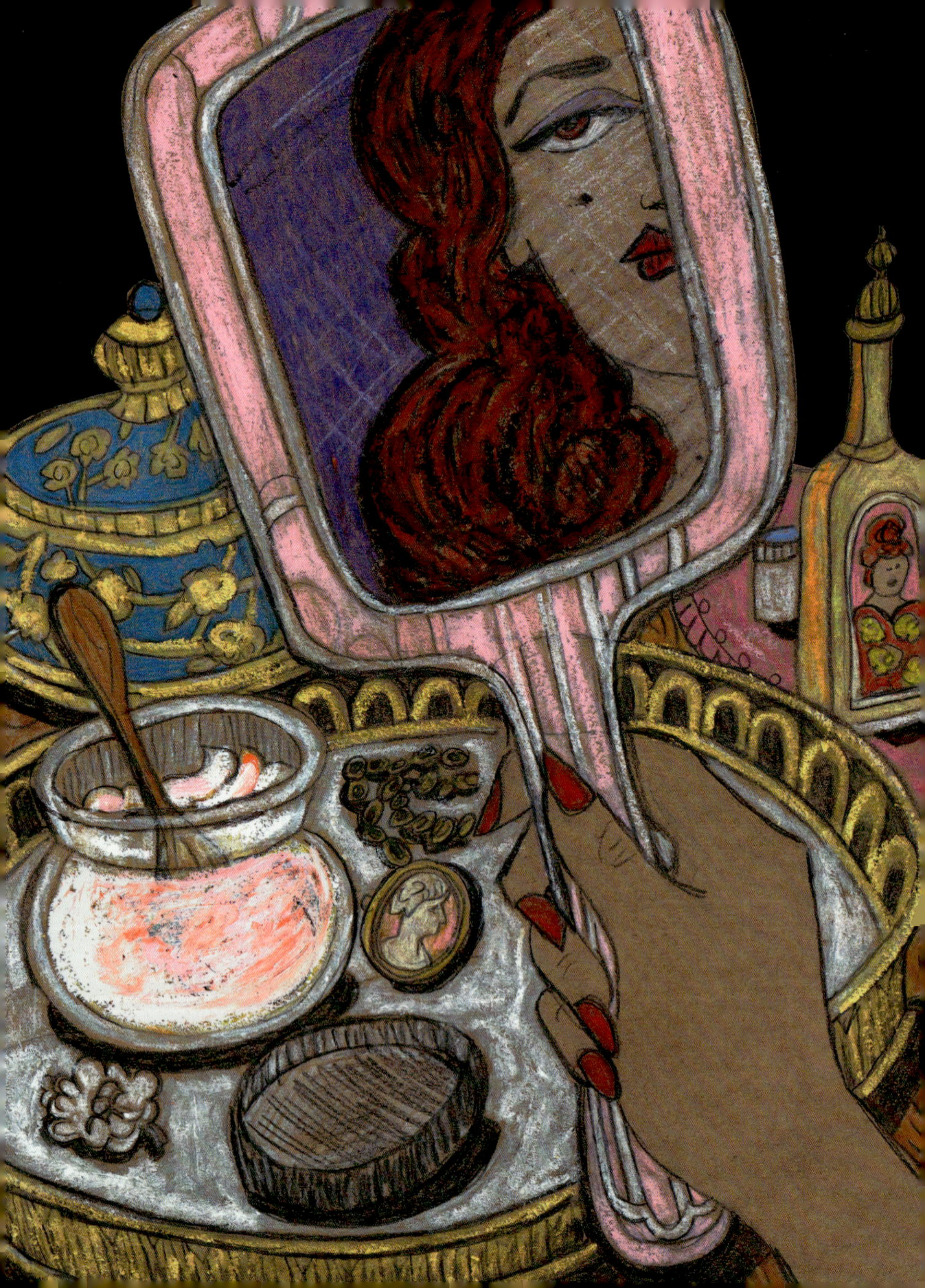

Peaches and Herbs Hand Lotion

(Makes about 6 ounces—enough for 1 small jar or 2 travel-size tins)

This soothing lotion hydrates and restores the skin's natural glow.

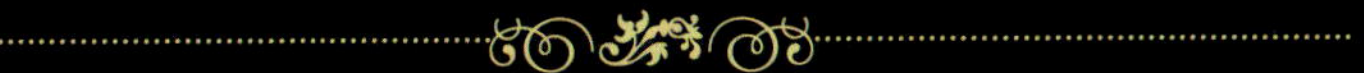

¼ cup shea butter
¼ cup coconut oil
5 drops peach essential oil
3 drops chamomile essential oil
1 tablespoon aloe vera gel
1 tablespoon rose water
1 teaspoon vitamin E oil

In a double boiler, combine the shea butter and coconut oil. Heat gently over a low simmer, stirring until fully melted. Remove from the heat.

Stir in peach essential oil, chamomile essential oil, aloe vera gel, rose water, and vitamin E oil.

Allow the mixture to cool for about 10 to 15 minutes, then use a whisk to whip vigorously until it becomes light and fluffy.

Spoon the lotion into a clean glass jar and allow it to cool completely before sealing the jar.

Massage the cream into your hands as needed. Take a moment to remind yourself that caring for your skin is a small act of gratitude for all you do each day.

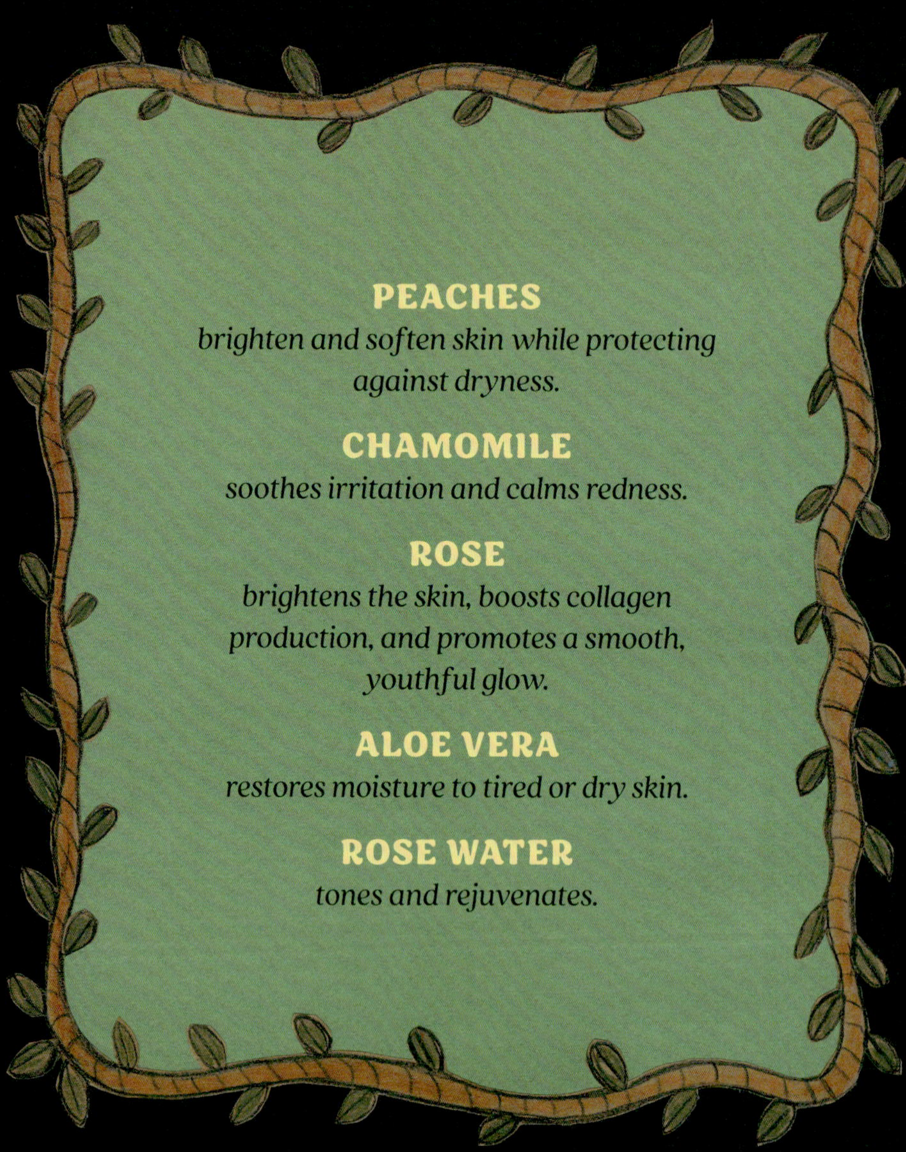

PEACHES
brighten and soften skin while protecting against dryness.

CHAMOMILE
soothes irritation and calms redness.

ROSE
brightens the skin, boosts collagen production, and promotes a smooth, youthful glow.

ALOE VERA
restores moisture to tired or dry skin.

ROSE WATER
tones and rejuvenates.

Did You Know?

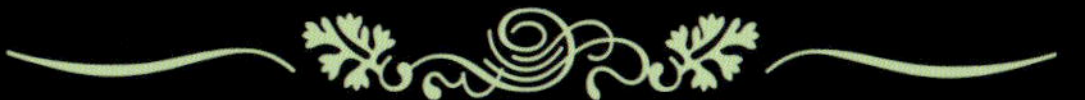

Peaches were cultivated in China more than 4,000 years ago, where they were treasured as symbols of immortality, vitality, and good fortune. Early Chinese writings depict peaches as a sacred fruit of the gods.

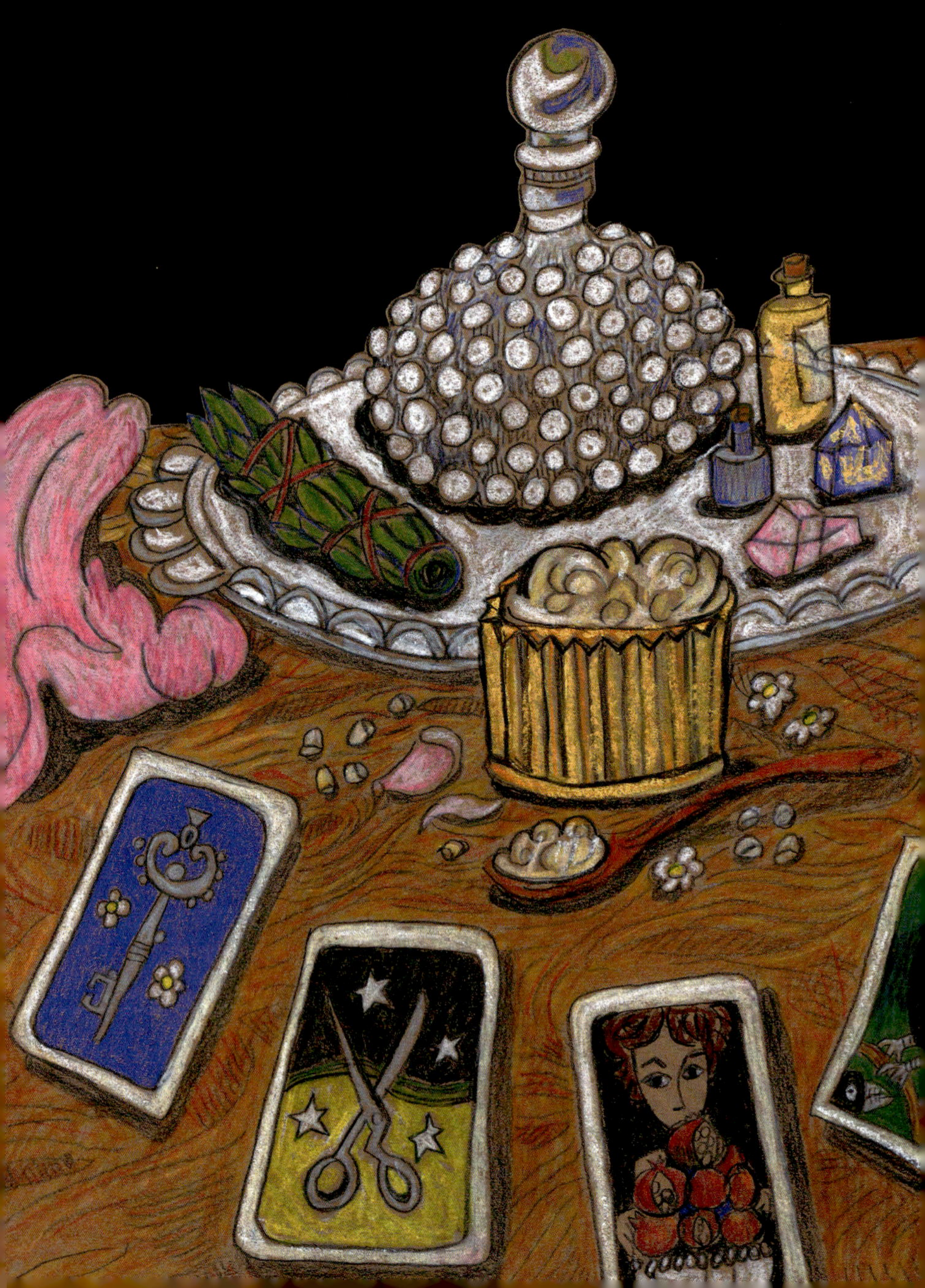

Nourishing Oatmeal Body Scrub

(Makes about 8 ounces—enough for 3–4 full-body applications)

A soothing scrub that softens, hydrates, and restores the skin's natural glow.

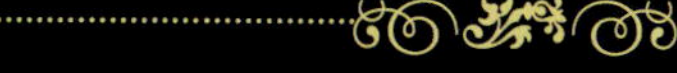

½ cup finely ground rolled oats
2 tablespoons brown sugar
2 drops chamomile essential oil
¼ cup coconut oil, melted
1 tablespoon maple syrup
½ teaspoon vanilla extract

In a medium bowl, combine the oats, brown sugar, and chamomile oil. Add the melted coconut oil, maple syrup, and vanilla, stirring until a thick, creamy texture forms.

Spoon the mixture into a clean glass jar with a tight lid—we love to recycle pickle or jelly jars.

To use, scoop a handful and gently massage onto damp skin in circular motions. As you exfoliate, breathe deeply and imagine releasing what no longer serves you—letting softness and calm return to your skin and spirit. Rinse with warm water.

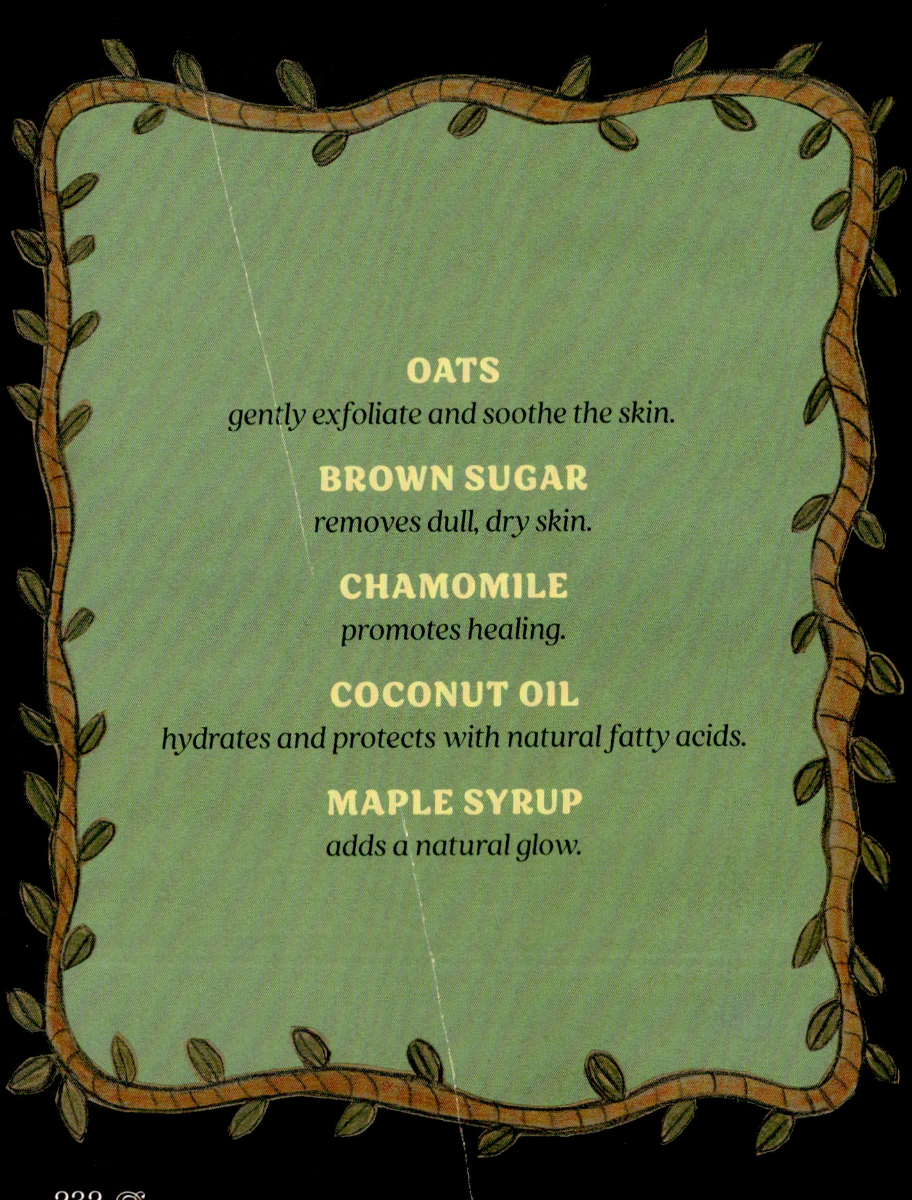

OATS
gently exfoliate and soothe the skin.

BROWN SUGAR
removes dull, dry skin.

CHAMOMILE
promotes healing.

COCONUT OIL
hydrates and protects with natural fatty acids.

MAPLE SYRUP
adds a natural glow.

Did You Know?

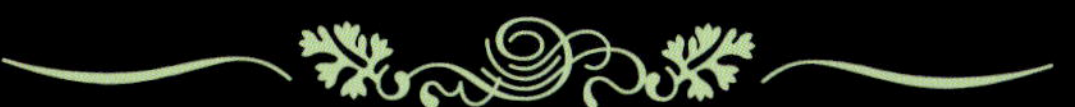

Long before we were buying pricey body scrubs at beauty supply stores, Indigenous cultures all around the world were using natural exfoliants like clay, cornmeal, or crushed shells to cleanse and renew the skin before important ceremonies.

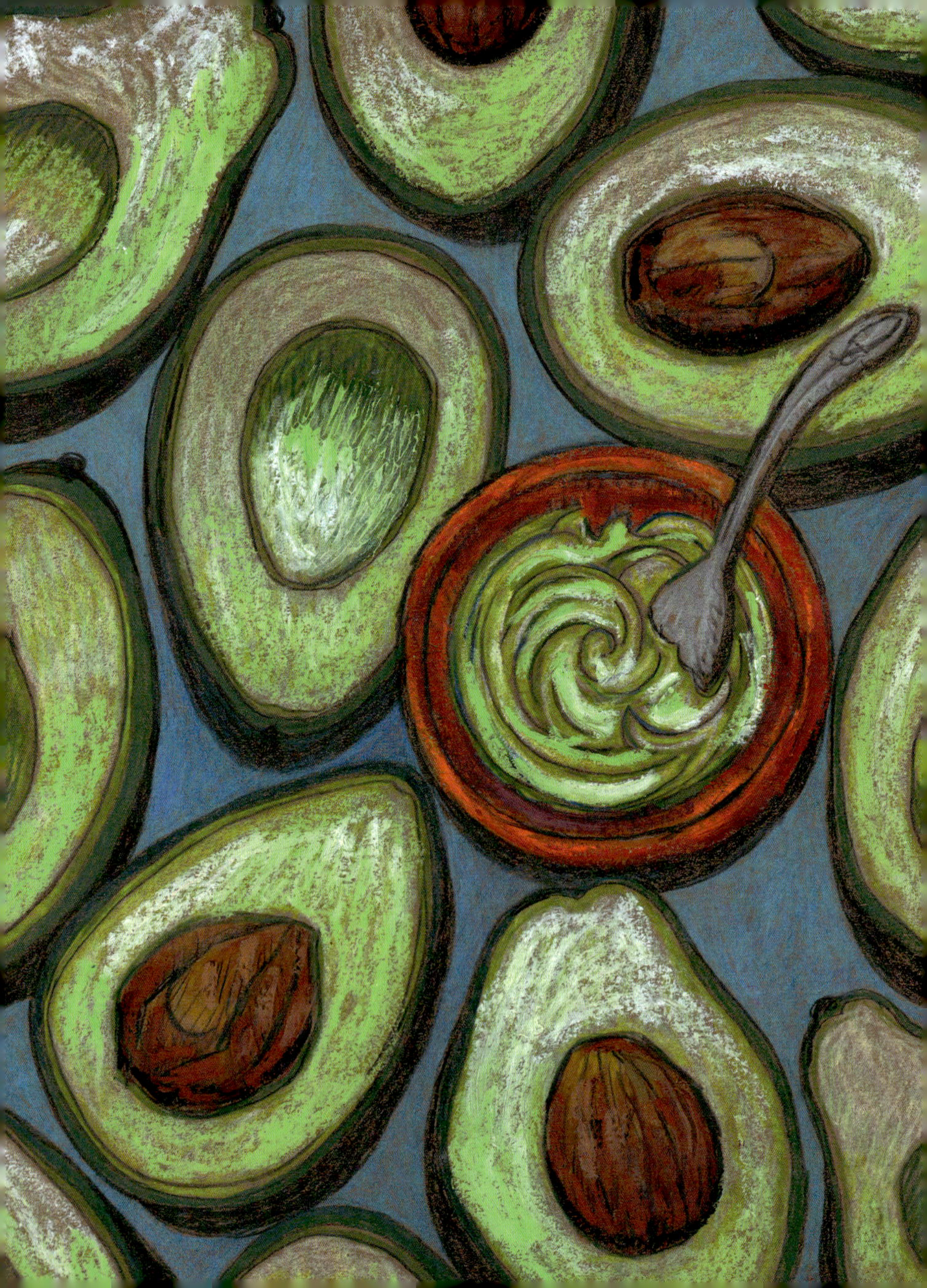

Avocado Hair Mask

This nourishing hair mask deeply hydrates, strengthens, and restores shine, leaving hair soft and revitalized.

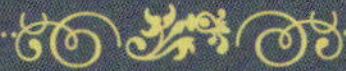

1 ripe avocado
1 tablespoon olive oil
1 teaspoon lemon juice

Cut the avocado in half, remove the pit, and scoop the flesh into a medium bowl. Use a fork to mash the avocado until it's smooth and free of lumps. Add the olive oil and lemon juice to the mashed avocado. Mix well.

Apply the mask to damp hair, focusing on the ends. Breathe deeply and slowly. Take your time as you apply. You're being kind to yourself—there is no need to rush!

Leave the hair mask on for 30 minutes. Rinse the mask out with warm water and then shampoo and condition your hair as usual.

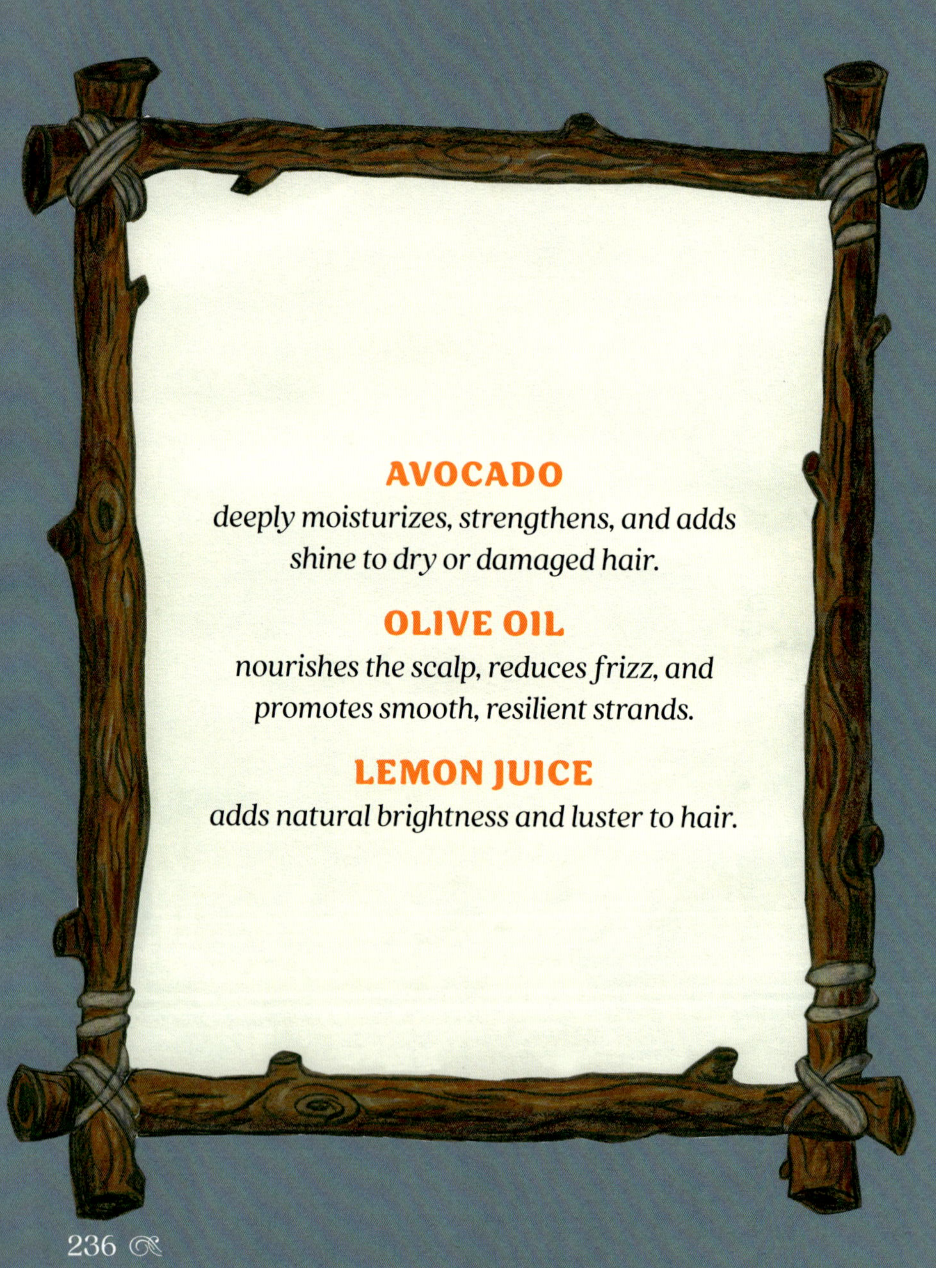

AVOCADO

deeply moisturizes, strengthens, and adds shine to dry or damaged hair.

OLIVE OIL

nourishes the scalp, reduces frizz, and promotes smooth, resilient strands.

LEMON JUICE

adds natural brightness and luster to hair.

Did You Know?

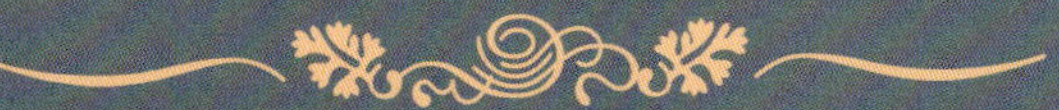

Avocados were discovered growing in south-central Mexico more than 5,000 years ago, where they were cultivated by ancient civilizations such as the Aztecs and the Maya. Avocados were valued for their rich flavor and nourishing oils.

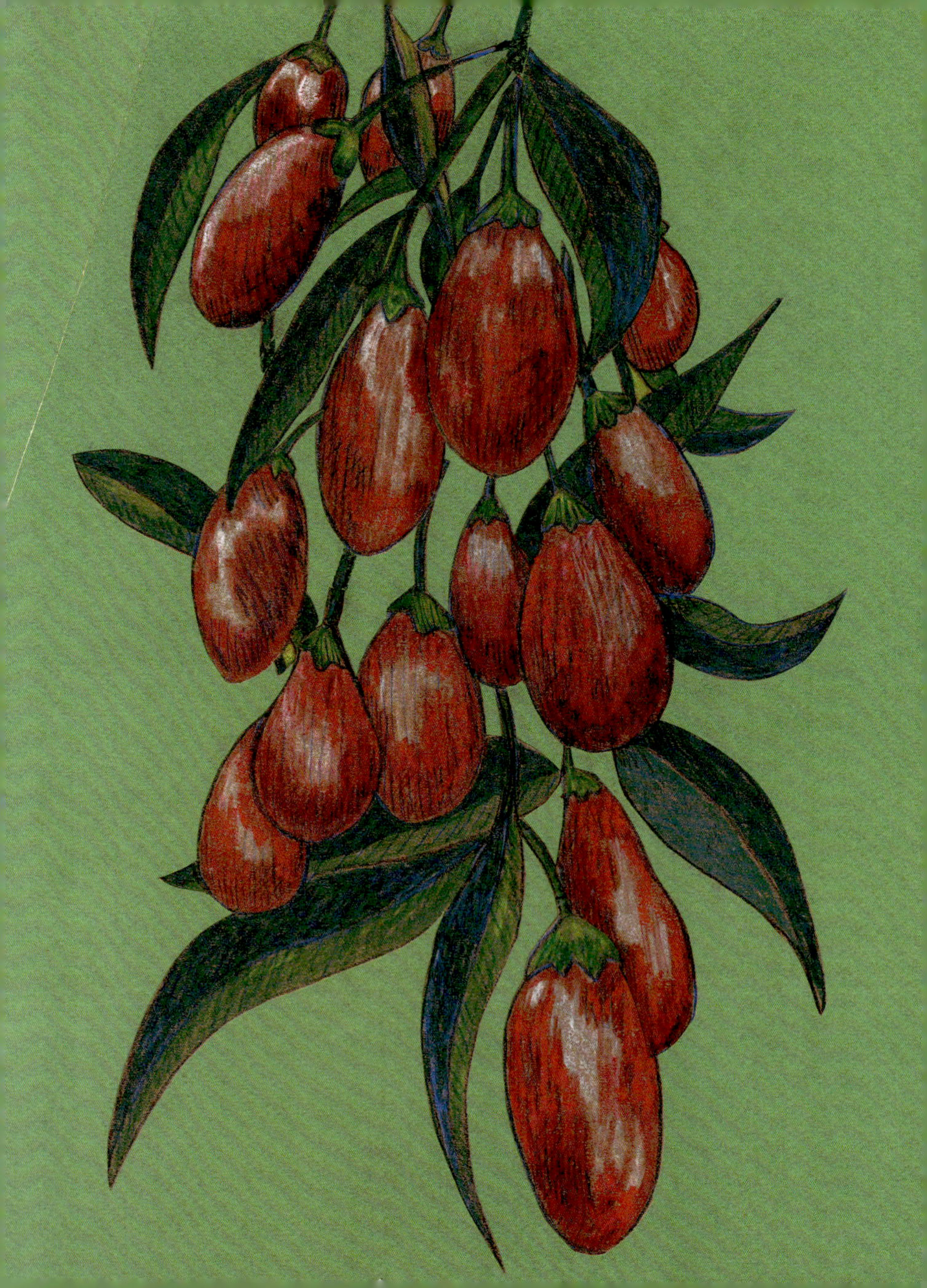

Goji Berry Trail Mix

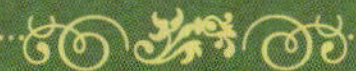

(Makes 4–5 servings)

Enjoy as a healthy snack or as a topping for salads, oatmeal, or yogurt.

½ cup raw almonds, chopped
½ cup walnuts, chopped
½ cup roasted pumpkin seeds
½ cup dried goji berries
½ cup dried cranberries
½ cup unsweetened coconut flakes
Pinch of sea salt

Place all ingredients into a large bowl. Gently toss until combined.

As you mix, take a second to notice the textures and aromas of each ingredient. Give a moment of thanks for how they will nourish you.

Transfer the trail mix to an airtight container such as a glass jar with a tight-fitting lid. It can be stored at room temperature for up to 2 weeks.

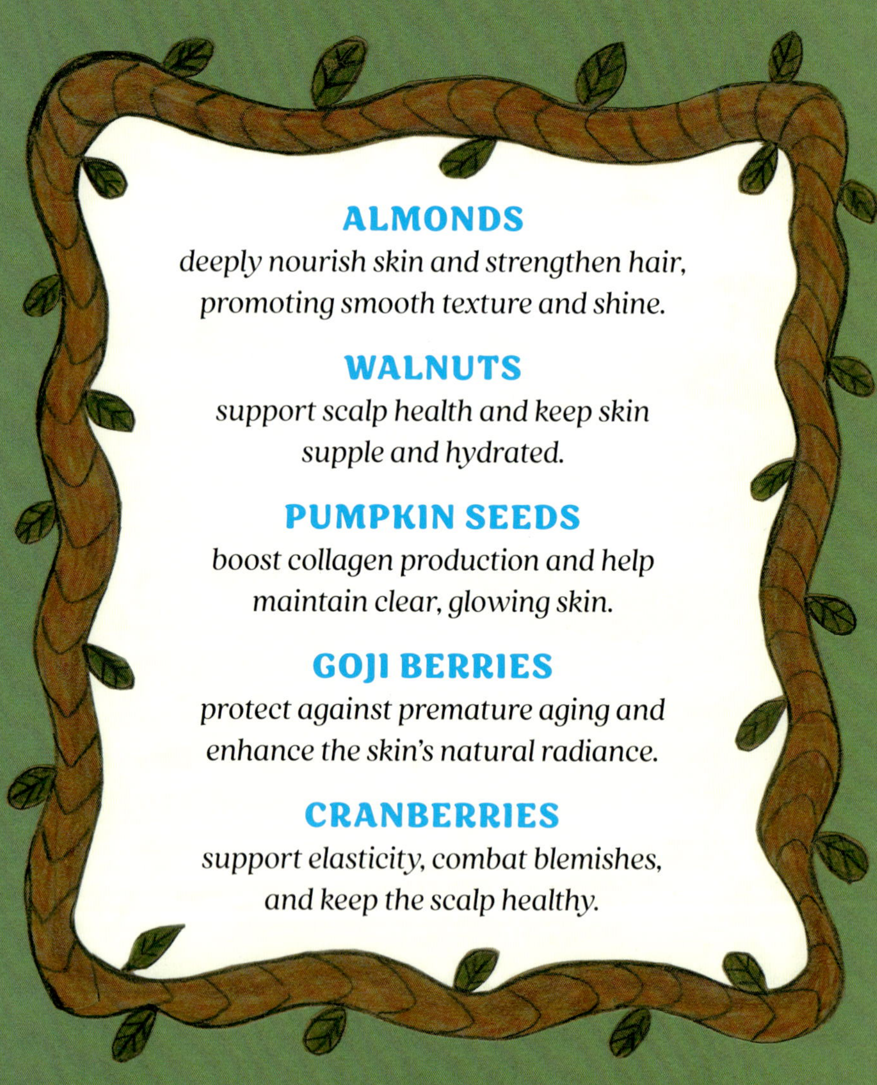

ALMONDS

deeply nourish skin and strengthen hair,
promoting smooth texture and shine.

WALNUTS

support scalp health and keep skin
supple and hydrated.

PUMPKIN SEEDS

boost collagen production and help
maintain clear, glowing skin.

GOJI BERRIES

protect against premature aging and
enhance the skin's natural radiance.

CRANBERRIES

support elasticity, combat blemishes,
and keep the scalp healthy.

Did You Know?

Trail mix originated as a convenient, energy-boosting snack for outdoor adventurers. Its earliest versions have roots in Indigenous cultures. Dried fruits, nuts, and seeds were used for portable nourishment during long journeys.

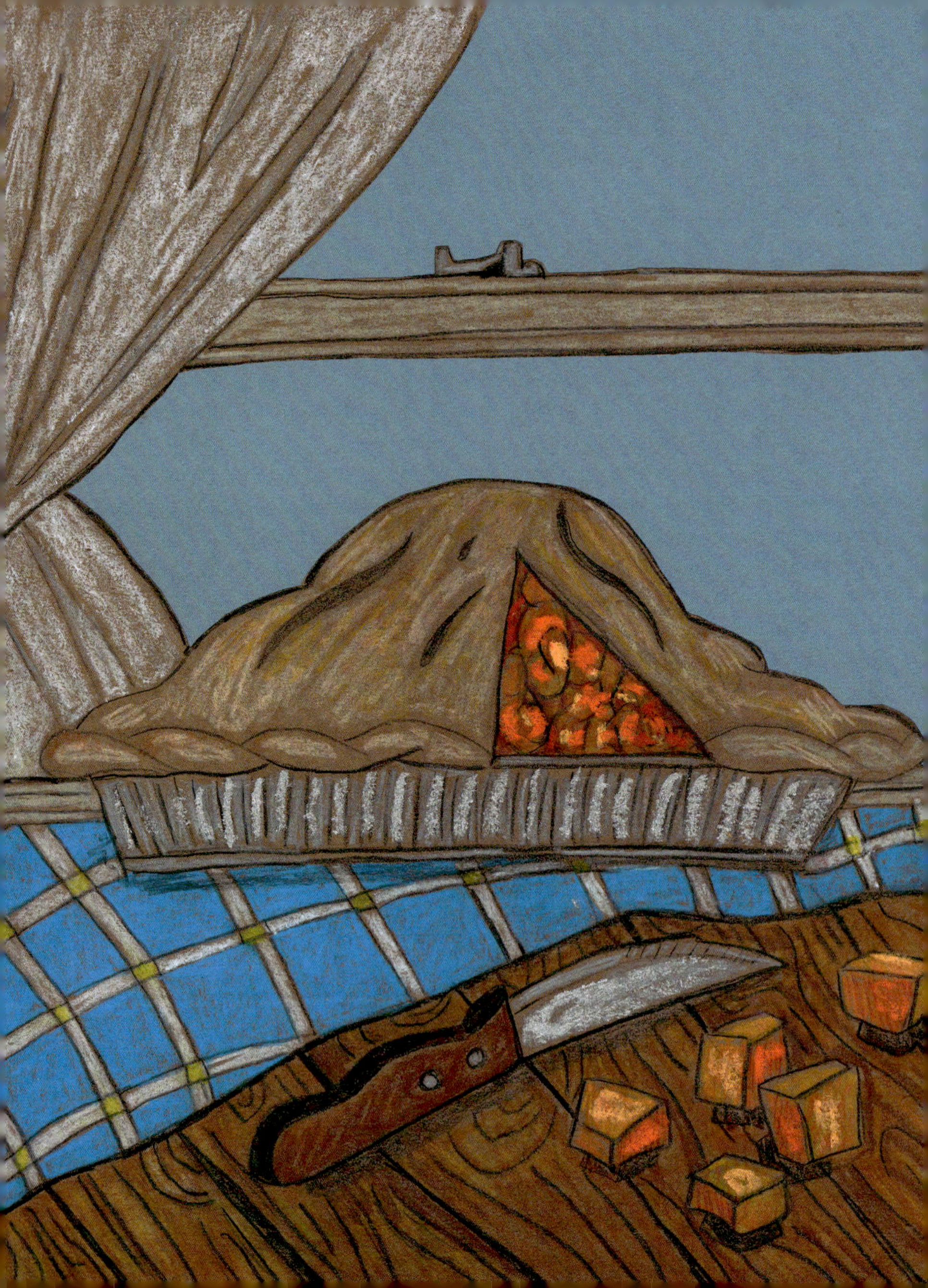

Sweet Potato Pie

(Serves 6–8)

This nourishing pie is rich in vitamins, antioxidants that support glowing skin and strong, vibrant hair. It's also delicious!

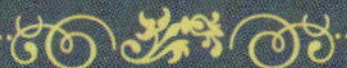

3 medium sweet potatoes, peeled and cubed
1 cup almond milk, plus 1 tablespoon for brushing the top crust
¾ cup brown sugar
¼ cup maple syrup
1 teaspoon vanilla extract
1 teaspoon ground cinnamon
½ teaspoon ground nutmeg
½ teaspoon ground ginger
¼ teaspoon salt
1 tablespoon flour
2 (9-inch) store-bought vegan pie crusts

Bring a large pot of water to a rolling boil. Add sweet potatoes and cook until tender, about 15 to 20 minutes. Drain, cool slightly, transfer to a large bowl, and mash until smooth. You should have about 2 cups mashed sweet potato.

Heat oven to 350°F.

Add almond milk, brown sugar, maple syrup, vanilla extract, cinnamon, nutmeg, ginger, salt, and flour to sweet potatoes. Mix until smooth. As you stir, inhale the comforting aroma of spices rising from the bowl. Appreciate what a delicious treat you are creating!

Tuck one pie crust into a pie dish and spoon in the sweet potato filling, smoothing the top. Cover with the second crust and seal by crimping the edges. Cut several steam vents in the top crust. Using a pastry brush, swipe a thin coat of remaining almond milk across the top crust.

Bake for 45 to 50 minutes, or until the crust is lightly golden. Allow the pie to cool for at least 1 hour before slicing.

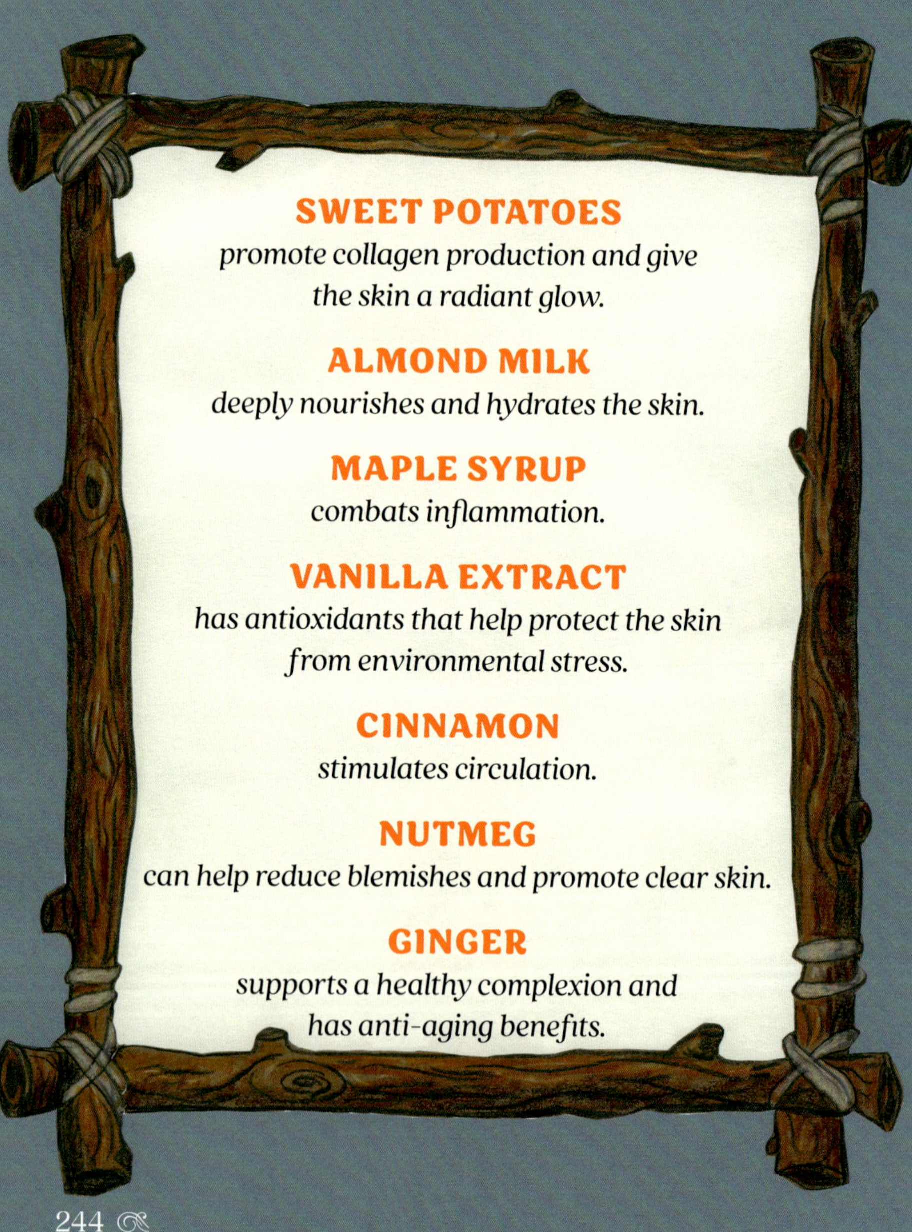

SWEET POTATOES
promote collagen production and give
the skin a radiant glow.

ALMOND MILK
deeply nourishes and hydrates the skin.

MAPLE SYRUP
combats inflammation.

VANILLA EXTRACT
has antioxidants that help protect the skin
from environmental stress.

CINNAMON
stimulates circulation.

NUTMEG
can help reduce blemishes and promote clear skin.

GINGER
supports a healthy complexion and
has anti-aging benefits.

Did You Know?

The origin of sweet potato pie is in African-American culinary history. It can be traced back to West Africa, where yams, which are similar in texture and flavor to sweet potatoes, were a dietary staple often mashed, seasoned, and baked. After enslaved Africans were transported to the Americas, they created new recipes inspired by traditions from Africa but using local ingredients. Soon, the sweet potato pie we know today was born. We give thanks to those souls for creating this delicious treat.

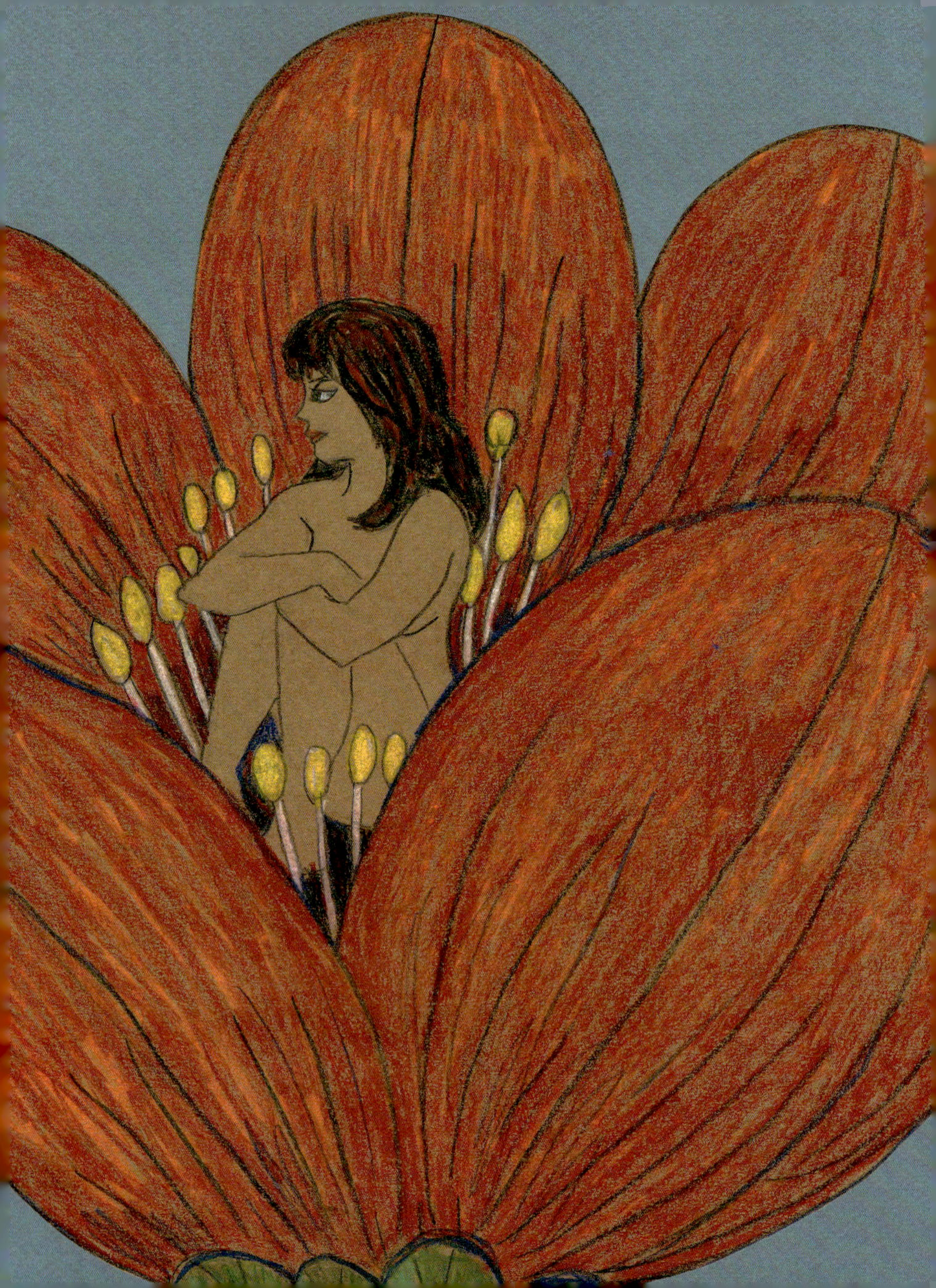

CHAPTER 8

HEAL YOUR SOUL

To heal your soul is to remember you are more than busy days and endless lists; you are someone who longs for grounding and calm. Wellness here is a soft practice such as lighting a candle, opening a window to let in the night air, or sipping a warm tea.

Throughout time, people have cared for their spirits through rituals like tying ribbons to wishing trees, collecting shells and stones for comfort, and scattering rose petals for love. Each simple act reminds us to pause, breathe, and smile.

In this chapter, we have teas to ease sorrow and bring joy, mists to refresh the spirit, and simmer pots to bring warmth to a room. Never rush as you make your recipes.

We'll weave mindfulness into every step and invite nature in. Maybe put some rosemary by the sink for courage, a stone on your desk for grounding, or a bowl of lemons on the kitchen table for joy.

Now raise a cup to the night, with our soothing *Full Moon Tea*.

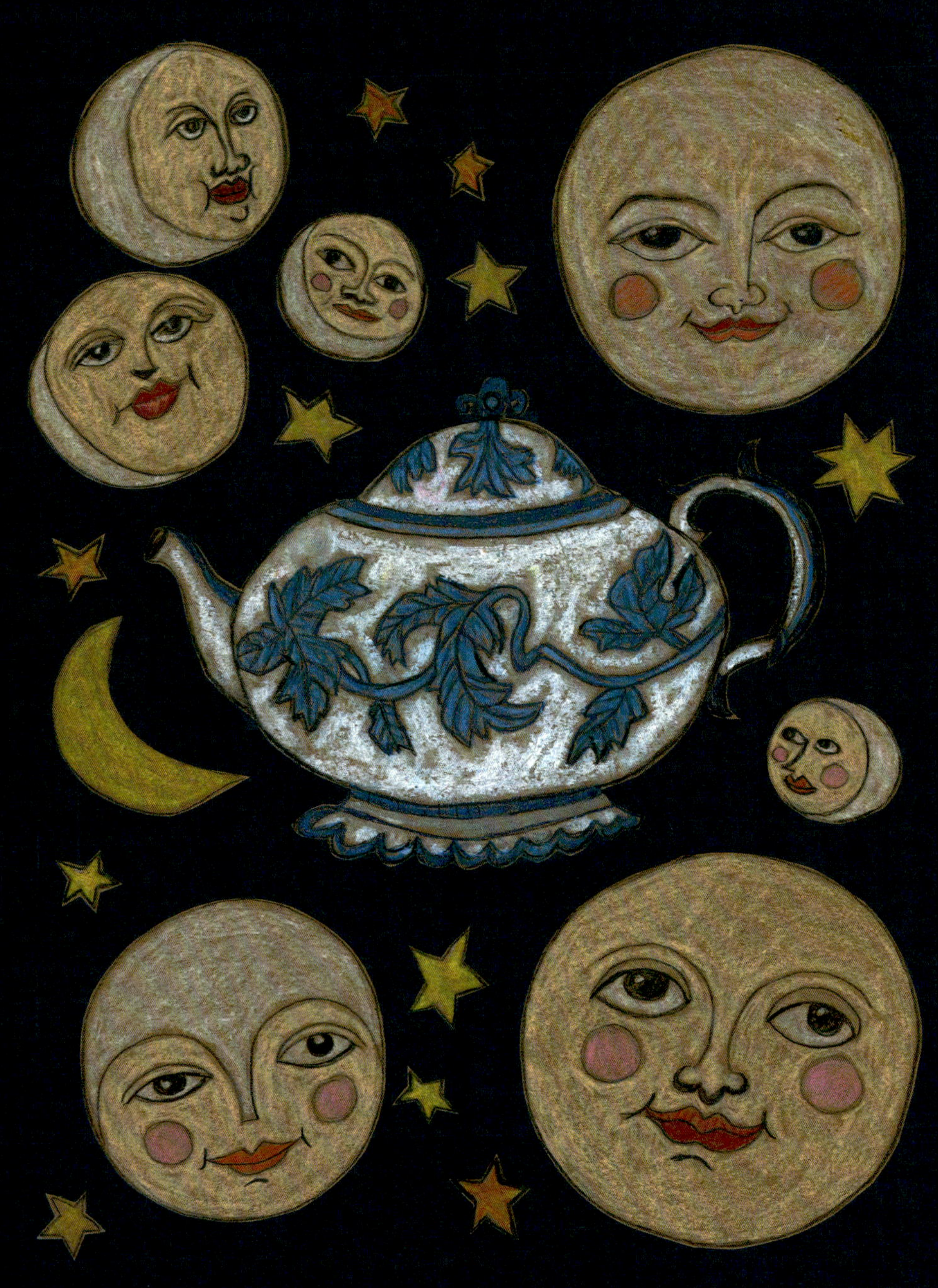

Full Moon Tea

A soothing blend to sip beneath the glow of the moon.

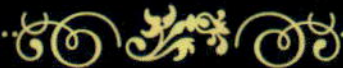

1 teaspoon dried chamomile flowers
1 teaspoon dried lavender buds
1 teaspoon dried lemon balm leaves
1 teaspoon dried rose petals
1 piece fresh ginger, about the size of a quarter
2 cups water

Combine the chamomile flowers, lavender buds, lemon balm leaves, rose petals, and fresh ginger in a small bowl.

Bring water to a boil.

Place 1 tablespoon of the herbal mixture into a tea infuser or teapot. Pour hot water over the herbs and cover to steep for 7 to 10 minutes. While the tea steeps, step outside or look out a window to admire the moon. Take a few slow breaths, imagining the moonlight filling you with calm energy.

Strain the tea into cups through a fine mesh sieve. Discard the spent herbs into the compost bin. Sip and enjoy this calming tea.

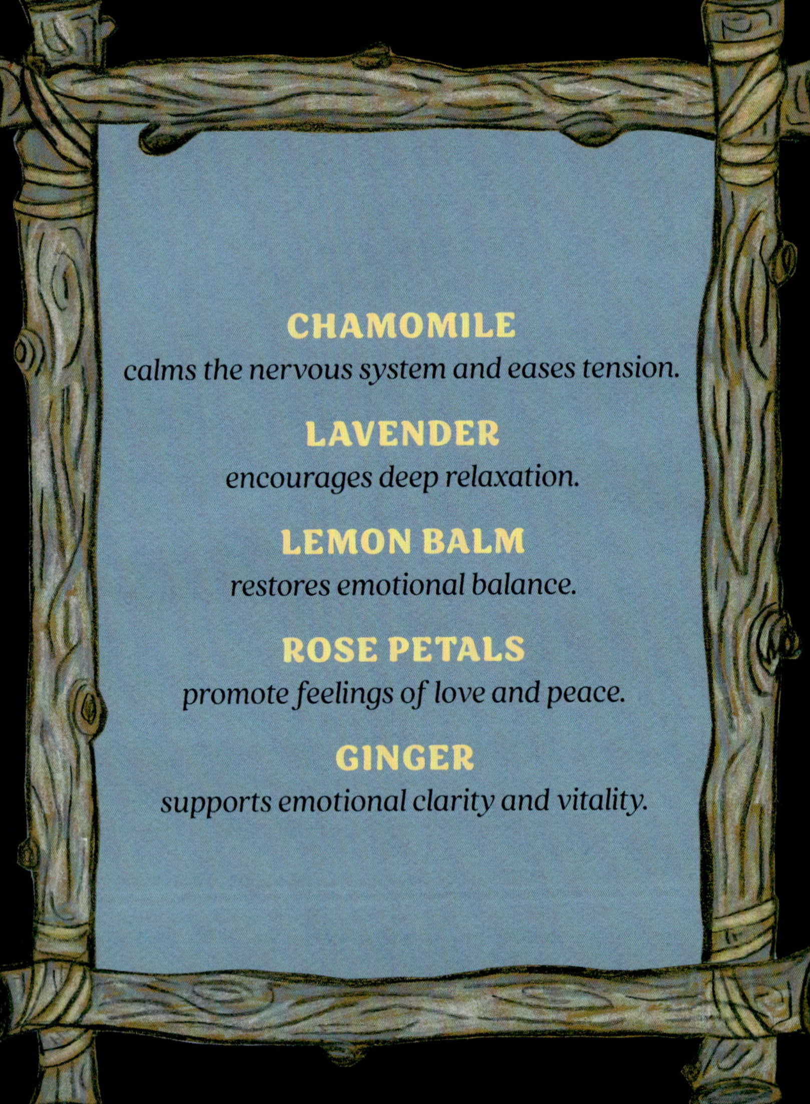

CHAMOMILE
calms the nervous system and eases tension.

LAVENDER
encourages deep relaxation.

LEMON BALM
restores emotional balance.

ROSE PETALS
promote feelings of love and peace.

GINGER
supports emotional clarity and vitality.

Did You Know?

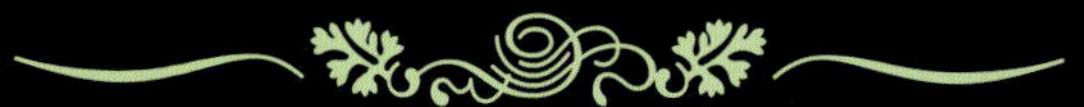

Spending time under a full moon can be deeply healing, as its light brings renewal, reflection, and emotional release. The moon's calming energy helps the mind quiet and the heart open. The full moon offers a moment to let go of what no longer serves you. So breathe in the night air and enjoy the beauty and healing power of the full moon with your tea!

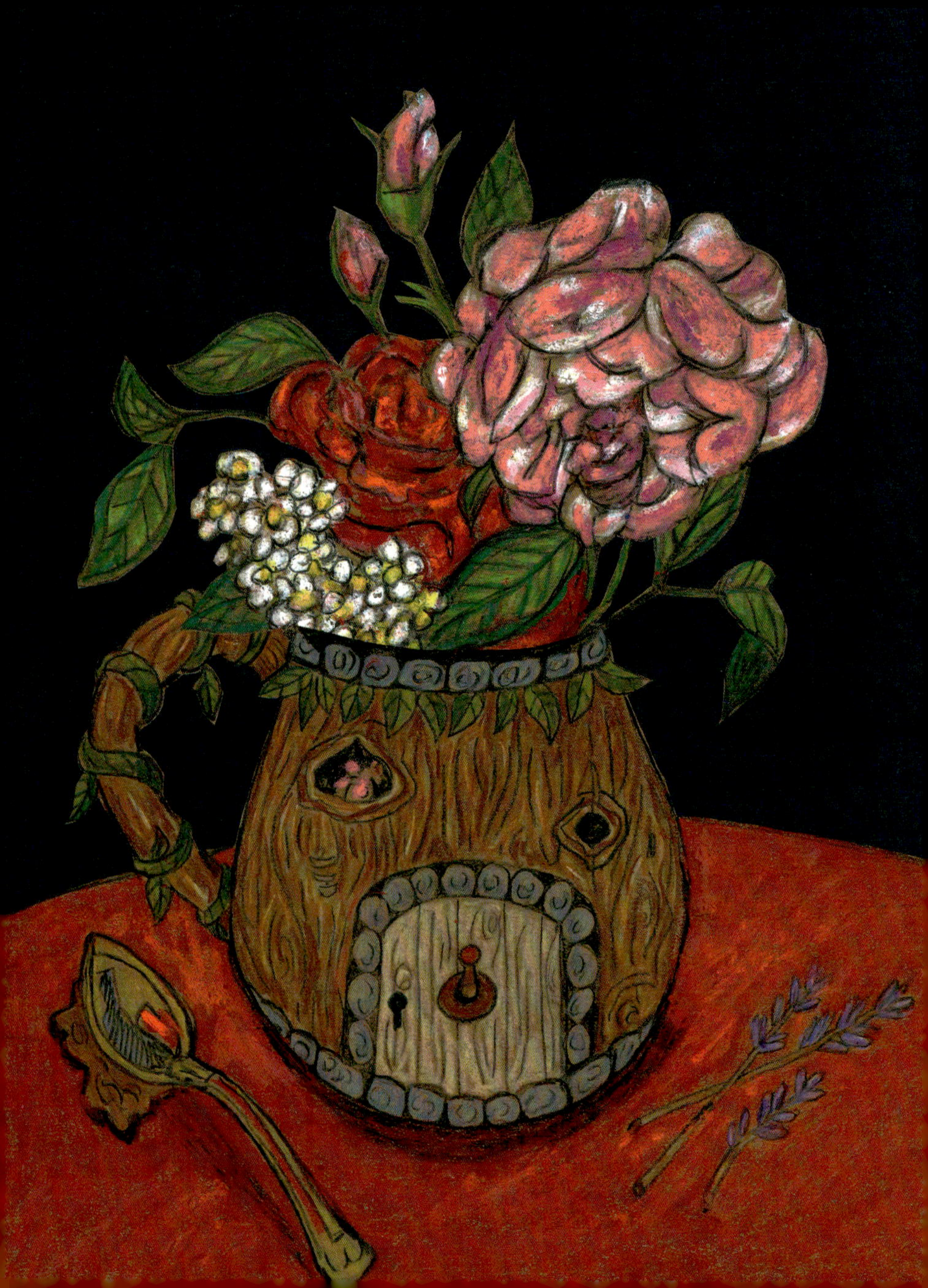

Titania's Nature Spirits Tea

(Serves 2)

Sit quietly with your tea, sipping slowly and enjoying the peaceful atmosphere you've created with the wee folk. Yes, we believe in fairies!

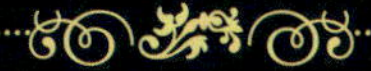

2 cups water
1 teaspoon dried chamomile flowers
1 teaspoon dried lavender flowers
1 teaspoon dried mint leaves
1 teaspoon dried rose petals
1 teaspoon agave sweetener (adjust to taste)

Bring water to a boil.

Place chamomile, lavender, mint, and rose petals into a teapot or infuser. Pour hot water over and allow tea to steep for 5 to 10 minutes.

Strain the tea into cups through a fine mesh sieve. Stir a spoonful of agave into each cup. Imagine that tiny sparks of inspiration and delight have gathered to share this moment with you.

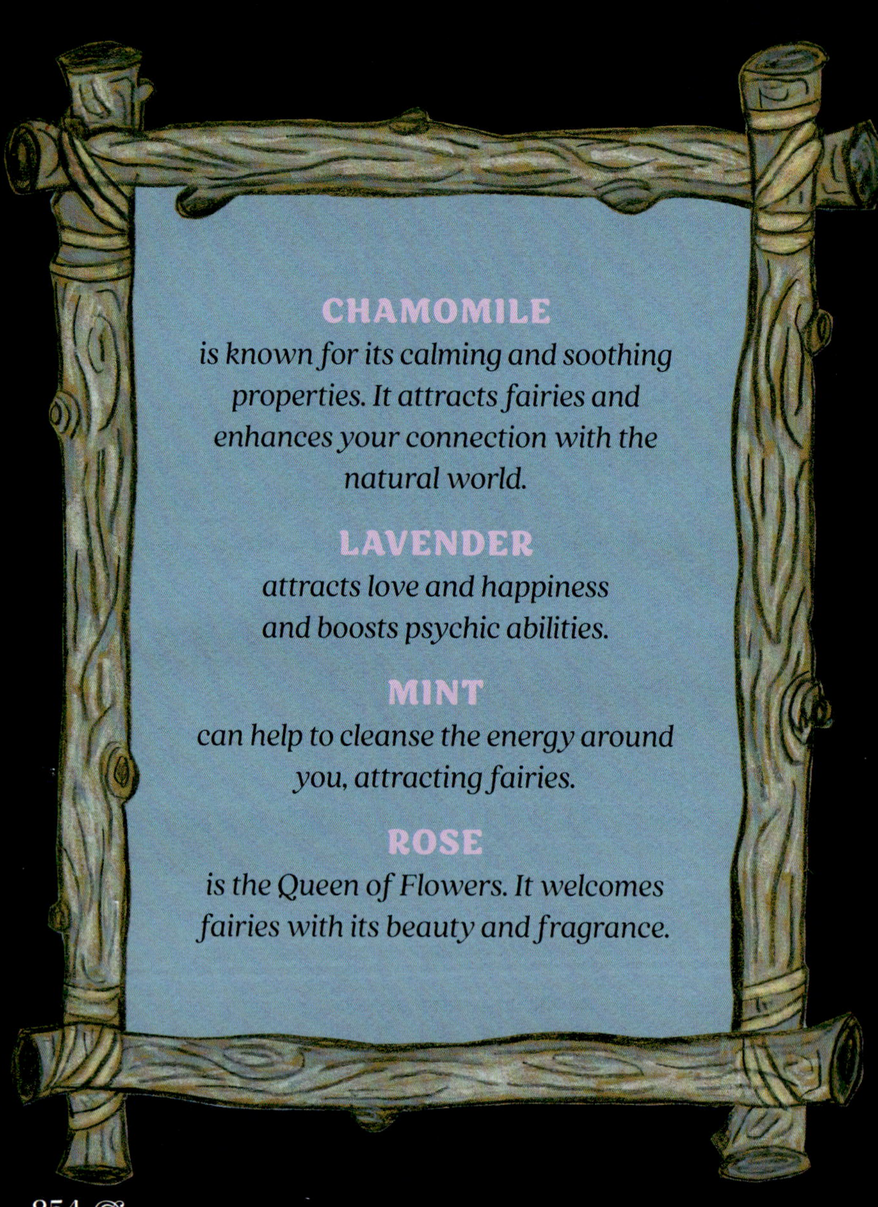

CHAMOMILE

is known for its calming and soothing
properties. It attracts fairies and
enhances your connection with the
natural world.

LAVENDER

attracts love and happiness
and boosts psychic abilities.

MINT

can help to cleanse the energy around
you, attracting fairies.

ROSE

is the Queen of Flowers. It welcomes
fairies with its beauty and fragrance.

Did You Know?

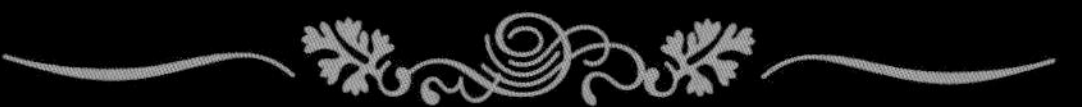

The title *Queen of the Fairies* belongs to Titania, who appears in Shakespeare's *A Midsummer Night's Dream*. Fairies are known as protectors of the home, warding off negative energies while attracting good luck and prosperity.

Ginseng Body Spritzer

(Makes one 8-ounce bottle)

A revitalizing mist to awaken and refresh your skin.

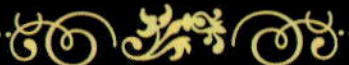

1 cup distilled water
1 tablespoon dried ginseng root
   (or the contents of 1 ginseng tea bag)
1 teaspoon dried chamomile flowers
1 teaspoon rose water
3-4 drops lavender essential oil
Small spray bottle (preferably glass)

Set water to boil.

Combine the ginseng root and chamomile flowers in a bowl. Pour hot water over them to steep for 15 minutes. As the herbs steep, take a few deep breaths and visualize the infusion absorbing energy that will bring calm and vitality.

Strain the mixture into a bowl through a fine mesh sieve. Allow to cool to room temperature. Discard the spent herbs into your compost bin.

Stir the rose water and lavender essential oil into the cooled liquid. Transfer to a clean spray bottle.

While filling the bottle, set an intention that each misting will be an act of self-care, refreshing both the body and the mind.

Store the spritzer in the refrigerator for a cooling effect. Shake gently before spraying. This spritzer can be used all over your body for a refreshing boost!

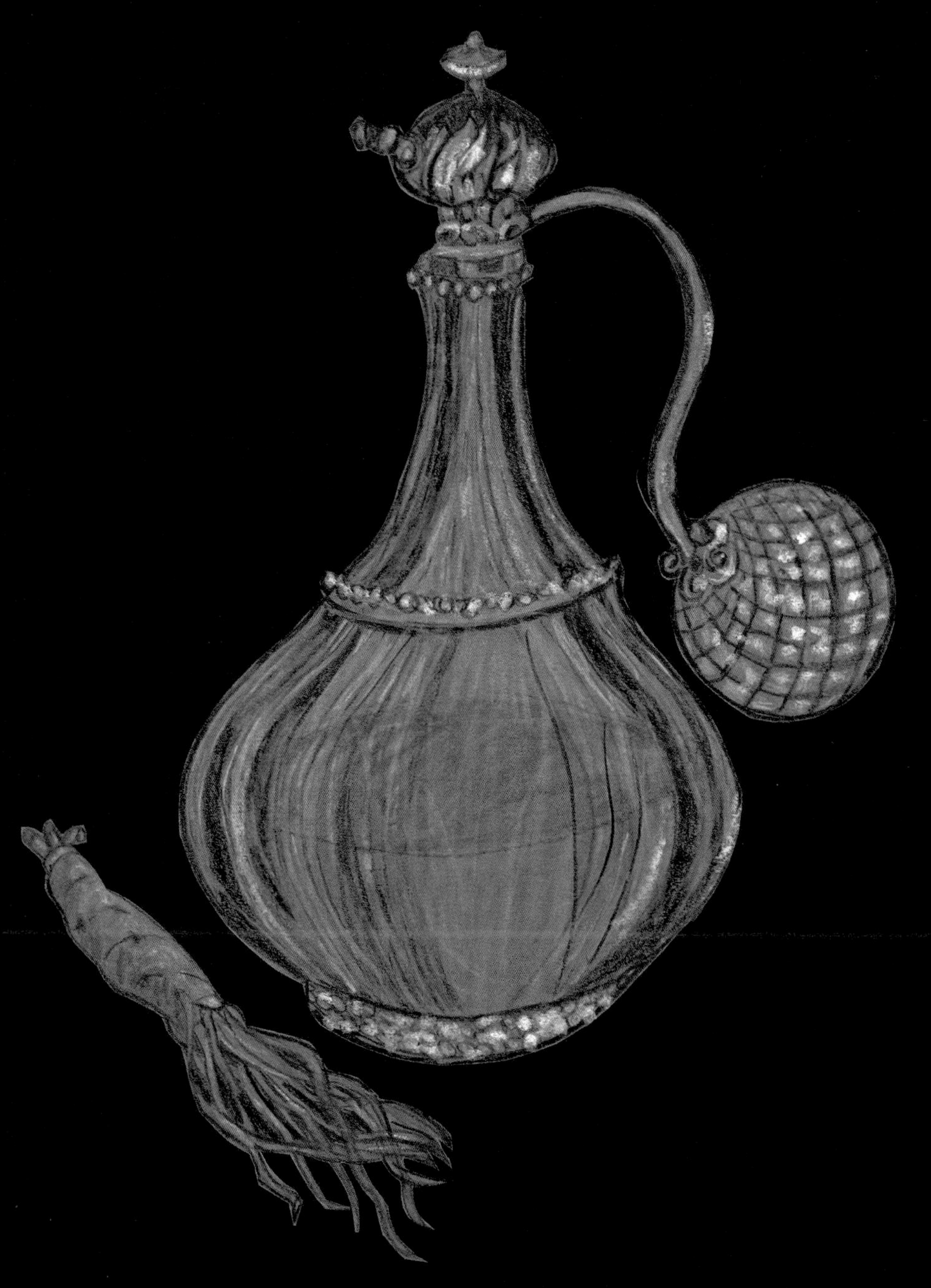

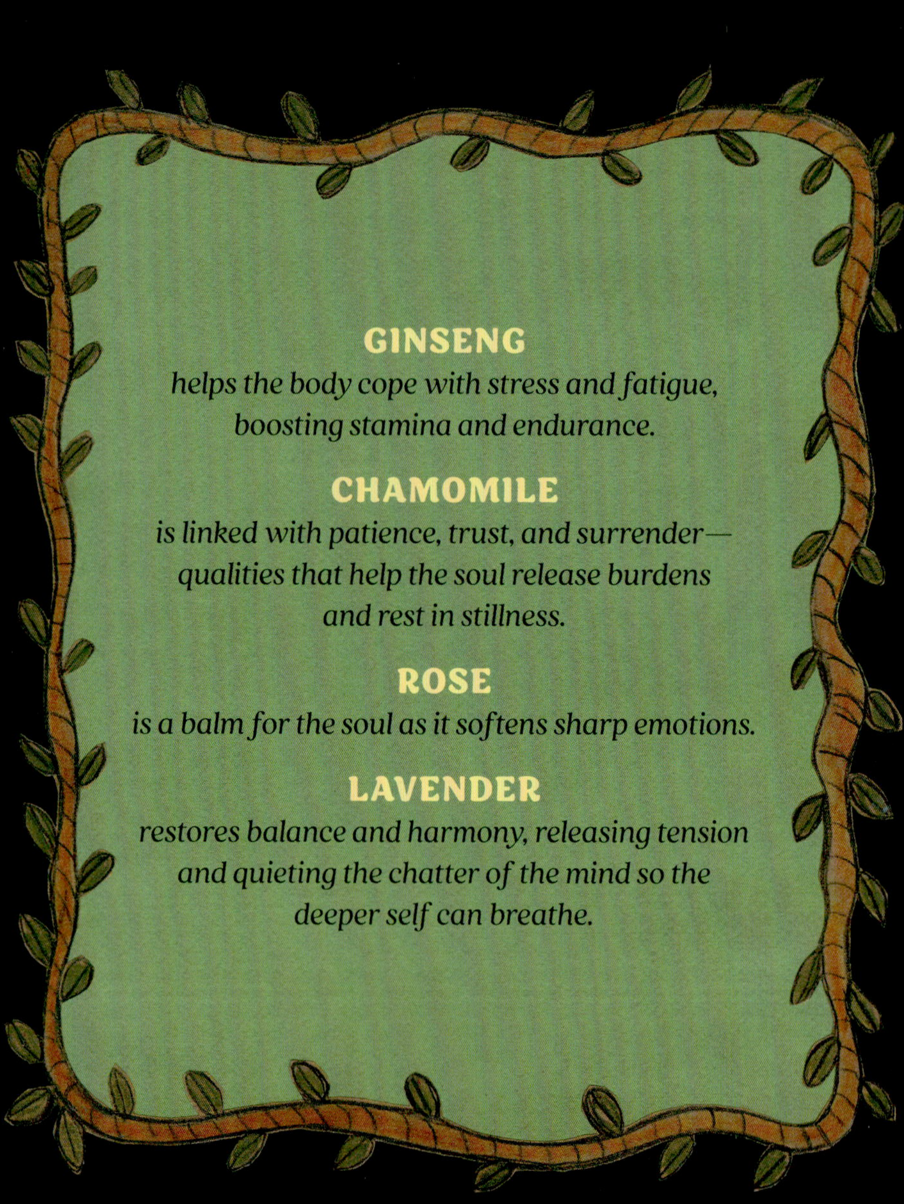

GINSENG

helps the body cope with stress and fatigue, boosting stamina and endurance.

CHAMOMILE

is linked with patience, trust, and surrender— qualities that help the soul release burdens and rest in stillness.

ROSE

is a balm for the soul as it softens sharp emotions.

LAVENDER

restores balance and harmony, releasing tension and quieting the chatter of the mind so the deeper self can breathe.

Did You Know?

In Chinese mythology, ginseng is often called the "root of heaven." It is said to have been discovered by the farmer Shennong, who tasted hundreds of plants to learn their healing powers.

Energy and Focus Simmer Pot

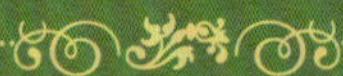

(Makes 1 simmer pot)

This simmer pot is a wonderful way to create a vibrant and uplifting atmosphere in your home or workspace.

2-3 lemons, sliced into rounds
1-2 oranges, sliced into rounds
3-4 sprigs fresh rosemary
1 vanilla bean
1 tablespoon sliced fresh ginger
2 sprigs fresh mint
9 black peppercorns
4 cups water

Place all ingredients into a medium pot. As you add each ingredient, notice its color, shape, and scent. Let each one invite you into the moment.

Bring the mixture to a boil. Once boiling, reduce the heat to a gentle simmer for at least 30 minutes, adding more water as needed to keep the water level consistent.

While it simmers, pause to enjoy the rising steam. Use it as a reminder to exhale tension and breathe in calm energy.

The delightful aroma will energize and refresh your space. You can keep the pot on the stove for a few hours, refreshing the water as necessary.

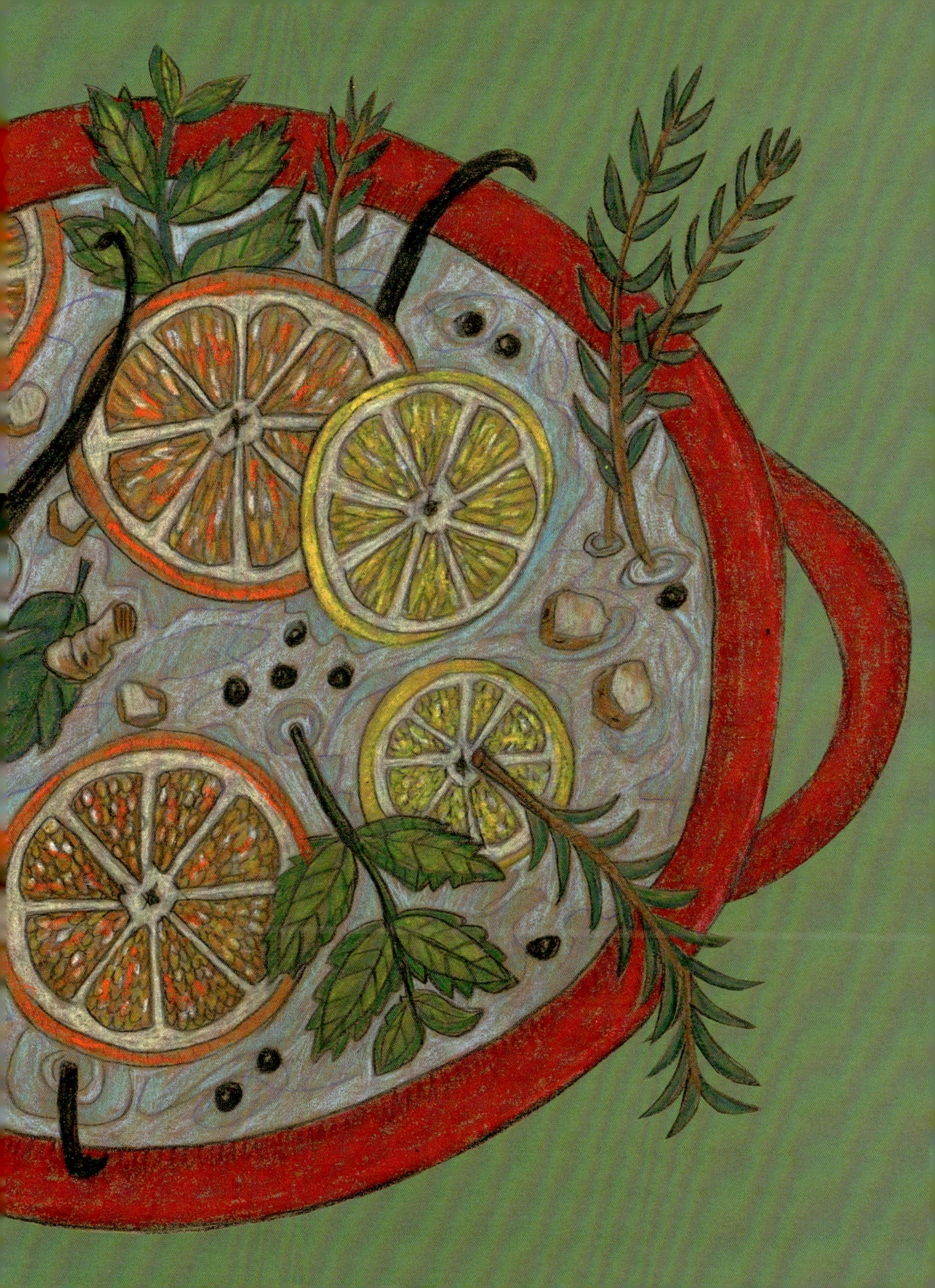

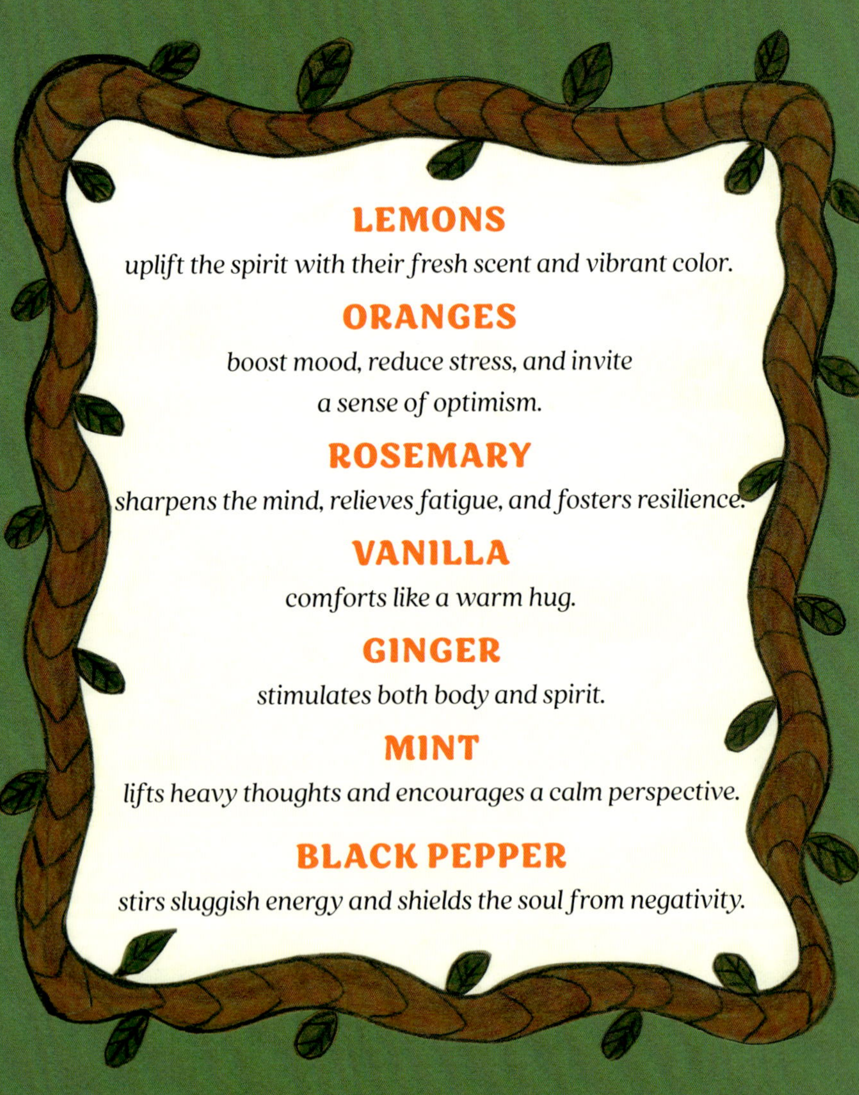

LEMONS
uplift the spirit with their fresh scent and vibrant color.

ORANGES
boost mood, reduce stress, and invite
a sense of optimism.

ROSEMARY
sharpens the mind, relieves fatigue, and fosters resilience.

VANILLA
comforts like a warm hug.

GINGER
stimulates both body and spirit.

MINT
lifts heavy thoughts and encourages a calm perspective.

BLACK PEPPER
stirs sluggish energy and shields the soul from negativity.

Did You Know?

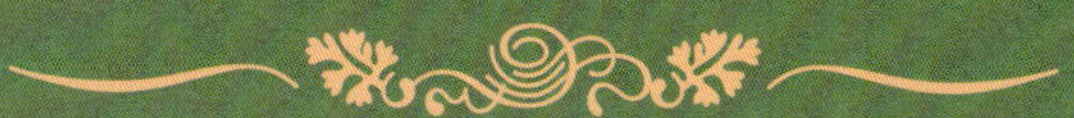

A simmer pot fills your space with soothing aromas that calm the mind and invite warmth, comfort, and balance. The simple act of preparing it can become a mindful ritual, reminding you to slow down and ground yourself in the present moment.

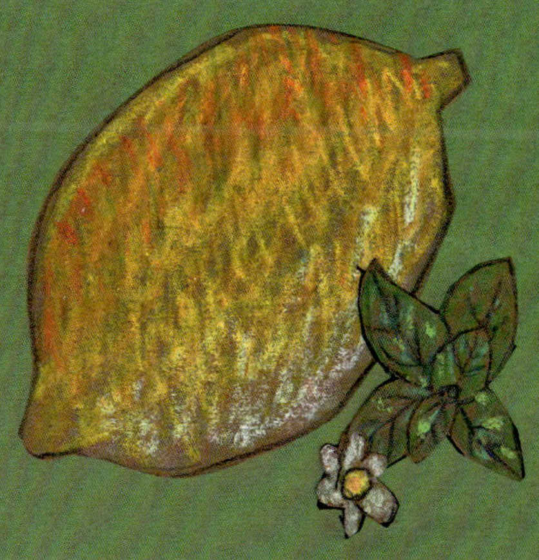

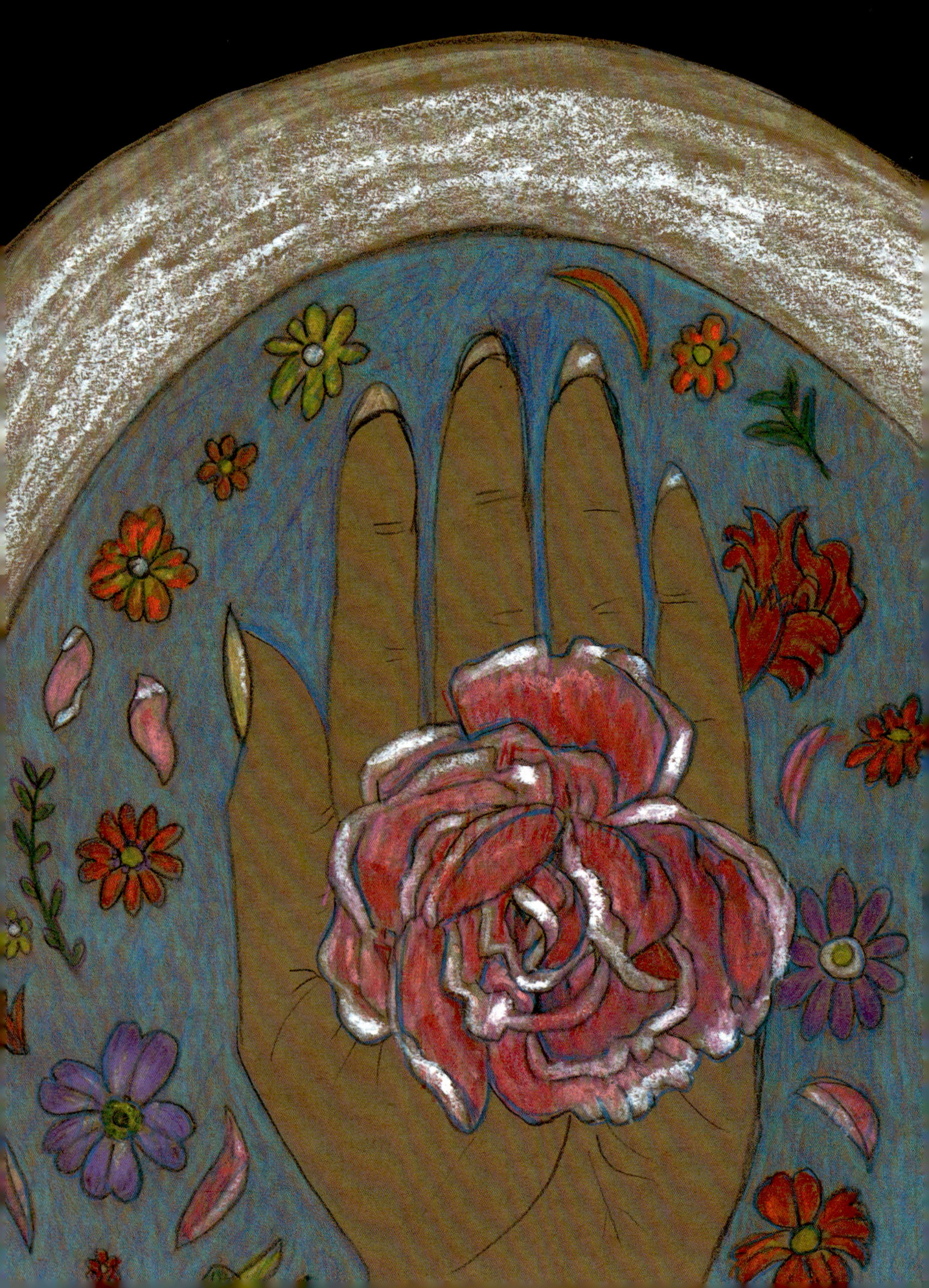

A Soulful Staycation

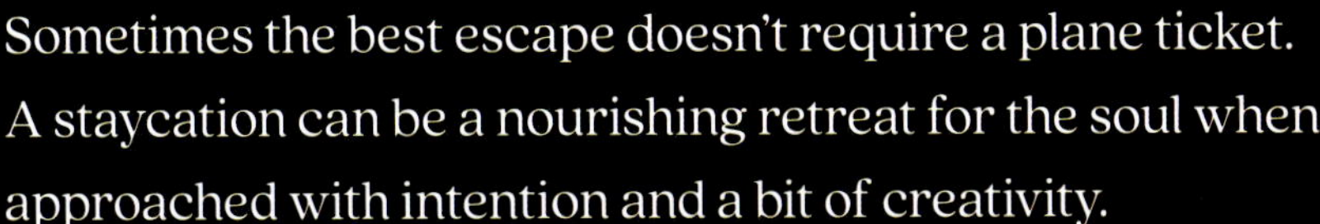

Sometimes the best escape doesn't require a plane ticket. A staycation can be a nourishing retreat for the soul when approached with intention and a bit of creativity.

Begin by tidying your space. Then light a candle and play your favorite music—tunes that make you smile. Plan activities that feel indulgent yet easy. Draw a bath with soothing salts, indulge in a slow skincare ritual (perhaps with *Aphrodite's Rose Face Mist*), or create a picnic on your living room floor with your favorite food and drink, and a good book.

Let wellness flow naturally through the day. Do some gentle stretching or take a mindful walk. Enjoy moving slowly, without deadlines or distractions. Leave your smartphone behind! Make time for a leisurely nap.

A soulful staycation is about permission to unplug, to play, and to step away from routine. By making your home a sanctuary, you can return to daily life with a fresh spirit.

Take a deep breath, and enjoy your well-deserved staycation.

Top 10 List of Fun Things to Do on Your Soulful Staycation

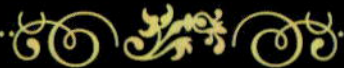

1. Have a movie marathon with healthy snacks and a cozy blanket on the couch.

2. Visit your local bookstore. Take your time looking. Pick out a book to read that piques your interest. Maybe get an art book to keep by your bedside to glance through before sleep.

3. Visit an art supply store for colored pencils or watercolors so you can try your hand at drawing or painting. Don't worry about being a great artist, just enjoy the colors and try to capture something at home (maybe your pet) in your sketchbook.

4. Have a spa day at home. Take a long bath with a bath tea or bath salts. Light a candle and play some soothing music. Then use all those beauty products you made from this book!

5. Take a no-phones-allowed nature walk in your favorite botanical garden. Spend time enjoying the colors, shapes, and scents of the plants. If you don't have a botanical garden nearby, visit a plant nursery and enjoy the plants there. Maybe pick up a lavender plant to keep next to your bed!

6. Have a tea ceremony at home with your favorite tea. Add small personal touches like your favorite music, a candle, or a meaningful object on the table. Write out a list of everything you're thankful for. Enjoy the comforting warmth of your tea.

7. Rearrange the furniture in your home. Maybe cut some flowers for your kitchen table. Sometimes a little change can really cheer you up!

8. If you have a dog, take them to a new place they've never been for a super fun walk. If you have a cat, spend time playing with them and doting on them. Most cats love to be brushed. All animals love attention, so why not spend a little extra time with them today?

9. Cook something new! Try a recipe you've never tried or always wanted to try. Have fun going to your local market and picking out all the ingredients you'll need.

10. Call that faraway friend or relative you've been meaning to call but have just been too busy. Ask them about how they're doing. You'll be so glad you did!

Did You Know?

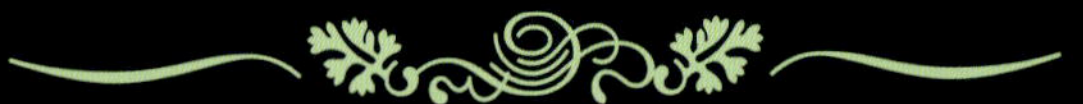

The term "staycation" originated in the early 2000s, gaining popularity during the 2008 financial crisis, when many people sought affordable alternatives to expensive travel. Instead of complicated vacations abroad, people began exploring leisure activities close to home—visiting local attractions, enjoying day trips, or simply transforming their homes into restful retreats.

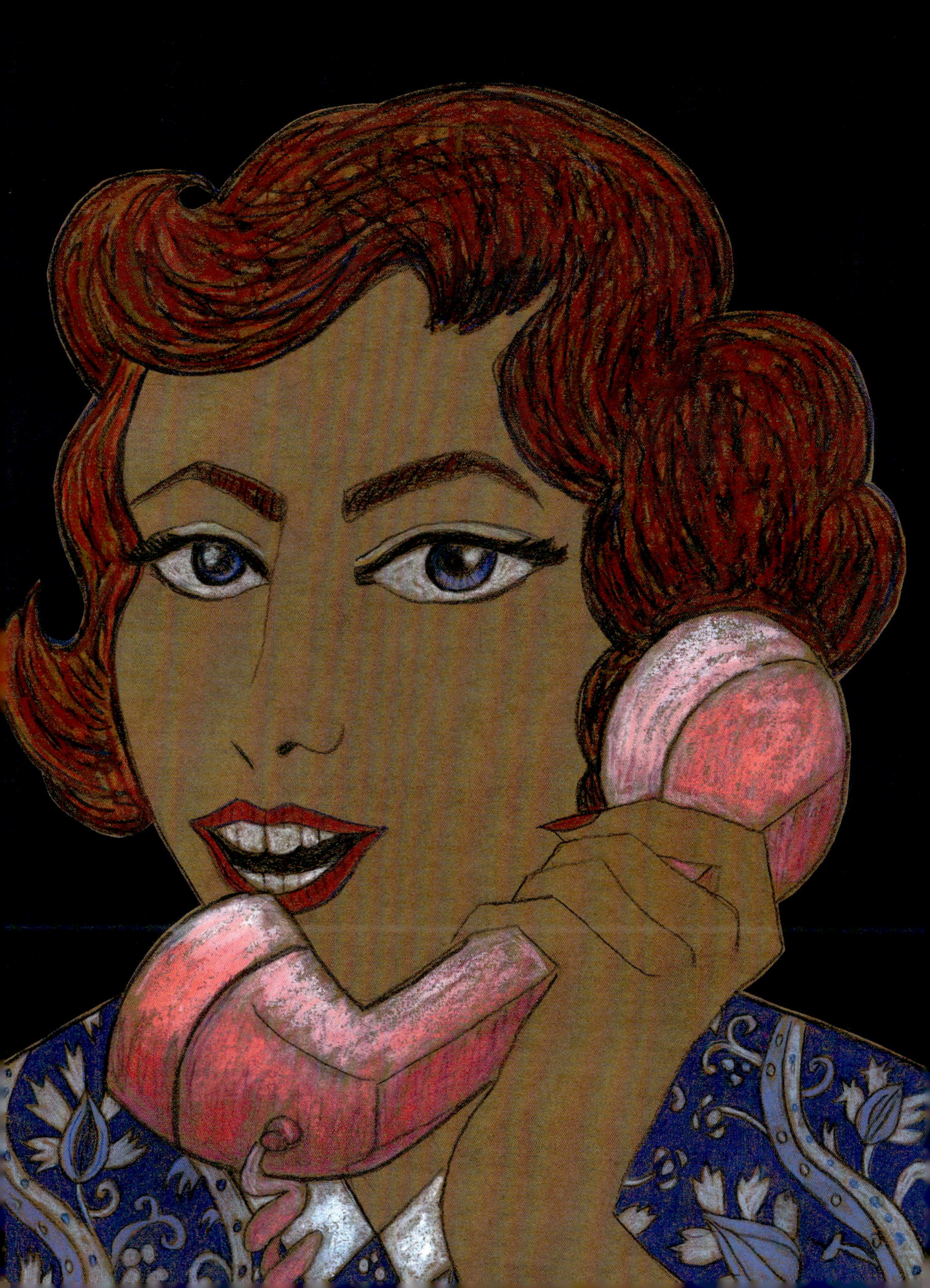

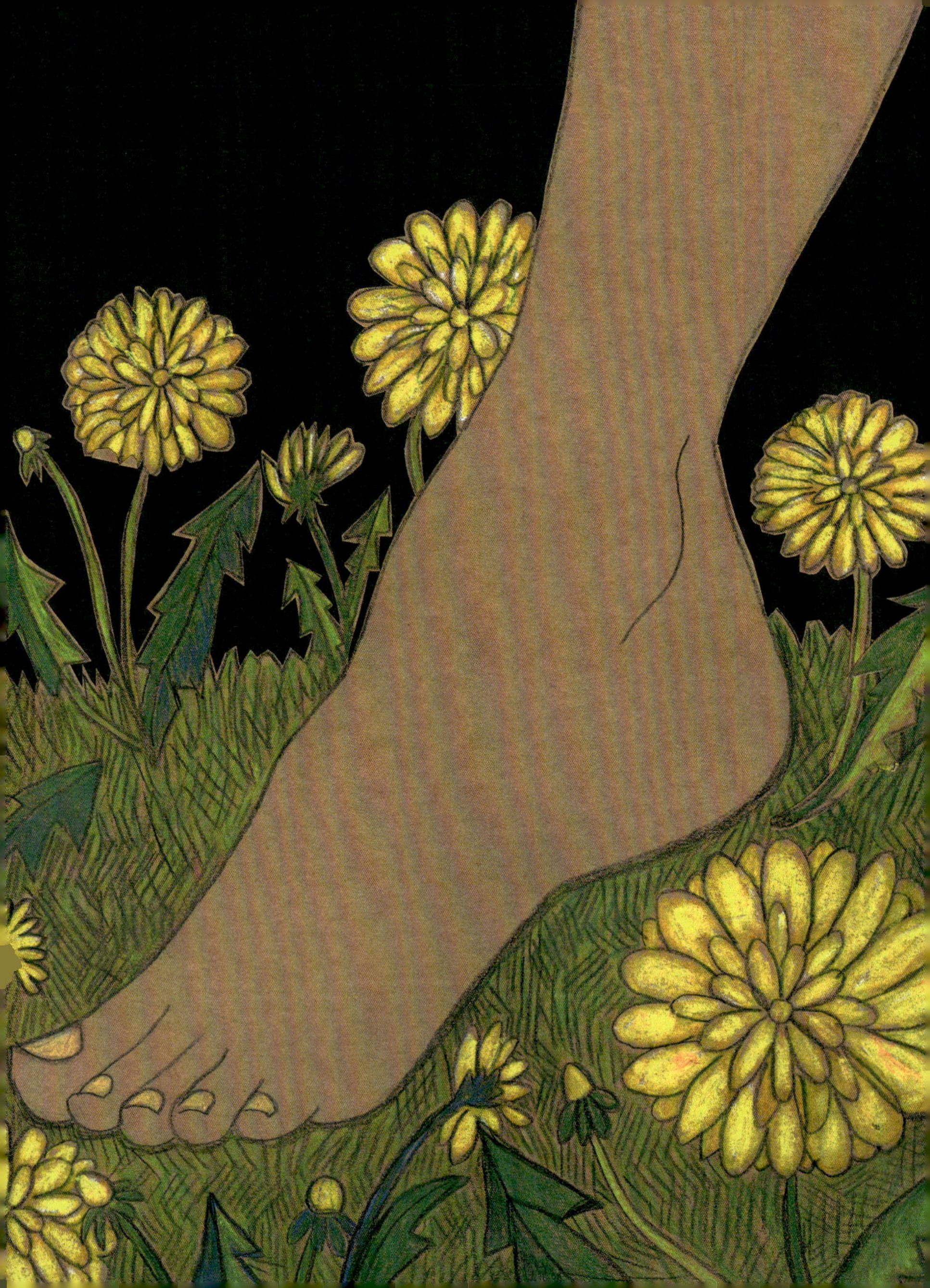

Earthing

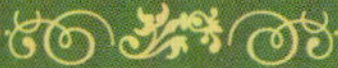

Earthing, also known as grounding, is the simple practice of walking barefoot on natural surfaces like grass, soil, or sand. This direct connection with the earth allows your body to absorb its natural energy, which many believe helps restore balance to the nervous system.

Scientific studies suggest that earthing can reduce stress, support better sleep, and decrease inflammation. On a wellness level, it encourages you to step outside, slow down, and reconnect with the present moment.

Feeling the cool grass under your feet or the warm sand between your toes can calm the mind, ease tension, and bring a sense of peace. One favorite kind of earthing is gardening. We love using bare hands to press seeds into the soil! A few minutes each day spent getting your hands in the dirt or your feet on the ground can serve as a mindful reset, helping you feel more centered and more relaxed.

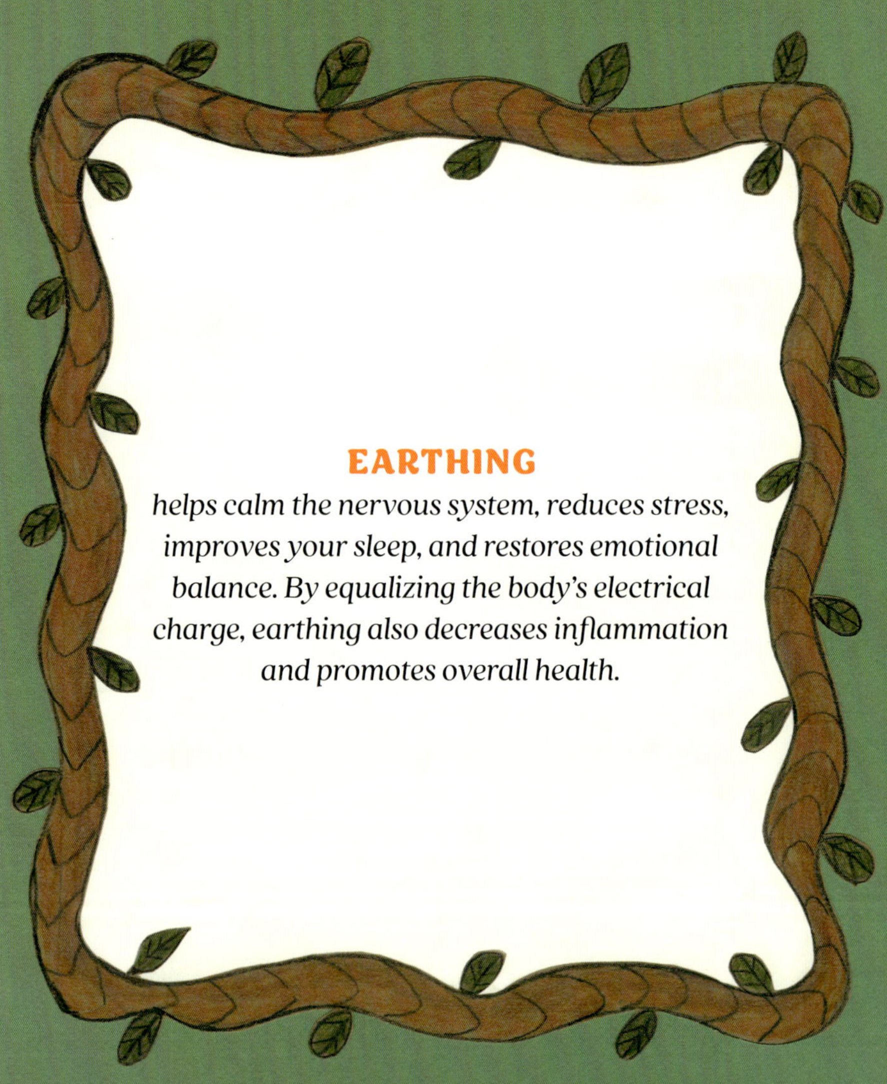

EARTHING

helps calm the nervous system, reduces stress, improves your sleep, and restores emotional balance. By equalizing the body's electrical charge, earthing also decreases inflammation and promotes overall health.

Did You Know?

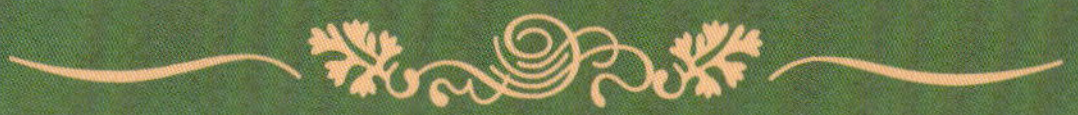

The modern concept of "earthing" began in the late 1990s when Clint Ober, a cable television pioneer, began researching the health effects of humans reconnecting with the Earth's natural electrical energy. Inspired by noticing how electrical systems require grounding, he wondered if people, insulated by shoes and modern living, were missing a vital connection. Ober's work popularized the term "earthing."

Forest Bathing

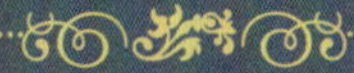

This is a wonderful, immersive, nature-centered salve for your soul!

Find a quiet forest where you can walk or sit without distraction. Perhaps there is a quiet wooded park in your area. (If possible, plan . . . park!). It should be a place that feels comfortable and safe.

Keep your smartphone silenced. As you step into the trees, pause and take a few deep breaths, letting the fresh air clear your mind and signal to your body that you are moving into peace.

Notice the colors of leaves, the textures of bark, the songs of birds, and the scents of nature. Let your senses guide you rather than your thoughts. Walk slowly because for now you have no destination, no reason to rush.

Stay there for a while, simply observing.

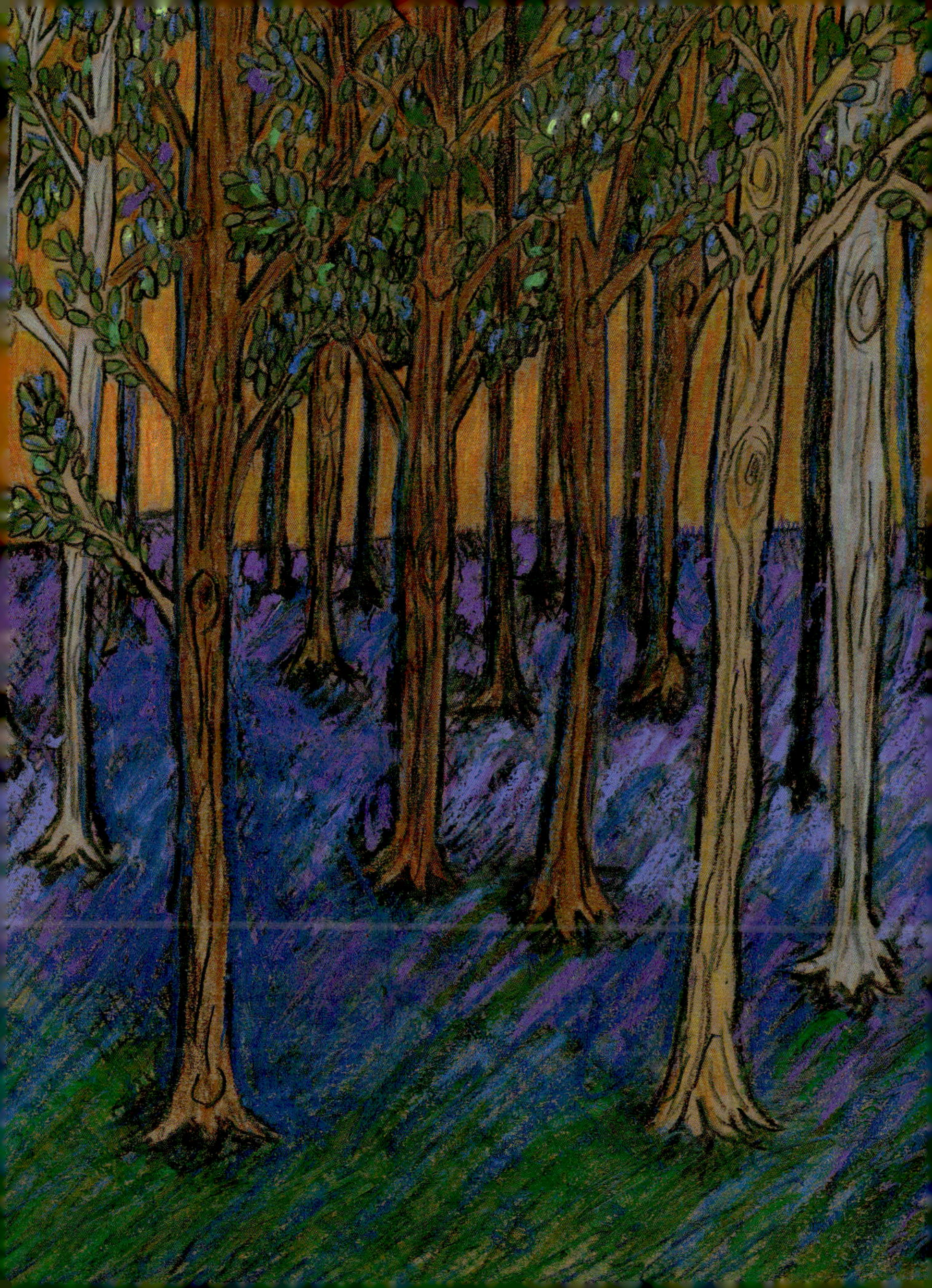

Place your hand on your chest as you breathe deeply, imagining the forest breathing with you—this shared rhythm can soothe the soul, dissolve feelings of isolation, and restore a sense of belonging. Find a tree that appeals to you in some way and hug it! If you hold tightly, you can feel the tree's energy pulsing into your hands and arms. It's incredible!

Now allow the silence, beauty, and timelessness of the forest to wash over you. Imagine roots growing from your feet into the earth, grounding and steadying your spirit. In this moment, the forest becomes a sanctuary that heals not only the body and mind but the soul as well.

Before leaving, offer gratitude to the forest and your tree friend, silently or aloud, for the calm, clarity, and renewal it has given you. Carry this sense of peace with you into your daily life.

Did You Know?

Forest bathing, known as *Shinrin-yoku* in Japanese, originated in Japan in the 1980s as a response to rising stress and health problems from urbanization and technology-driven lifestyles. The Japanese Ministry of Agriculture, Forestry, and Fisheries promoted it as a form of "ecotherapy," encouraging people to immerse themselves in nature for improved well-being. Scientific studies soon confirmed its benefits, showing that spending mindful time in forests can lower cortisol (the stress hormone), strengthen the immune system, improve cardiovascular health, enhance mood, and nourish the spirit.

Blackberry Vinegar

(Makes one 18-ounce bottle)

**Blackberry vinegar can be used in salad dressings, in marinades,
or as a refreshing addition to beverages. Truly nourishment for the soul!**

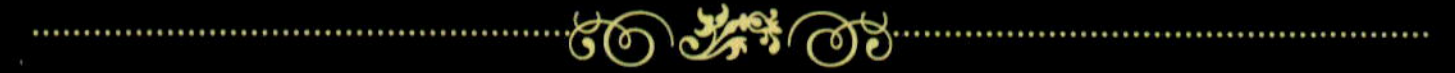

2 cups fresh blackberries
2 cups apple cider vinegar
Large glass jar with lid

In a medium-sized bowl, combine the blackberries and apple cider vinegar. Using a fork, gently mash the blackberries to release their juices. This will help infuse the vinegar with flavor.

As you mash, notice the rich color and aroma—pause to appreciate the beauty of nature's offering.

Transfer the mixture to a jar and seal the container tightly. Let the mixture sit in a cool, dark place for 2 weeks. Shake it gently every few days to stimulate the infusion. Each time you shake the jar, take a deep breath and set a simple intention—such as patience, gratitude, or clarity.

After 2 weeks, strain the mixture through a fine mesh sieve into a clean bottle or jar, pressing gently on the blackberries to extract as much liquid as possible. Discard the spent blackberries into the compost bin. Seal the bottle tightly and store in a cool, dark place for up to 1 year.

Use your vinegar in dressings or simply drizzled over vegetables for an invigorating pop of energy.

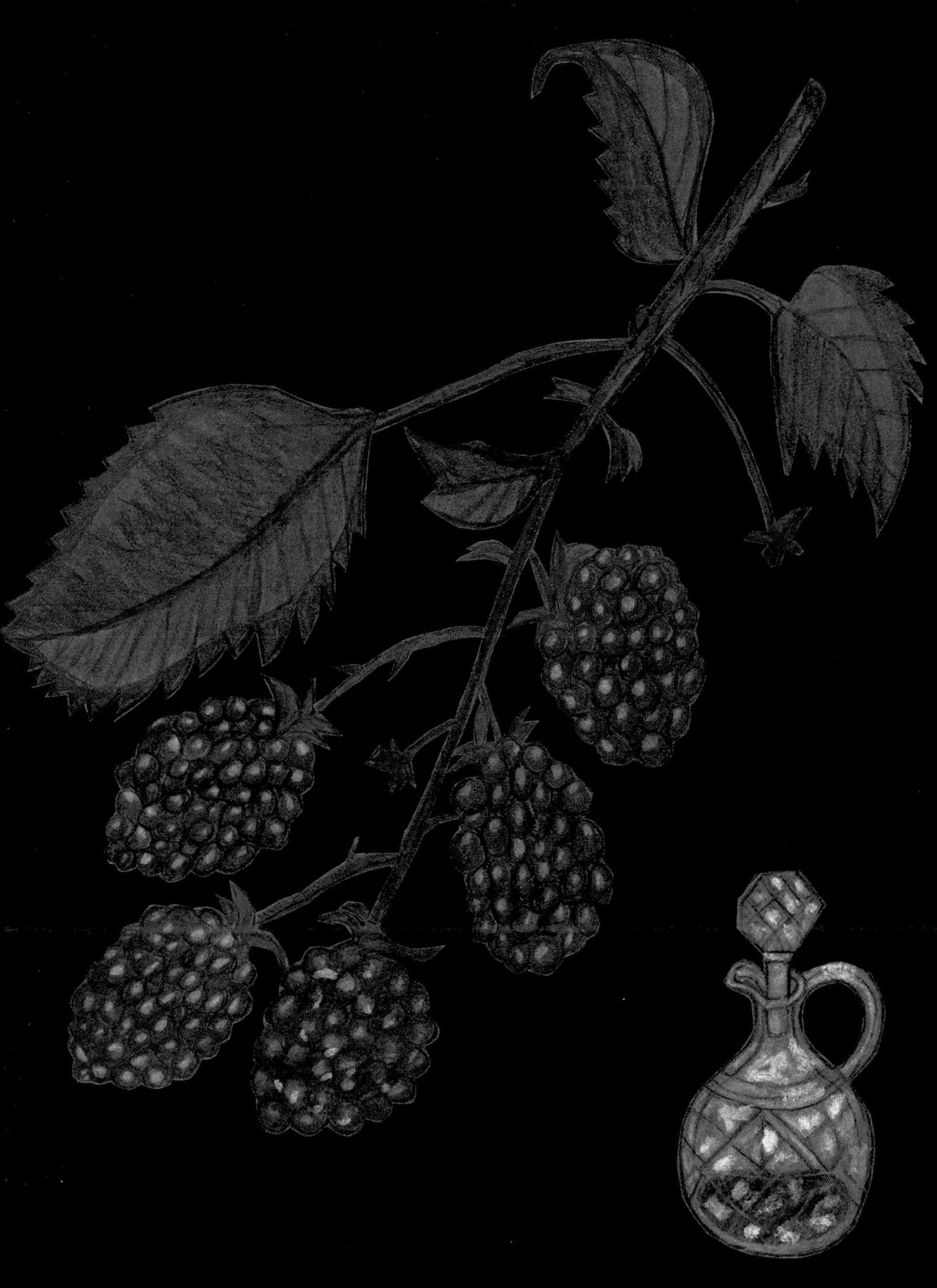

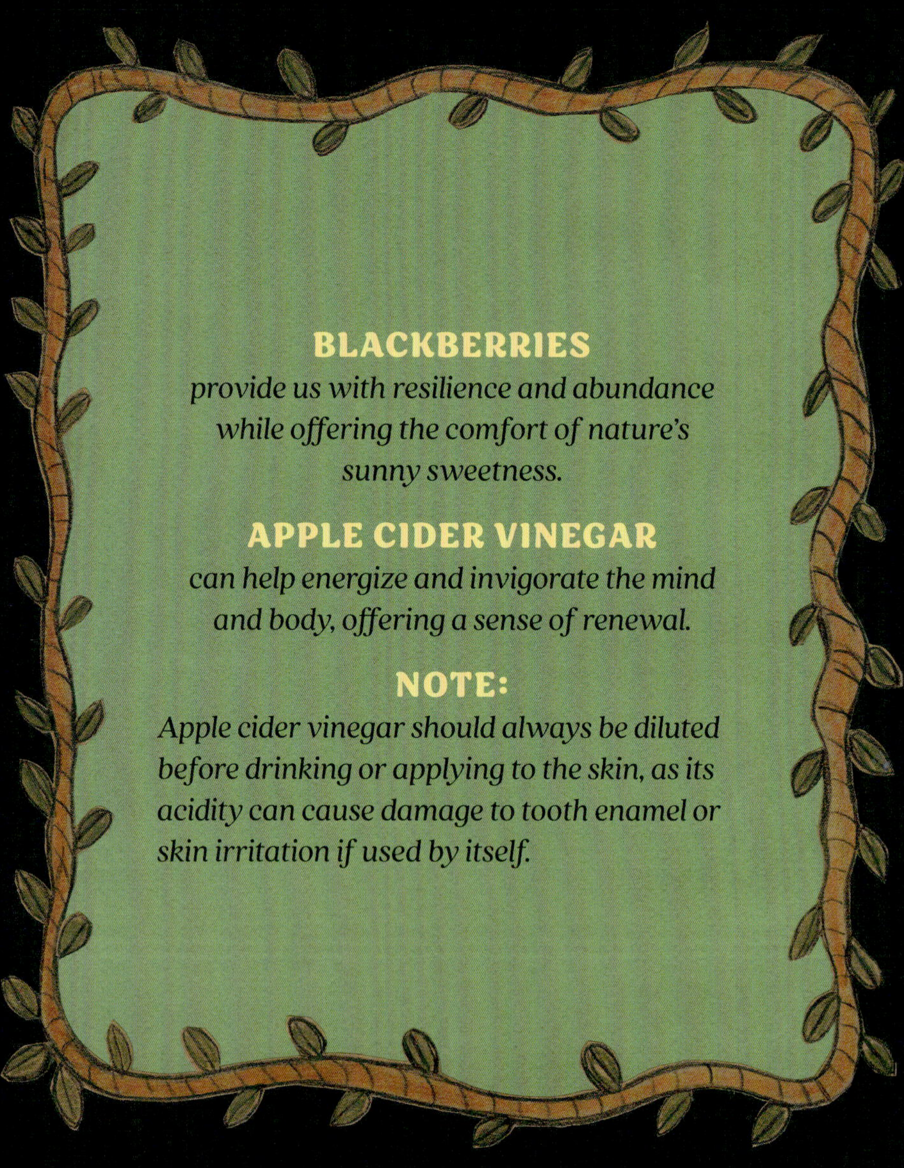

BLACKBERRIES

provide us with resilience and abundance while offering the comfort of nature's sunny sweetness.

APPLE CIDER VINEGAR

can help energize and invigorate the mind and body, offering a sense of renewal.

NOTE:

Apple cider vinegar should always be diluted before drinking or applying to the skin, as its acidity can cause damage to tooth enamel or skin irritation if used by itself.

Did You Know?

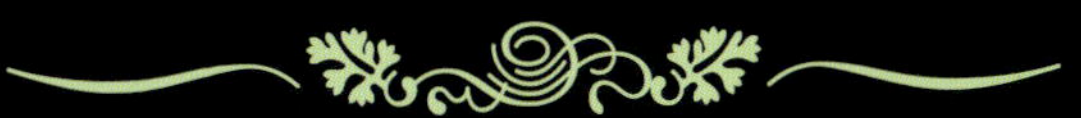

In Celtic folklore, blackberries were believed to hold the last warmth of the summer sun, and gathering them before Samhain (the end of harvest season) was said to bring strength to last through the darker months of winter. In early America, apple cider vinegar was a staple in colonial households, sipped daily with water as a tonic to cleanse the body.

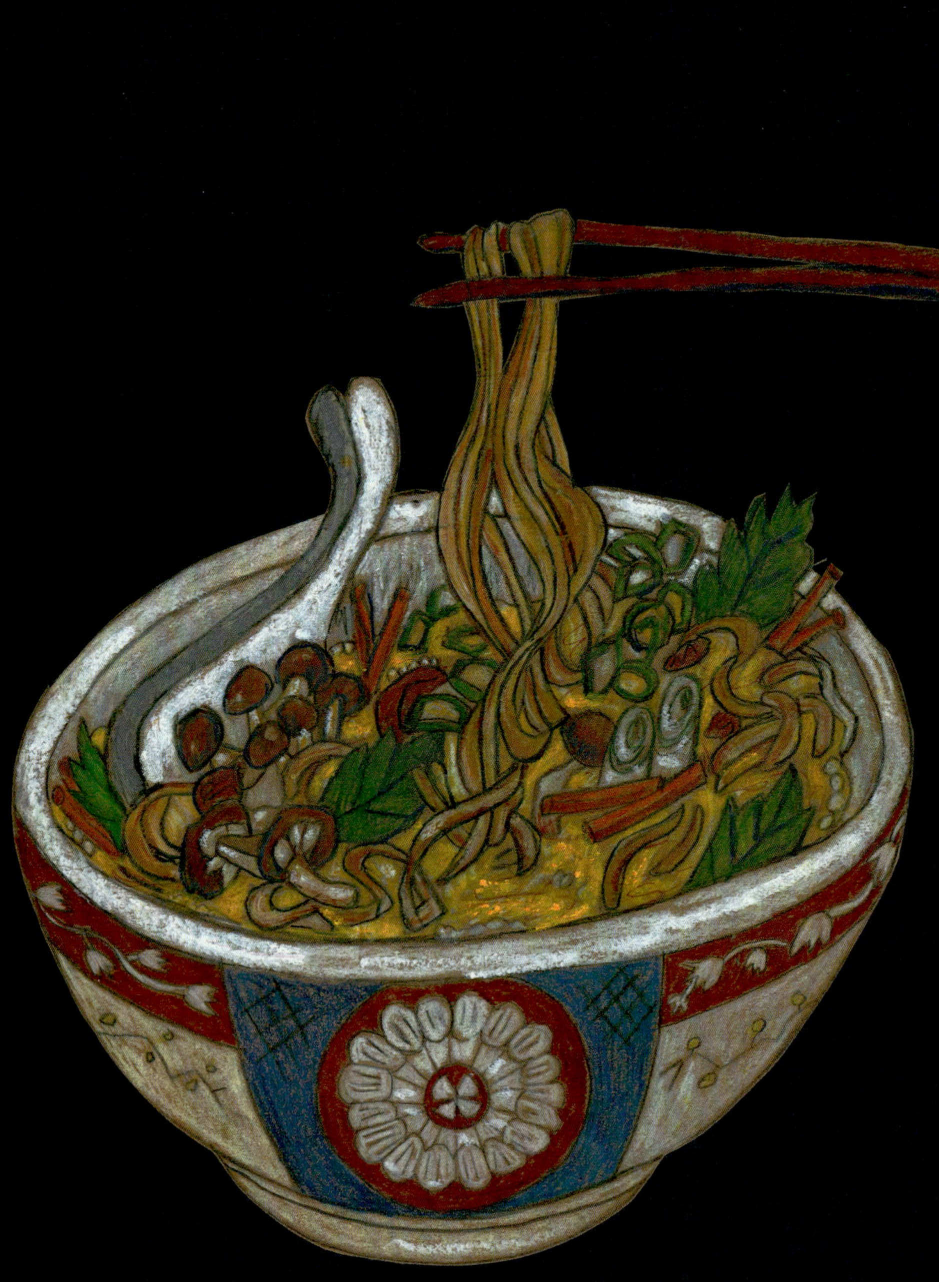

Veggie Ramen Soup with Sun-Dried Tomatoes and Mushrooms

(Makes 3–4 servings)

**Nothing warms the soul quite like a delicious hot bowl
of lovingly made ramen soup!**

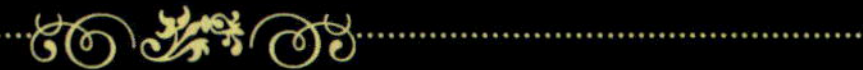

1 tablespoon sesame oil
2 cloves garlic, minced
1-inch piece ginger, minced
1 cup mushrooms, sliced
½ cup chopped sun-dried tomatoes
4 cups vegetable broth
2 cups water
2 tablespoons soy sauce
1 tablespoon miso paste
½ pound frozen ramen noodles (not instant)
1 cup spinach, chopped
1 carrot, cut into very thin matchsticks
Chopped scallion, sesame seeds, and red pepper flakes for garnish

Heat sesame oil in a large pot over medium heat. Sauté garlic and ginger for 1 minute until fragrant. Add mushrooms and cook for 3 to 4 minutes until softened. Stir in sun-dried tomatoes, then add vegetable broth and water.

Bring mixture to a simmer, then add soy sauce and miso paste. Stir until dissolved.

Add ramen noodles and cook for 3 minutes. Add spinach and carrots and simmer for 2 minutes more. As your soup simmers, pause and breathe deeply, imagining each ingredient infusing the broth with calm, nourishment, and healthfulness.

Ladle soup into bowls and garnish with chopped scallion, sesame seeds, and red pepper flakes. Serve hot and enjoy your soulful vegetarian ramen soup!

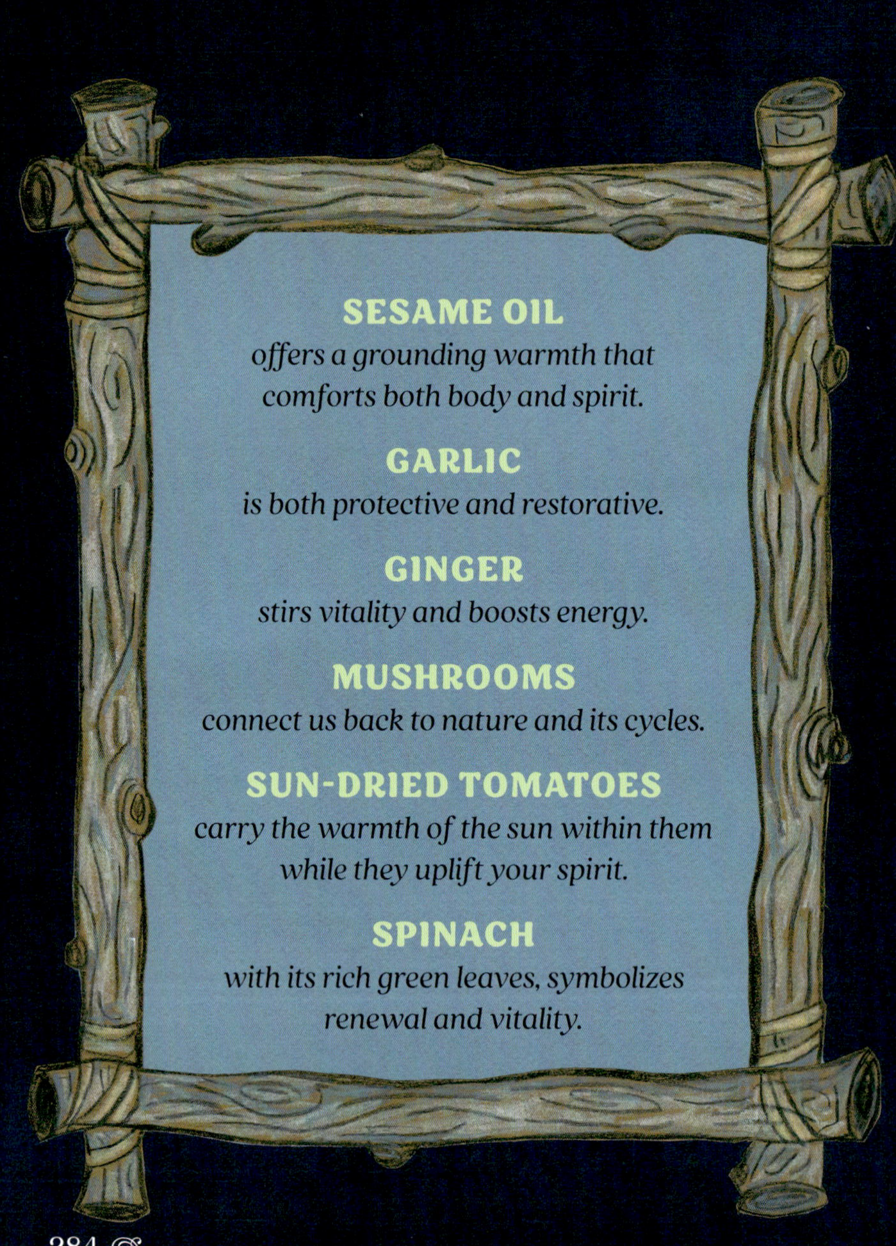

SESAME OIL

offers a grounding warmth that comforts both body and spirit.

GARLIC

is both protective and restorative.

GINGER

stirs vitality and boosts energy.

MUSHROOMS

connect us back to nature and its cycles.

SUN-DRIED TOMATOES

carry the warmth of the sun within them while they uplift your spirit.

SPINACH

with its rich green leaves, symbolizes renewal and vitality.

Did You Know?

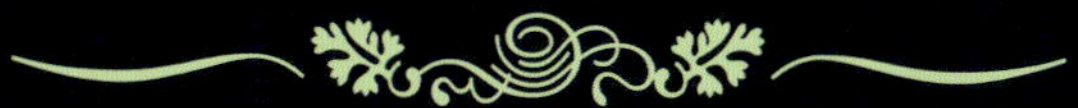

Ramen originated in Japan in the late 19th to early 20th century, inspired by Chinese wheat noodles brought over by Chinese immigrants. It evolved as a quick, affordable, and nourishing dish.

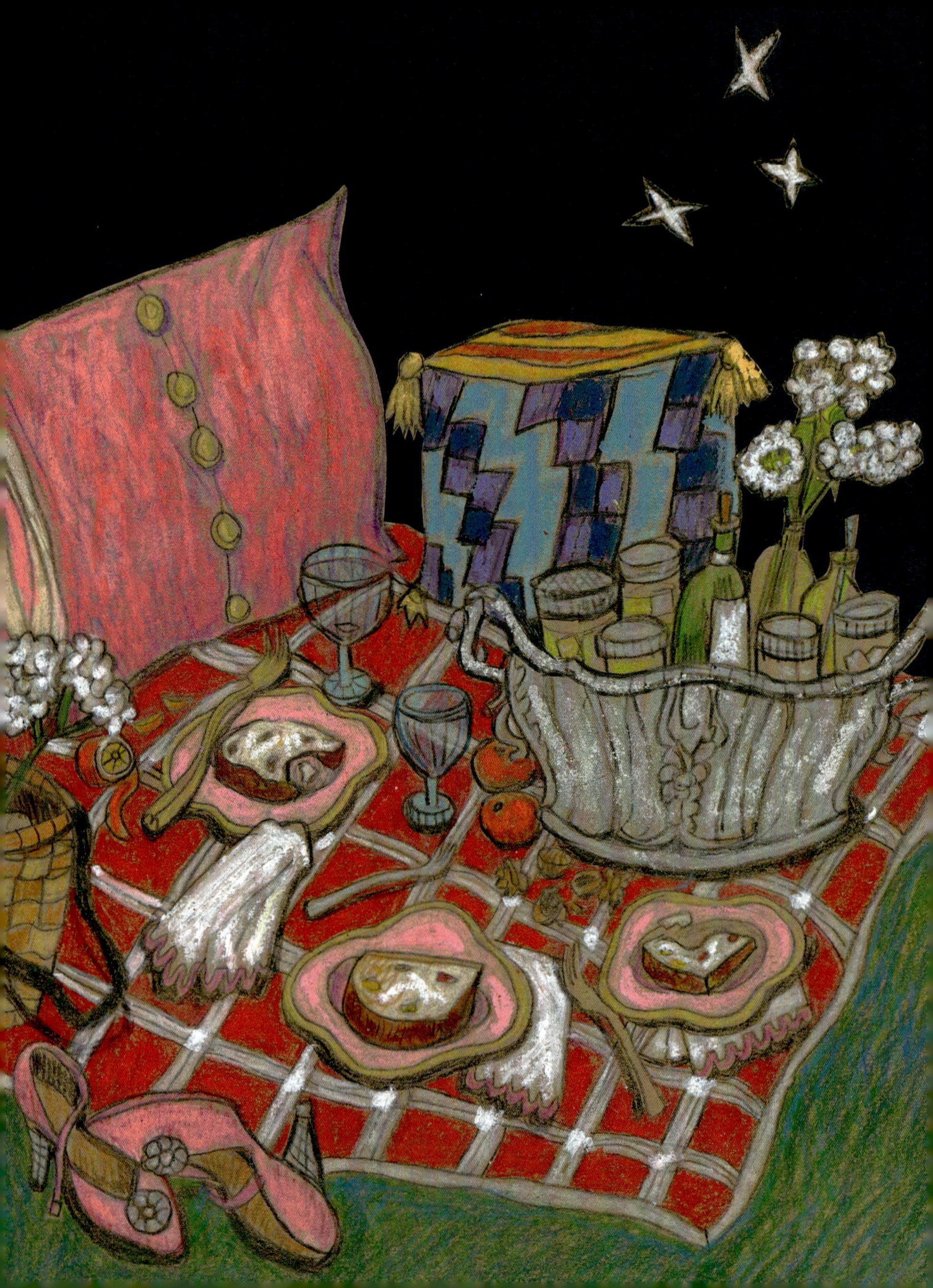

CHAPTER 9

THE HEALING GARDEN PICNIC

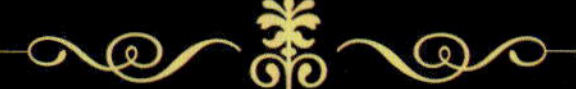

MENU

Rhubarb Lemonade

Garden Gin and Tonic Jars

Garden Goddess Dip with Crudité

Vietnamese Summer Rolls

Roasted Potato Salad with Rosemary

Cucumber Salad with Red Onion, Dill, and Flaxseeds (page 113)

Friendship Fruit Cake

In the golden hush of late afternoon, the healing garden welcomes guests with the scent of freshly gathered herbs drifting on a soft warm breeze. On the ground under a big tree is a red-and-white checkered tablecloth scattered with wildflowers, and on that is chilled *Rhubarb Lemonade* and platters of vibrant plant-based treats. As twilight approaches, the candlelight begins to dance around the feast, casting a warm glow over the *Friendship Fruit Cake*.

Laughter mingles with conversation until the sky turns a velvety dark blue as it heads into night. The air is filled with soft, joyful music, the candles flicker in harmony with the fireflies, and your garden becomes a celebration—an evening where food and spirit combine in joyful abundance.

Before you take your first bites, pause for a moment of gratitude for the privilege of being all together on this beautiful evening. Feel the earth beneath you, take in the lilting music and the sounds of the birds settling in for the evening. Let your senses awaken completely to the beauty around you. Enjoy your healing picnic!

Rhubarb Lemonade

(Serves 4)

This refreshing beverage combines the tartness of rhubarb with the crispness of lemonade.

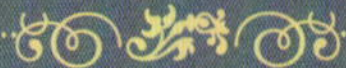

2 cups rhubarb, chopped
1 cup sugar
4 cups water, divided
Juice squeezed from 6 lemons (about 1¼ cups)
Lemon slices and mint sprigs for garnish

In a saucepan, combine rhubarb, sugar, and 1 cup of water. Bring to a boil over medium heat, then reduce heat and simmer for about 10 minutes until the rhubarb is soft. Strain the mixture through a fine mesh sieve into a bowl. Discard the rhubarb into the compost bin.

In a pitcher, mix the strained rhubarb liquid with the remaining 3 cups of water and the lemon juice. Stir well. Refrigerate for several hours.

Fill glasses with ice. Pour in lemonade and garnish each glass with a lemon slice and a mint sprig. Enjoy the refreshment and sense of vitality your lemonade provides!

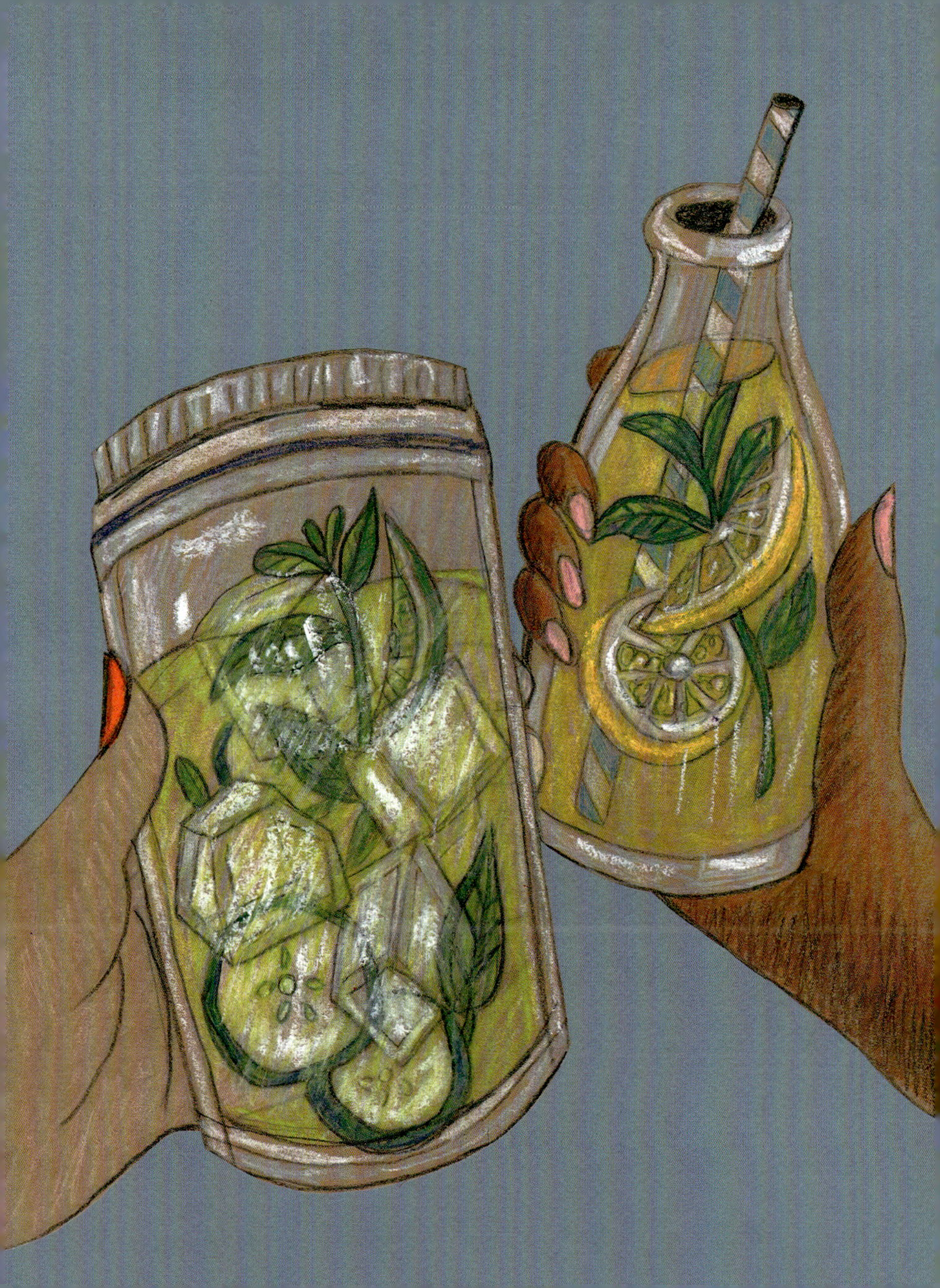

Garden Gin and Tonic Jars

(Serves 4)

These adorable cocktail jars are not only easy to transport to your picnic, but you can simply place them in a bucket of ice and let your guests serve themselves. No bartender needed!

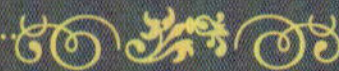

1 cup gin
1 cup fresh mint leaves, torn
1 medium cucumber, unpeeled, sliced thinly
Ice cubes
4 cups tonic water
Extra mint leaves, cucumber slices, and lime wedges for garnish
4 glass jars with lids, about 12 ounces each, for serving

In a large glass jar or container with a lid, combine the gin, mint leaves, and sliced cucumber, saving a few cucumber slices for garnish. Seal the container tightly and let it infuse in the refrigerator for at least 4 hours, or overnight for a stronger flavor.

Strain the mixture through a fine mesh sieve. Add the solids to your compost bin.

Fill each glass with ice cubes. Divide the gin mixture evenly between the four jars. Top each with 1 cup tonic water and swirl gently to combine.

Add a few fresh mint leaves, a slice of cucumber, and a lime wedge to each drink. Seal the jars and keep them very cold until you're ready to serve. If you are traveling to a picnic, keep the jars in an insulated cooler to prevent the ice from melting. Enjoy your garden cocktails!

Garden Goddess Dip with Crudité

Bursting with veggie goodness, this dip is a vibrant conversation starter.

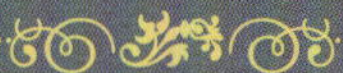

1 (8-ounce) container of plain vegan soy or coconut yogurt
1 avocado, peeled, pitted, and diced
1 cup fresh parsley leaves, chopped
1 cup fresh mint leaves, chopped
2 scallions, thinly sliced
1 medium garlic clove, minced
1 tablespoon olive oil
1 tablespoon lemon juice
Dash hot sauce, to taste
Salt and pepper to taste
Fresh vegetables for serving, such as sliced carrots, red and yellow
   bell peppers, radishes, cucumbers, and celery

Add yogurt, avocado, parsley, mint, scallions, garlic, olive oil, lemon juice, hot sauce, salt, and pepper to a food processor and blend for 2 to 3 minutes or until smooth. As the mixture blends, appreciate the colors and aromas they impart.

Transfer mixture to a bowl. Cover the bowl and chill in the refrigerator for at least 30 minutes to allow the flavors to develop.

Serve with fresh vegetables.

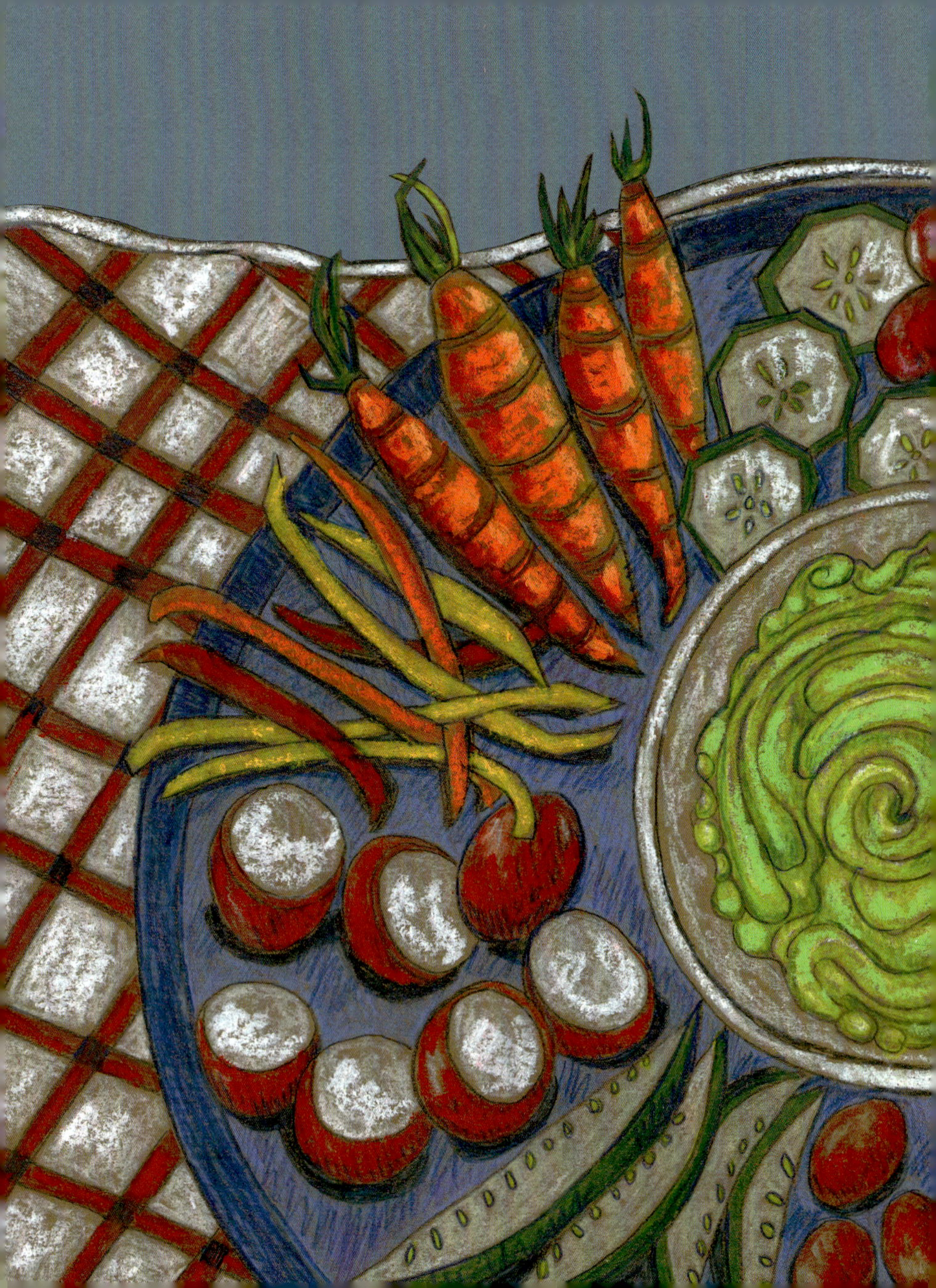

Vietnamese Summer Rolls

(Serves 4)

Paired with a creamy peanut butter dipping sauce, these summer rolls offer a delightful combination of textures and flavors. The edible flowers are a stunning touch!

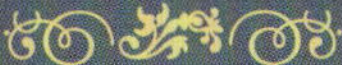

For the sauce:
¼ cup peanut butter
2 tablespoons soy sauce
1 tablespoon maple syrup
1 tablespoon rice vinegar
1 teaspoon sesame oil

For the rolls:
8 rice paper wrappers
1 cup vermicelli noodles, cooked
1 cup shredded carrots
1 medium cucumber, cut into matchsticks
1 red bell pepper, cut into matchsticks
1 cup lettuce leaves (butter or romaine), torn into pieces
1 cup fresh herbs, such as mint, basil, or cilantro
Some edible flowers, such as nasturtiums or violets

In a bowl, whisk together peanut butter, soy sauce, maple syrup, rice vinegar, and sesame oil until thoroughly combined. Set aside.

Fill a shallow dish or pie plate with warm water. Working with one rice paper wrapper at a time, dip wrapper into the water to soften, about 10 to 15 seconds. Place the wrapper on a clean, dry surface. Lay ⅛ of the vermicelli noodles in the center, then add ⅛ each of the carrots, cucumber, bell pepper, lettuce, and fresh herbs on top. Finish with some edible flowers. Pause to give gratitude for the beauty of your ingredients.

Fold the sides of the wrapper over the filling and then roll it up tightly from the bottom to the top. Repeat with the remaining wrappers and fillings, ensuring as you go that you have enough to fill each summer roll equally.

Serve summer rolls on a decorative platter with the peanut dipping sauce.

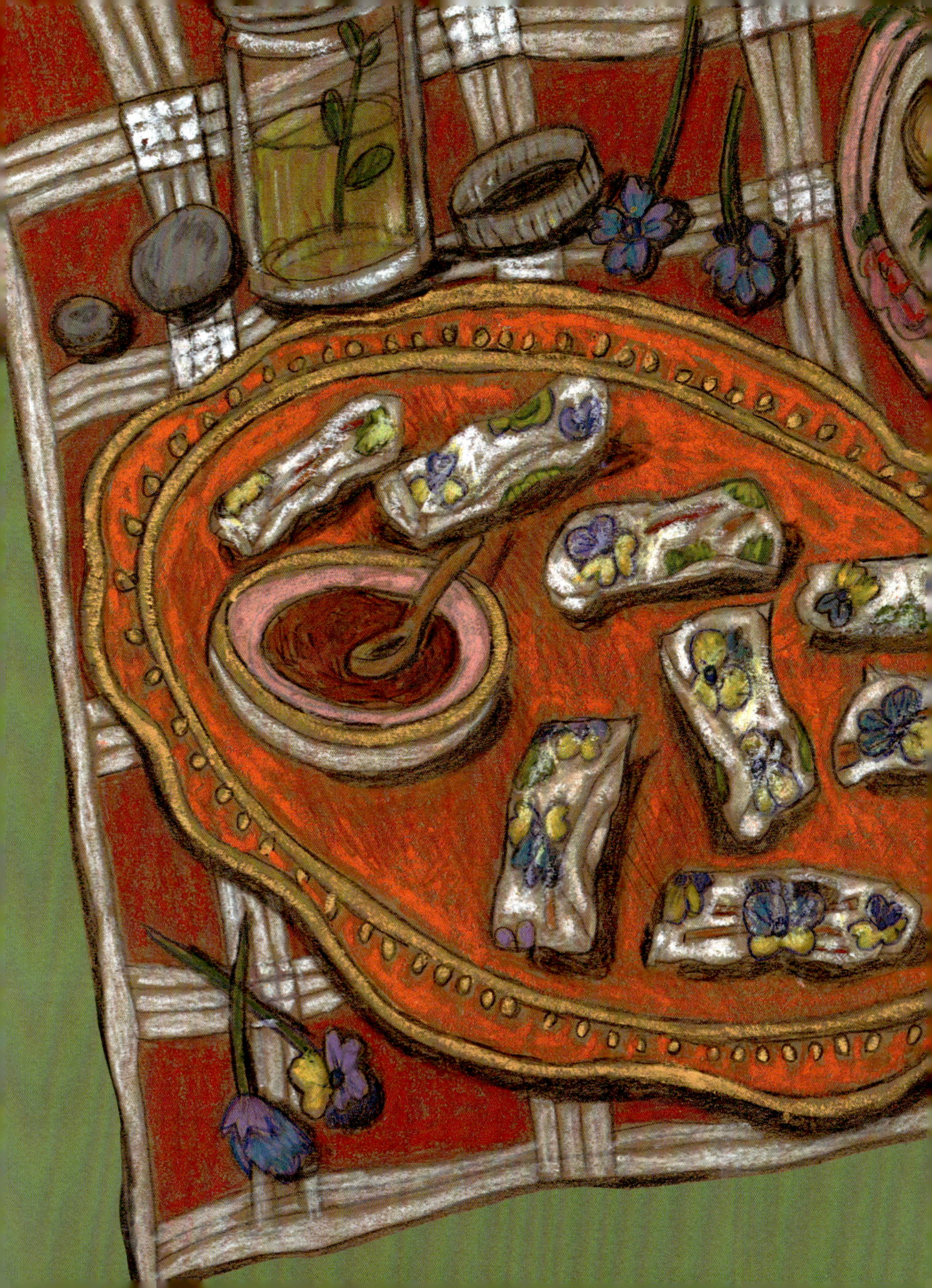

Roasted Potato Salad with Rosemary

(Serves 4)

This tangy potato salad will be a wonderful addition to your picnic. It can be made ahead and is delicious served warm or at room temperature.

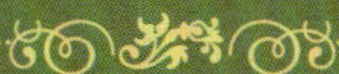

2 pounds baby or new potatoes, halved (or quartered if large)
4 tablespoons olive oil
2 tablespoons fresh rosemary, chopped
2 cloves garlic, finely chopped
Salt and pepper, to taste
1 small red onion, finely chopped
1 tablespoon Dijon mustard
2 tablespoons lemon juice

Heat oven to 400°F.

In a large mixing bowl, toss the potatoes with olive oil, chopped rosemary, garlic, salt, and pepper until well coated.

Spread the potatoes on a baking sheet in a single layer. Roast for about 25 to 30 minutes, or until potatoes are golden brown, turning once halfway through. Let potatoes cool slightly. Inhale their earthy aroma, letting the scent ground you.

In a large serving bowl, mix together the roasted potatoes, red onion, and Dijon mustard. Drizzle with lemon juice and toss to ensure all the flavors combine.

Serve salad warm or at room temperature.

Cucumber Salad with Red Onion, Dill, and Flaxseeds

(See recipe on page 113.)

Friendship Fruit Cake

(Serves 4–6)

This cake is perfect to make for a gathering with friends. The spices are chosen for their ability to nurture relationships!

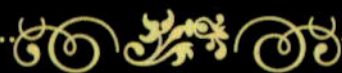

1 cup raisins
½ cup dried cranberries
½ cup dried apricots, chopped
1 cup whole-grain cereal (such as bran flakes)
1 cup unsweetened applesauce
½ cup maple syrup
⅓ cup vegetable oil, plus more for greasing the pan
1 teaspoon vanilla extract
1 cup whole-wheat flour
1 teaspoon baking powder
1 teaspoon baking soda
1 teaspoon ground cinnamon
½ teaspoon ground nutmeg
¼ teaspoon ground ginger
Pinch of salt

Heat oven to 350°F and lightly grease a loaf pan with vegetable oil.

In a small bowl, combine the dried fruit and cereal. Set aside.

In a medium bowl, whisk together the applesauce, maple syrup, vegetable oil, and vanilla.

In a large bowl, whisk together the flour, baking powder, baking soda, cinnamon, nutmeg, ginger, and salt. Gradually add the applesauce mixture to the flour mixture and stir until just combined. Fold in the cereal mixture.

Scrape the batter into the prepared loaf pan and smooth the top. Bake for 45 to 55 minutes or until a toothpick inserted into the center comes out mostly clean. Inhale its beautiful aroma as it bakes.

Allow the cake to cool for 10 minutes in the pan before transferring it to a wire rack to cool completely. Slice and serve.

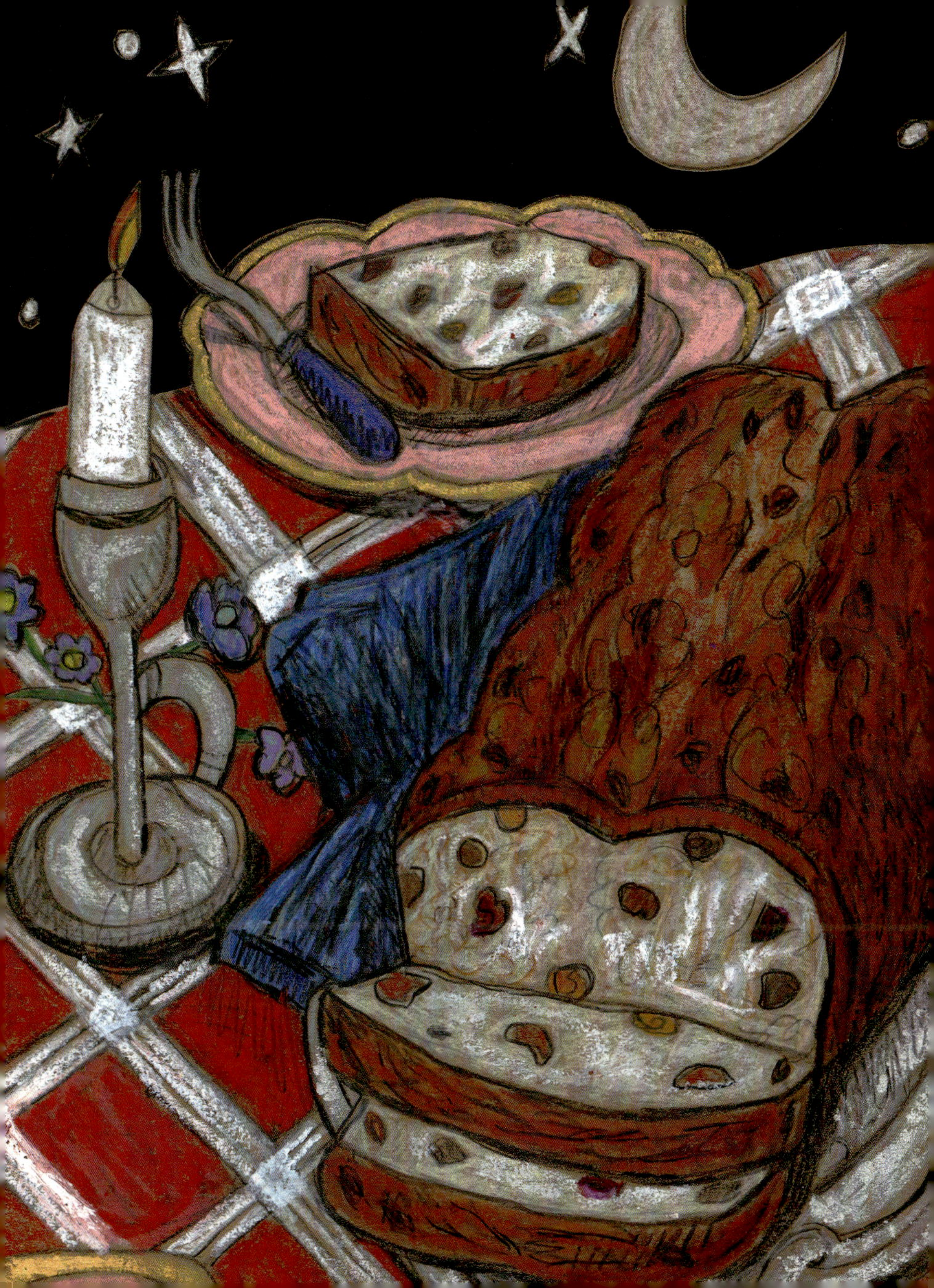

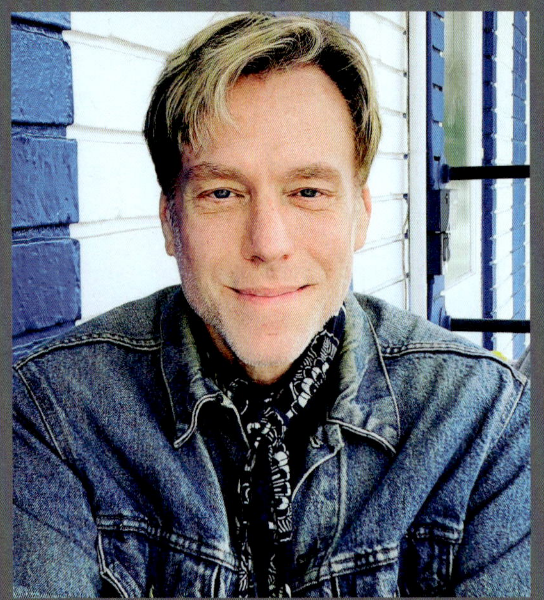

CHRIS YOUNG

is a passionate self-taught gardener who believes in the power of the flower. His written work has appeared in *Country Living*, *WestCoast*, and *Martha Stewart Living*. In 2023 Chris and his creative partner Susan Ottaviano produced *The Green Witch's Guide to Magical Plants and Flowers*, an in-depth illustrated exploration of botany-based recipes, spells, and folklore. (Photo by Jon Kinnally.)

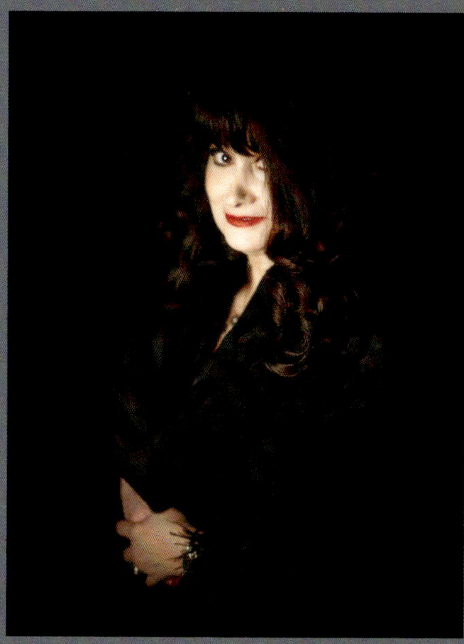

SUSAN OTTAVIANO

Artist, performer, and author, Susan co-created and illustrated *The Green Witch's Guide to Magical Plants and Flowers* with Chris Young. When not making music with her band Book of Love, Susan works as a recipe developer and food stylist for magazines, cookbooks, and international brands. (Photo by Noah Fecks.)

PLEASE FOLLOW CHRIS AND SUSAN ON INSTAGRAM @2greenwitches

Thanks to:

Tucker Shaw, Jade Lee, Jon Kinnally, Lisa Hagan, Abigail Gehring, Ted Ottaviano, Steven Kolb, Noah Fecks, Paul Zakris, Sarah Hall, Yardayna Zuller, Nora Burns, Deborah Harry, Norma Kamali, Scooter LaForge, Tonya Hurley, Alex Tubero, John Bartlett, PJ Smith, Chloe Coscarelli, Blair Fell, and Julie Pochron.

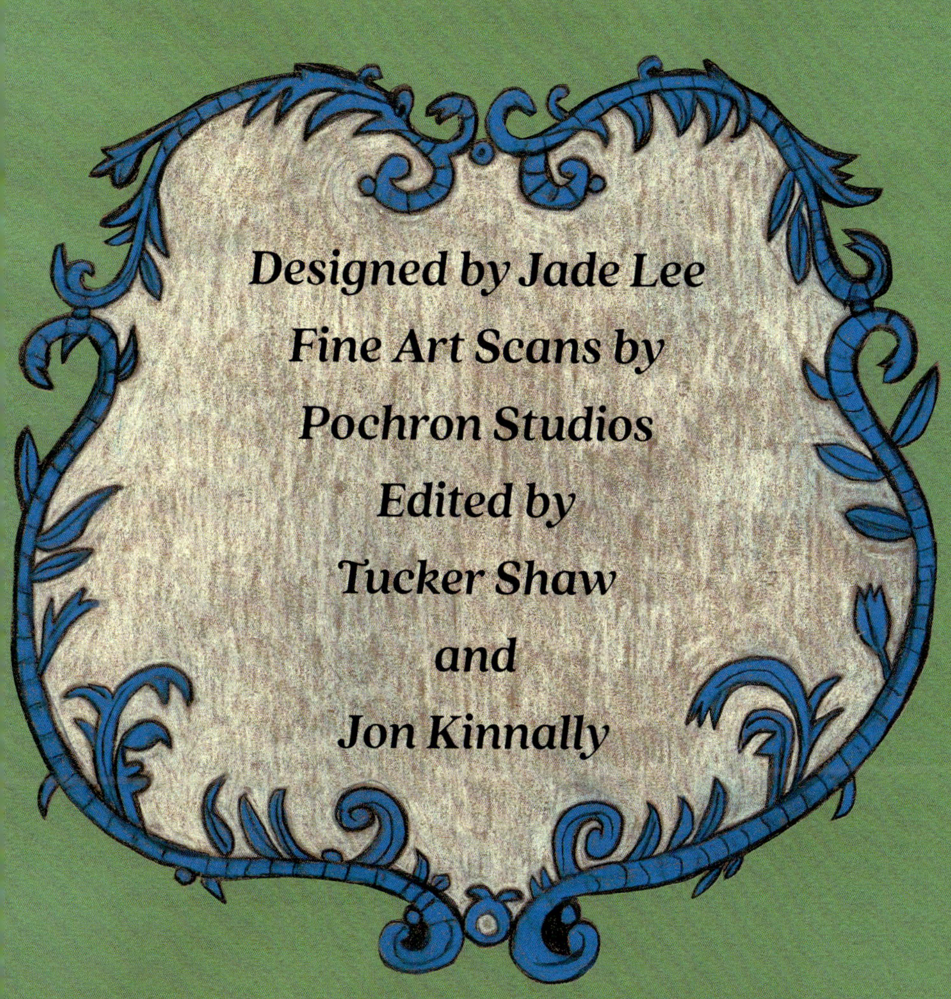

Designed by Jade Lee
Fine Art Scans by
Pochron Studios
Edited by
Tucker Shaw
and
Jon Kinnally

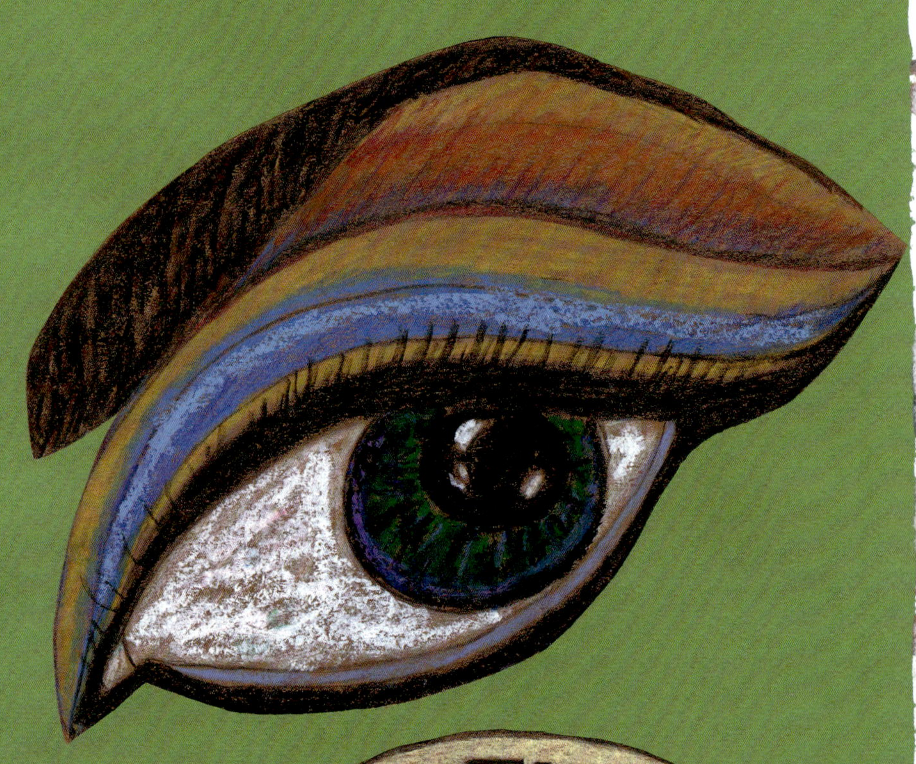

THE END
SEE YOU NEXT TIME!

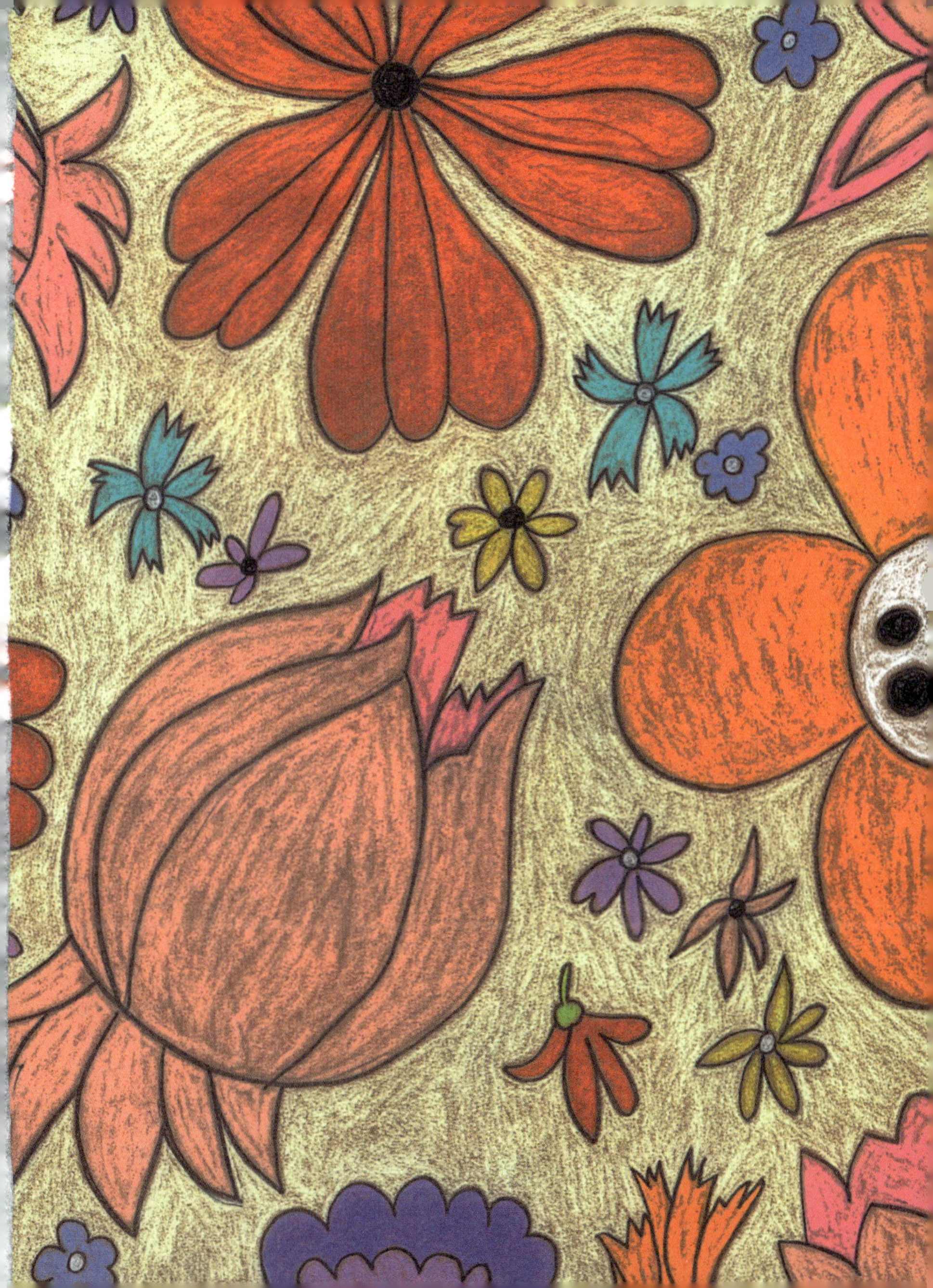

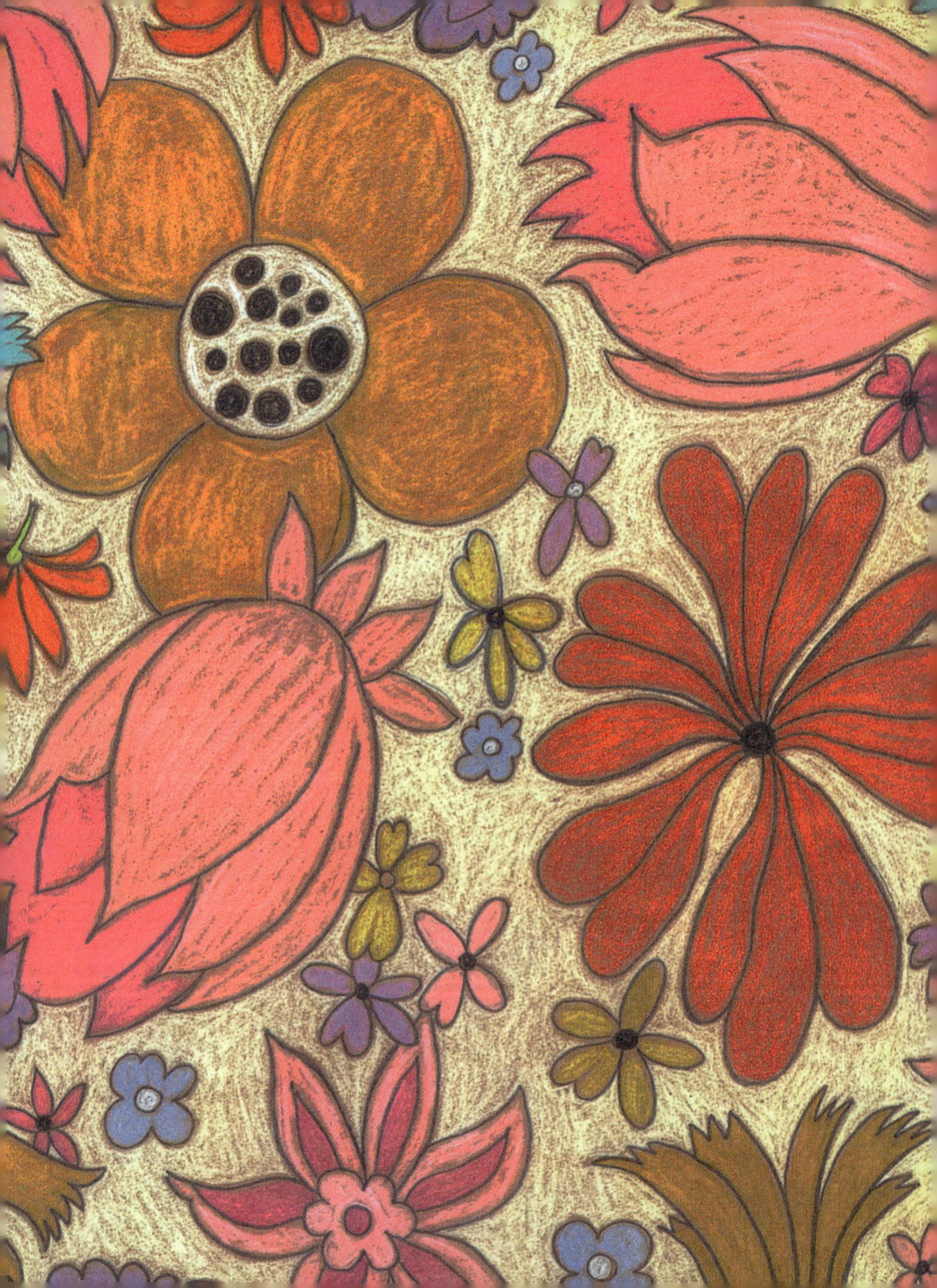